Arrhythmias

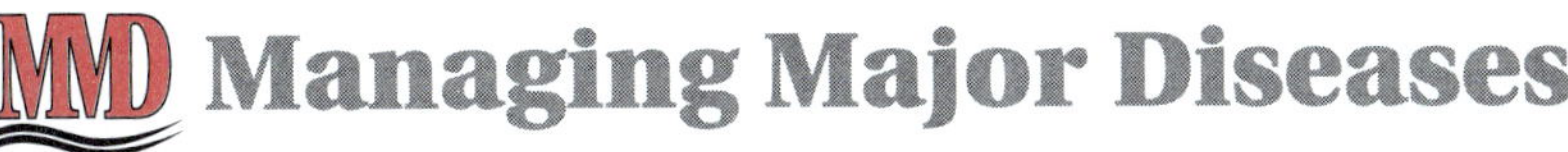

Arrhythmias

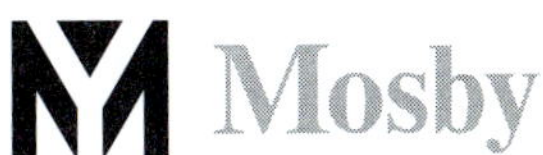

St. Louis Baltimore Boston Carlsbad Chicago Minneapolis New York Philadelphia Portland
London Milan Sydney Tokyo Toronto

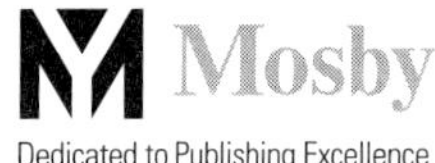

Publisher Stanley Loeb
Editorial Director William J. Kelly
Clinical Director Cindy Tryniszewski, RN, MSN
Associate Editor Kevin D. Dodds
Clinical Project Manager Aleesa M. Mobley, RN,CS, MS, CCRN, ANP
Editors Catherine E. Harold, Laura J. Ninger, Marcia Ringel, Gale Sloan Thompson
Clinical Editors Marlene Ciranowicz, RN, MSN, CDE; Sammie Justesen, RN, BSN; Colleen Seeber-Combs, RN, MSN, CCRN
Copy Editor Stacey Ann Follin
Production Editor Anthony F. Trioli
Manufacturing Manager William A. Winneberger, Jr.
Art and Design Manager Guy Jacobs
Designers Lynn Foulk, Jennifer Marmarinos
Illustrators Graphic World Illustration Services, Michael Reingold, Rolin Graphics, Inc.
Composition Specialist Robert Galindo
Indexer Barbara Hodgson

Printing and binding by R.R. Donnelley & Sons, Inc./CTP
Printed in the United States of America

Mosby, Inc.
11830 Westline Industrial Drive
St. Louis, Missouri 63146

Library of Congress Cataloging-in-Publication Data
Arrhythmias.
p. cm. — (Managing major diseases)
Includes bibliographical references and index.
ISBN 0-323-00854-2
1. Arrhythmia. 2. Arrhythmia—Nursing. I. Series.
[DNLM: 1. Arrhythmia. WG 330 A7743 1999]
RC685.A65A773 1999
616.1'28—dc21
DNLM/DLC
for Library of Congress 98-47836
CIP

99 00 01 02 03 04 / 9 8 7 6 5 4 3 2 1

Contents

Advisory Board

Contributors and Consultants

Contributors

Nezam A. Al-Nsair, RN, MSN
Doctoral Student, College of Nursing
Jordan University of Science and Technology
Irbid, Jordan

Linda S. Baas, RN, PhD, CCRN
Assistant Professor
College of Nursing and Health
University of Cincinnati Medical Center
Cincinnati, Ohio

Theresa A. Beery, RN, PhD, CCRN
Assistant Professor
College of Nursing and Health
University of Cincinnati Medical Center
Cincinnati, Ohio

Marcy Caplin, RN,CS, MSN
Independent Nurse Consultant
Hudson, Ohio

Christine Lind Colella, RN,CS, MSN
Clinical Instructor
College of Nursing and Health
University of Cincinnati Medical Center
Cincinnati, Ohio

Anita S. Desimone, RN, BS, MPH
Adult Nurse Practitioner
Occidental College, Student Health Center
Pasadena, Calif.

Melissa M. Dikeman, RN, MSN, CCRN, CRNP
Adult and Geriatric Nurse Practitioner
Veterans Administration Medical Center
Philadelphia, Pa.

Annemarie N. Elder, RN, BSN, CCRN
Administrative Supervisor, Critical Care
Jefferson University Health System, Bryn Mawr Hospital
Bryn Mawr, Pa.

Sheree M. Fitzgerald, RN,C, BSN
Program Coordinator
Ancora Psychiatric Hospital
Ancora, N.J.

Maryann Foley, RN, BSN
Independent Nurse Consultant
Flourtown, Pa.

Deborah L. Green, RN,CS, MSN
Director, Medical Telemetry and CHF Program
Moses H. Cone Health System
Greensboro, N.C.

Linda LaCharity, RN, PhD
Instructor
College of Nursing and Health
University of Cincinnati Medical Center
Cincinnati, Ohio

Mary Ann Siciliano McLaughlin, RN, MSN
Independent Nurse Consultant
Magnolia, N.J.

Susan M. Noonan, RN, BSN
Staff Nurse, ICU
Saint Luke's Hospital, East
Fort Thomas, Ky.

Teresa J. Schleimer, RN, BSN, CCRN
Staff Nurse
Jewish Hospital
Kenwood, Ohio

Ginny Wacker-Guido, RN, MSN, JD
Professor and Chair, Department of Nursing
Eastern New Mexico University
Portales, N.M.

Maria Wilson, RN, MSN, CCRN
Staff Nurse
Abington Memorial Hospital
Abington, Pa.

Consultants

Janice M. Fitzgerald, RN, BSN, MS
Independent Nurse Consultant
Glassboro, N.J.

Brenda M. Reap-Thompson, RN, MSN
Consultant, Chauncey, Inc.
Educational Testing Service
Princeton, N.J.

Joseph P. Zbilut, RN,C, PhD, DNSc
Adult Nurse Practitioner
Professor, Adult Health Nursing, College of Nursing
Associate Professor, Molecular Biophysics and Physiology
Rush University
Chicago, Ill.

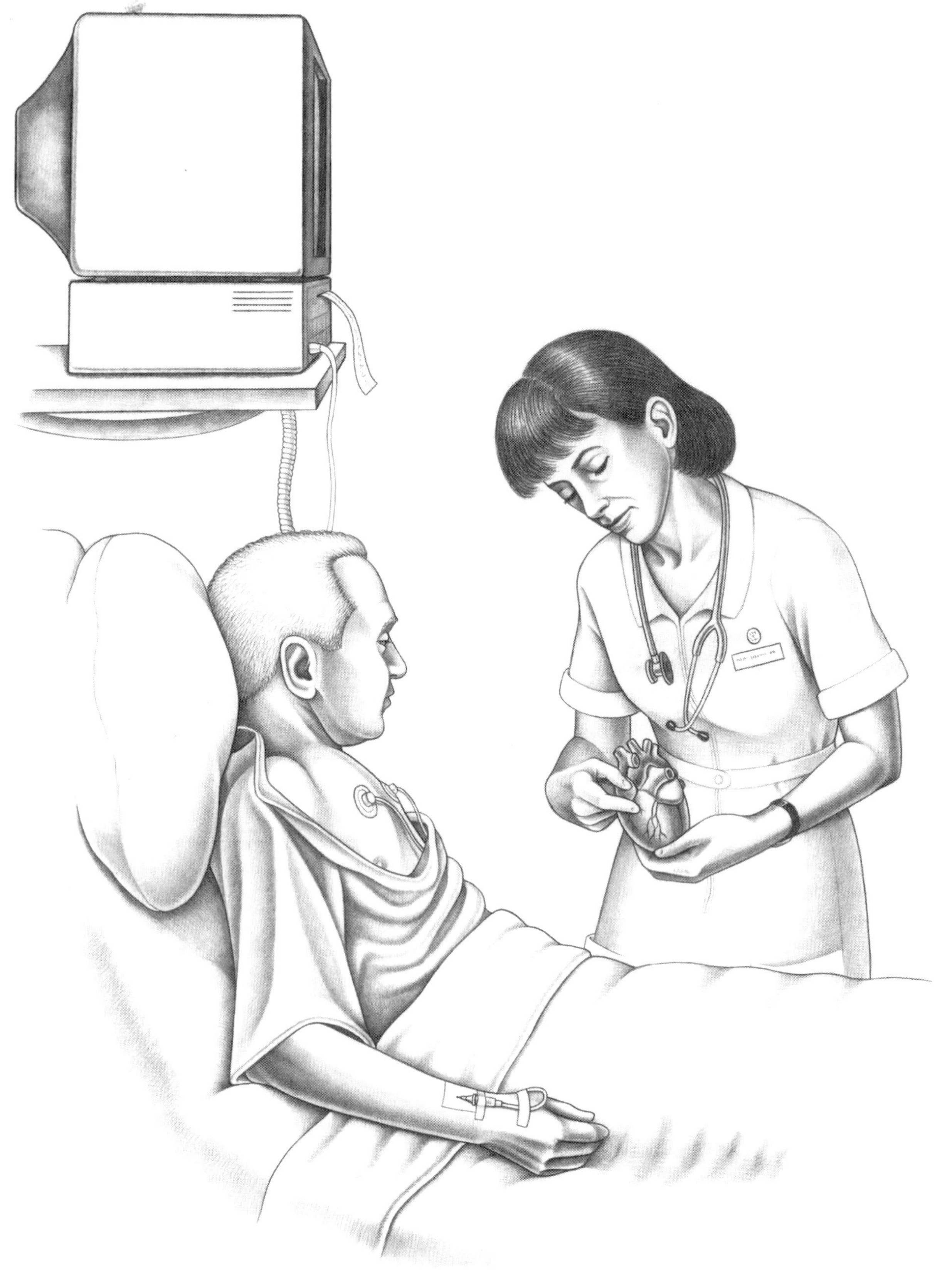

1

Anatomy and Physiology Review

In today's health care environment, nurses—all nurses—need more sophisticated skills than ever before. Take electrocardiogram (ECG) interpretation. In the past, only critical care nurses needed to know how to read rhythm strips. But now, nearly all nurses need not only to interpret ECGs but also to understand the underlying causes of arrhythmias and, most important, to provide expert patient care based on that understanding.

This chapter reviews the fundamental information you need to hone these essential skills. You'll find a pertinent review of the structure and function of the heart, a succinct discussion of the electrophysiology of the cardiac conduction system, and a clear explanation of the role of the autonomic nervous system.

Cardiac anatomy

The heart—a cone-shaped, muscular organ—lies in the central region of the thorax, just above the diaphragm. About two-thirds of the heart, including the apex, lies to the left of the midline (see *Inside the heart,* page 2).

Heart wall

The heart wall consists of three layers: the pericardium, the outermost layer; the myocardium, the middle layer; and the endocardium, the innermost layer (see *Layers of the heart wall,* page 3).

Pericardium

The pericardium, which surrounds the heart, slows ventricular dilation and helps prevent infection from spreading into the tissues of the heart. The pericardium is divided into three sublayers: the fibrous pericardium, the parietal layer of serous pericardium, and the epicardium, or visceral layer of serous pericardium.

The fibrous pericardium, the pericardium's outermost layer, is actually a loose-fitting sac that surrounds the entire heart. It's not attached to the heart directly but to the large blood vessels at the top of the heart. Beneath the heart's apex, the fibrous pericardium is also attached to the diaphragm, which helps to hold the heart in place.

The parietal layer of serous pericardium lines the inside of the fibrous pericardium. It's separated from the epicardium by the pericardial space, a fluid-filled cavity that cushions the beating heart against friction.

The epicardium adheres to the outside surface of the heart. This layer is made up of epithelium-covered connective tissue, which contains capillaries, small lymph vessels, and nerve fibers.

Myocardium

The myocardium, which makes up the bulk of the heart wall, consists of the cardiac cells that pro-

Inside the heart

This cross-sectional view of the heart shows you the four chambers, the four valves, and other key structures.

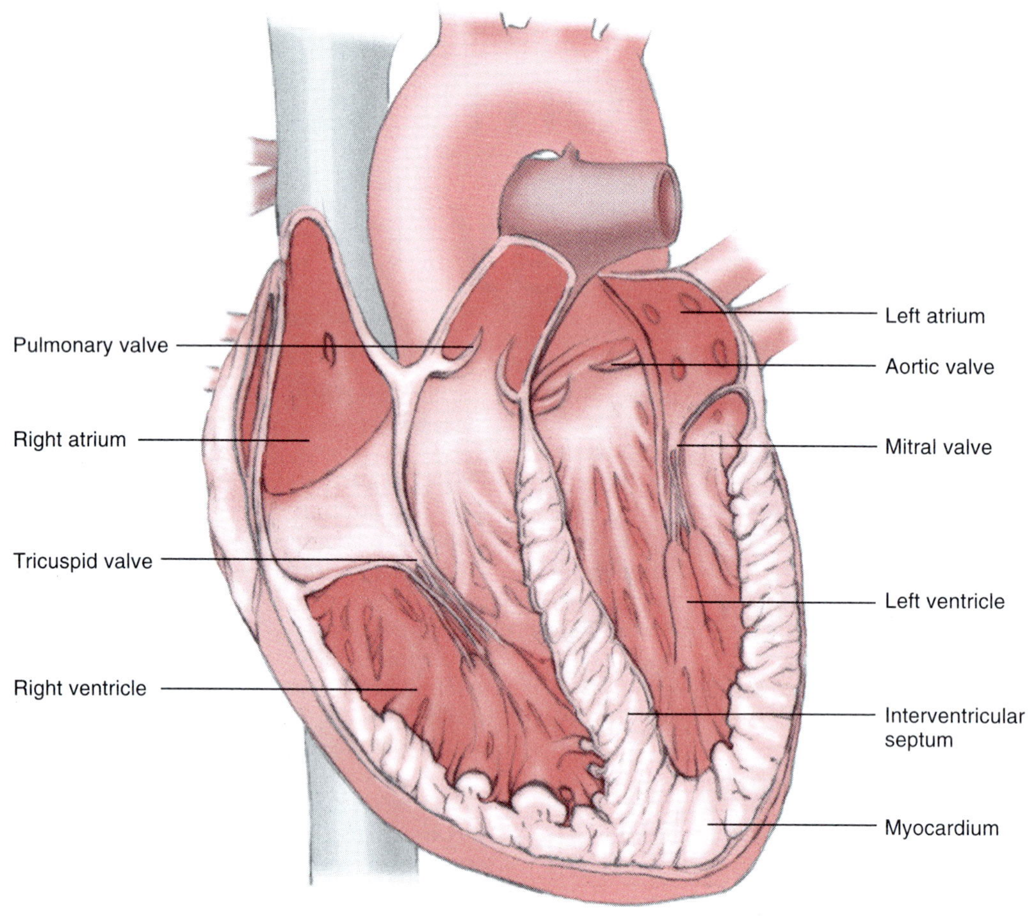

duce the heart's forceful contractions. These cardiac cells are separated by specialized cell membranes called intercalated disks. Because these intercalated disks have little electrical resistance, electrical impulses easily pass through them.

Cardiac cells are fused to each other by connections called gap junctions. Each gap junction allows electrically charged ions to move from one cardiac muscle cell to another without entering the extracellular fluid.

Endocardium

The endocardium, which lines the inside of the myocardium, is made up of endothelial tissue. This innermost layer of the heart wall comes into direct contact with the blood being pumped through the heart's chambers. Specialized folds

Layers of the heart wall

The heart wall has three main layers: the endocardium, myocardium, and pericardium. The pericardium is further divided into the parietal and visceral layers of the serous pericardium and the fibrous pericardium. The pericardial space, which is filled with about 15 ml of serous pericardial fluid, separates the parietal and visceral layers of the serous pericardium.

As the inset shows, the myocardium is made up of cardiac cells that are separated by specialized membranes called intercalated disks and joined together by gap junctions. The intercalated disks and gap junctions allow electrical impulses to pass easily from one cardiac muscle cell to the next.

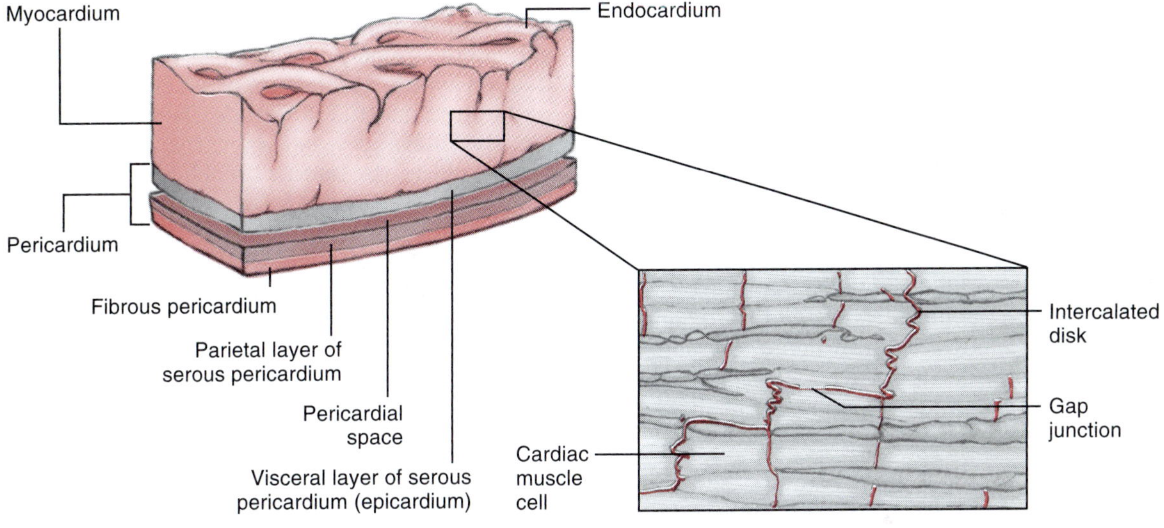

in the endocardium make up the functional parts of the heart's valves.

Heart chambers

The heart has four chambers—two upper chambers (the left atrium and the right atrium) and two lower chambers (the left ventricle and the right ventricle). The left and right atria are relatively thin-walled, low-pressure chambers. They function primarily as receptacles for blood before it moves into the two high-pressure pumping chambers, the left and right ventricles.

The right atrium receives deoxygenated blood from the superior and inferior venae cavae. Then it feeds the blood into the right ventricle, which pumps the blood out of the heart and through the pulmonary arteries to the lungs.

Oxygenated blood travels from the lungs to the heart through the pulmonary veins. The left atrium receives the blood and feeds it into the left ventricle, which then pumps the blood back into the body through the aorta.

Heart valves

The heart has two types of valves: atrioventricular (AV) valves, which separate the atria from the ventricles, and semilunar valves, which separate the ventricles from the pulmonary and systemic circulatory systems. Made of the endocardium's subendothelial connective tissue, both types of valves prevent blood from flowing backward into the heart's chambers after it passes through them.

No valves separate the superior and inferior venae cavae from the right atrium or the pulmonary veins from the left atrium. Only the continuous flow of blood through the vessels prevents excessive backflow with each atrial contraction.

Atrioventricular valves

The heart has two AV valves: a tricuspid valve and a mitral, or bicuspid, valve. Blood flows from the right atrium to the right ventricle through the tricuspid valve, which is made up of three leaflets of endocardium. The pointed ends of the leaflets project into the ventricle and are attached to the papillary muscles of the ventricle by cordlike structures, the chordae tendineae. The chordae tendineae and their papillary muscles keep the leaflets pointing in the direction of blood flow.

The mitral valve operates in a similar manner. Blood flows from the left atrium into the left ventricle through the mitral valve. Within the mitral valve, two leaflets of endocardium, which are attached by chordae tendineae to the papillary muscles of the left ventricle, point into the ventricle.

Semilunar valves

Two types of semilunar valves control blood flow from the ventricles: the pulmonary valve, which is formed from the lining of the pulmonary artery, and the aortic valve, which is formed from the lining of the aorta. Of course, the pulmonary valve lies between the right ventricle and the pulmonary artery; the aortic valve, between the left ventricle and the aorta.

Each semilunar valve has three fibrous, semilunar cusps. The cusps of the aortic valve are somewhat thicker than those of the pulmonary valve. The opening and closing of these valves depend on pressure gradient variations between the chambers and great vessels between which they lie.

Cardiac physiology

A series of muscular contractions pumps blood through the heart's chambers. These contractions are triggered by electrical impulses, which travel through the heart by way of the cardiac conduction system.

If this system works properly, the chambers of the heart contract rhythmically, a condition called AV synchrony. If the system works improperly, the chambers contract with an irregular rhythm, producing asynchrony.

Cardiac conduction system

The heart contains a complex system of specialized cardiac cells whose purpose is to generate and conduct electrical stimuli. This cardiac conduction system is made up of several connected parts: the sinoatrial (SA) node, Bachmann's bundle, the internodal pathways, the AV node, the bundle of His, the bundle branches, and the Purkinje fibers (see *Pathways of cardiac conduction*).

Sinoatrial node

The SA node, which is located in the posterior portion of the heart where the superior vena cava joins the right atrium, contains two different types of cardiac cells: round, pacemaker cells and slender, impulse-conducting cells.

The SA node acts as the heart's main pacemaker. Normally, it paces the heart at 60 to 100 beats per minute (bpm). The process of stimulating atrial and ventricular contractions begins when an electrical charge builds up in the pacemaker cells of the SA node. When one or more of these cells reach their electrical threshold, they discharge an electrical impulse into neighboring, impulse-conducting cells. And the electrical impulse spreads from cell to cell out of the SA node.

Bachmann's bundle and the internodal pathways

Bachmann's bundle, the cardiac conduction system's anterior interatrial pathway, conducts impulses from the SA node directly to the left atrium. These impulses cause the left atrium to contract, forcing blood into the left ventricle.

At the same time that an electrical impulse is traveling to the left atrium through Bachmann's bundle, other impulses are traveling through the right atrium by way of three internodal pathways: the anterior, middle, and posterior path-

Pathways of cardiac conduction

Beginning at the sinoatrial node, electrical impulses follow the pathways of cardiac conduction, first stimulating atrial contractions and then ventricular contractions.

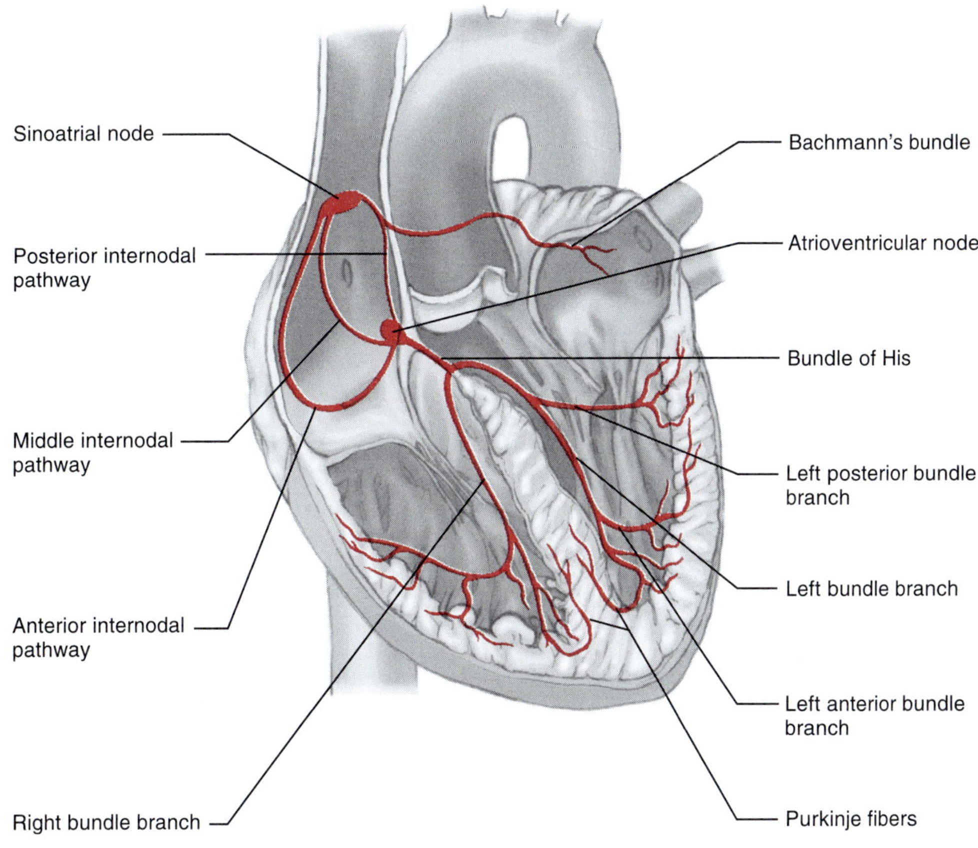

ways. The electrical impulses cause the right atrium to contract simultaneously with the left atrium. Then these impulses continue on through the internodal pathways to the AV node.

Atrioventricular node

The AV node, which sits on the right side of the interatrial septum, contains fewer pacemaker cells and more impulse-conducting cells than the SA node. So even though electrical impulses can travel through the AV node, it can't generate its own spontaneous impulses. However, tissue around the AV node, called the AV junction, can produce electrical impulses and pace the heart if the SA node becomes disabled. Any area of the heart other than the SA node that functions as the heart's main pacemaker is called an *ectopic pacemaker,* or an *ectopic focus.*

The AV junction generates spontaneous impulses more slowly than the SA node. Normally, electrical impulses are discharged from the AV junction at a rate of 40 to 60 times per minute.

As electrical impulses travel through the AV node, they generally slow down. This slowing gives the atria time to empty blood into the ventricles before ventricular contractions begin.

Bundle of His

The bundle of His, also called the AV bundle, conducts electrical impulses from the AV node into the ventricles. It begins as an anterior extension of the AV node and passes down the right side of the interventricular septum for about 12 mm before dividing into the right and left bundle branches.

Like the AV node, the bundle of His delays electrical impulses as they pass through. Usually, conduction in the bundle of His is unidirectional, so electrical impulses generated in the ventricles' cardiac cells don't reenter the atria.

Right and left bundle branches

After traveling through the bundle of His, electrical impulses move down the right and left bundle branches. The right bundle branch, a direct continuation of the bundle of His, proceeds down the right side of the interventricular septum. The left bundle branch, which is considerably thicker than the right one, is a sheath of conduction fibers that spreads along the septal subendocardium of the left ventricle. The left bundle branch splits into a thin anterior branch and a thick posterior branch.

Purkinje fibers

After traveling through the left and right bundle branches, electrical impulses are conducted through broad cardiac cells, the Purkinje fibers. Located in the left and right ventricles, the Purkinje fibers conduct impulses more quickly than any other cardiac cells. And the culmination of impulses in the Purkinje fibers results in contractions of the left and right ventricles simultaneously.

Accessory atrioventricular pathways

Some people have accessory AV pathways. These extra pathways can function as loops along which impulses travel from the ventricles back into the atria, triggering serious atrial arrhythmias.

Synchrony and asynchrony

Normally, electrical impulses are delayed as they move through the cardiac conduction system. These delays result in synchrony. The atria contract and relax simultaneously. And the action of the atria works in concert with the contraction and relaxation of the ventricles.

With a normal sinus rhythm, the atria contract (atrial systole) while the ventricles relax (ventricular diastole), and the ventricles contract (ventricular systole) while the atria relax (atrial diastole). This synchronous pattern of systolic and diastolic activity allows the heart to pump blood into the heart's chambers and out through the pulmonary and systemic circulatory systems.

Asynchrony, which results from a disturbance in the heart's normal rhythm, causes physiologic problems. If, for example, the atria don't contract at the proper time, ventricular filling becomes impaired, and cardiac output diminishes.

Electrophysiology

The electrical impulses that initiate the heart's muscular contractions move through the heart from cell to cell by way of electrically charged ions, which are exchanged across cell membranes. The cell's ability to exchange these charged ions results from its membrane potential. And as the charged ions are exchanged, the cells go through several phases of polarization and depolarization.

Membrane potential

Because the membrane of a cardiac muscle cell is semipermeable, sodium, potassium, and calcium ions can move into and out of the cell. This movement of positively and negatively charged ions across the cell membrane is called the cell's membrane potential.

Actually, the membrane potential has two phases: the resting potential, a period of electrical inactivity, and the action potential, a period of electrical activity. During the action potential, sodium and potassium ions change places across the cell membrane. After the action potential, the sodium-potassium pump moves ions back across the membrane, returning the cell to the resting potential.

Resting potential

When a cell is at rest, many negatively charged ions (anions) and a few positively charged ions (cations) lie just inside the cell membrane, and many cations lie just outside it.

In this resting state, the sodium cations, which are the predominant cation outside the cell, can't move through the membrane. However, the potassium cations that lie inside the cell can move across the membrane to the outside of the cell. As they do, the cell becomes more negatively charged with a higher ratio of anions to cations.

During the resting potential, no electrical activity occurs. The cell is said to be polarized—negatively charged inside and positively charged outside.

Action potential

The action potential of the cell membrane develops in response to an electrical stimulus from a neighboring cell. The permeability of the cell membrane changes, and cations move from outside the cell, through the membrane, to the inside of the cell. This action changes the electrical charge inside the cell because more cations are now inside the membrane. At this time, the cell is said to be depolarized, with a more equal distribution of cations on both sides of the cell membrane.

The speed at which the action potential takes place depends on whether the cardiac muscle cell is a fast or slow response cell.

Fast and slow response cells

Fast response cells are located throughout the conduction system in the myocardial fibers of the atria and ventricles and in the Purkinje fibers. Slow response cells are located in the heart's natural pacemaker regions, the SA and AV nodes.

Fast and slow response cells differ in several ways: the velocity of their electrical impulses, the voltage of their resting potentials, and the behavior of their response channels.

Conduction velocity

Fast response cells conduct electrical impulses at 0.3 to 0.4 m/second. Slow response cells conduct electrical impulses at 0.02 to 0.2 m/second. As fast and slow response cells conduct these electrical impulses, the voltage of their membrane potentials changes from a negative charge to a less negative charge.

Voltage of resting potential

Usually, the voltage of the resting potential in fast response cells is about −90 millivolts (mV). As the cells conduct an electrical impulse, the voltage of the resting potential changes to about −60 mV, at which point an action potential develops quickly, and the cells become depolarized. This depolarization causes myocardial contractions.

The voltage of the resting potential in slow response cells is about −60 mV, considerably less negative than in fast response cells. During the resting potential, the cell membrane becomes less permeable to potassium, so fewer cations leave the cell. With more sodium cations going out and more potassium cations staying in the cell, it gradually becomes depolarized.

Response channels

In fast and slow response cells, ions move across the cell membranes primarily through specific ion channels. Gates that open and close according to changes in voltage or certain chemical signals regulate these channels.

Particularly in a fast response cell, open potassium response channels are plentiful, so potassium tends to move easily from inside to outside the cell. However, the cell has fewer open sodium response channels. And sodium tends to move into the cell only when most of the sodium response channels are open, so sodium is less mobile.

During the resting membrane potential, very little sodium movement takes place because the cell membrane is relatively impermeable to sodium. But in response to electrical stimulation during the action potential, sodium response channels open, and sodium can move into the cell easily.

This complex system of opening and closing response channels is the cells' way of maintaining electrical potential. If all of a cell's response channels were opened and all ions moved across the cell membrane at one time, the cell would soon reach equilibrium, and the electrical potential would disappear.

Sodium-potassium pump

The sodium-potassium pump reestablishes the difference in charges across the cell membrane after ions have moved during the action potential. The pump moves two potassium cations back into the cell for every three sodium cations it moves back out of the cell. This ratio assures that the outside of the cell membrane remains more positive than the inside after the action potential.

Because the pump recreates the electrical potential difference between the positive and negative charges inside and outside the cell membrane, it's an electrogenic pump. The pump is an example of an active transport system, using energy to move a substance against its electrical or chemical gradient.

Basically, the sodium-potassium pump consists of a specialized carrier molecule, which is powered by an adenosine triphosphatase (ATPase) molecule created by the cell's mitochondria. Inside the cell, three sodium cations bind to sodium-binding sites on the carrier's inner face. At the same time, an energy-containing ATPase molecule binds to the carrier. Then the ATPase molecule breaks apart, transferring its stored energy to the carrier.

The carrier changes shape, releases the three sodium cations to the outside of the cell, and attracts two potassium cations to its potassium-binding sites. Then the carrier returns to its original shape, releasing the two potassium cations and the remnant of the ATPase molecule to the inside of the cell. After releasing the potassium cations and the ATPase molecule, the carrier is ready for another pumping cycle.

Phases of depolarization and repolarization

As described, a fast response cardiac cell is polarized during its resting potential. As an electrical impulse stimulates the cell, an action potential develops, and the cell becomes depolarized. Then, the sodium-potassium pump works to repolarize the cell, returning the cell to its resting potential.

This cycle of depolarization and repolarization is divided into five phases of activity, numbered 0 through 4. And these five phases can be grouped into two refractory periods based on whether a cell can or cannot respond to outside electrical stimuli (see *Action potential curve: A view of depolarization and repolarization*).

Phase 0

During phase 0, sodium response channels open, and sodium movement across the cell membrane increases rapidly. The incoming rush of sodium changes the charge inside the cell membrane, making the cell's interior much less negative. The resting membrane potential moves rapidly from −90 mV toward a less negative charge. When the membrane potential reaches a threshold of about −60 mV, an action potential occurs.

During an action potential, the electrical impulse travels over the entire cell membrane. Sodium continues to move into the cell, creating a brief period when the membrane potential becomes positively charged. This reversal of polarity from negative to positive is called the overshoot.

Phase 1

During phase 1, the sodium response channels close, allowing no more sodium to enter the cell. And potassium begins to leave the cell, causing a partial repolarization, in which the cell begins to return to its polarized state.

Phase 2

During phase 2, the plateau phase, calcium moves into the cell through open calcium response channels. And potassium begins to move out of the cell. The incoming calcium counteracts the exiting potassium, so the charge of the membrane potential remains about the same.

Phase 3

In phase 3, the calcium response channels close, allowing no more calcium to enter the cell. Potassium leaves the cell more rapidly, causing the cell to become quickly repolarized.

Toward the end of this phase, the sodium-potassium pump begins to work, moving three sodium cations out of the cell for every two potassium cations it brings back in. And the charge of the cell's membrane potential returns to nearly −90 mV.

Phase 4

During phase 4, the cell becomes fully repolarized. This is the cell's resting potential, which

Action potential curve: A view of depolarization and repolarization

The depolarization-repolarization cycle causes electrical changes to occur in fast response cardiac cells. The action potential curve shows you how the polarity of these cells changes from negative to positive, and then back to negative again.

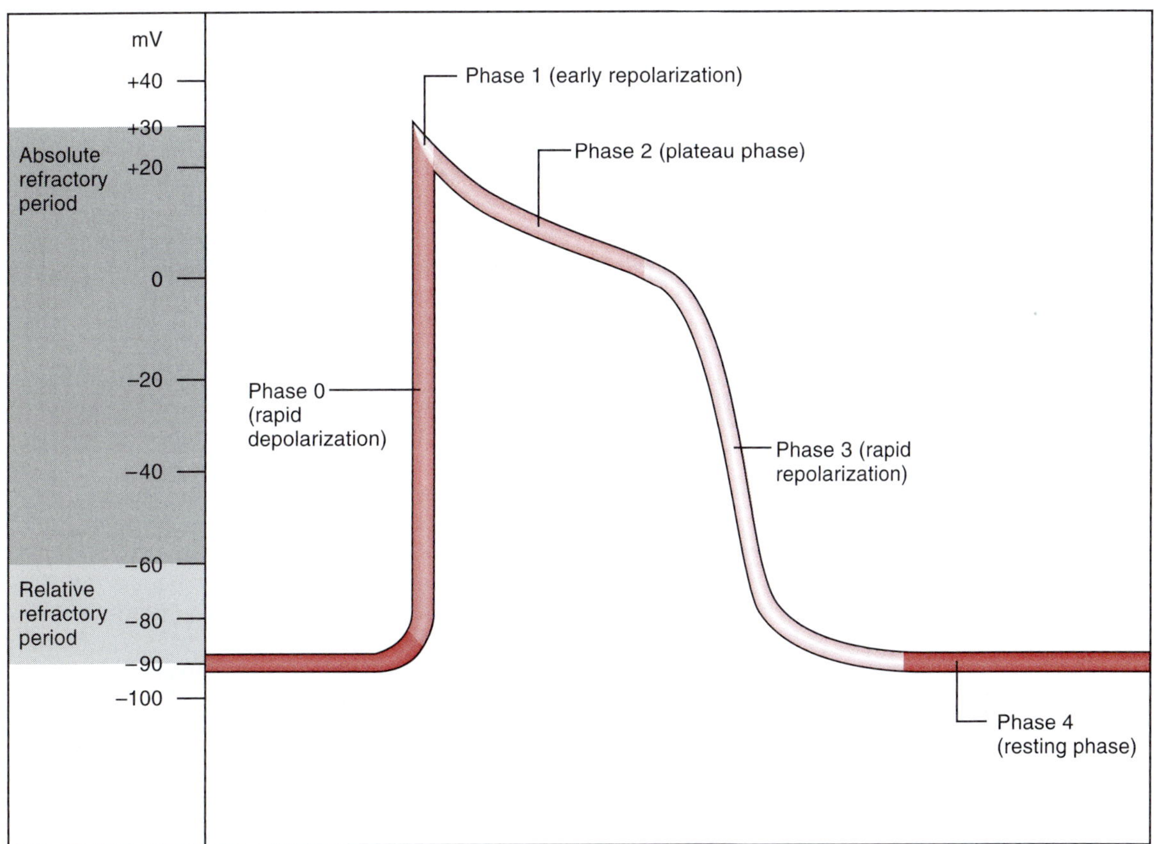

has a charge of about −90 mV. Calcium slowly leaks out of the cell. And the sodium-potassium pump continues moving sodium out and potassium back into the cell.

Refractory periods

The five phases of depolarization and repolarization can be grouped into two refractory periods: absolute and relative.

Usually, the absolute refractory period starts near the beginning of phase 0, when rapid depolarization brings the charge of the cell's membrane potential to about −60 mV. The period continues throughout phases 1 and 2 and ends about halfway through phase 3, when rapid repolarization brings the charge of the membrane potential back down to about −60 mV.

During the absolute refractory period, the cell is never completely polarized. It's saturated with sodium cations. And too few sodium response channels have been reset to permit the cell's reactivation by an outside electrical impulse.

The relative refractory period starts during the second half of phase 3. And it continues throughout phase 4 and into the beginning of phase 0. During this period, the charge of the cell's membrane potential is never more positive than about −60 mV.

In the beginning of the relative refractory period, the cell has achieved partial repolarization. It can respond to stronger-than-normal outside electrical impulses. Therefore, the early relative refractory period is a vulnerable time in the depolarization-repolarization cycle. During the second half of phase 3, an electrical impulse that stimulates the cell can induce serious arrhythmias. Only when the cell has become completely repolarized during phase 4 can an electrical impulse safely activate it.

Autonomic nervous system

The autonomic nervous system controls the rate at which the heart beats and the strength of its contractions. Normally, an adult's heart beats at a rate of about 70 bpm. However, during periods of physical activity or emotional distress, the autonomic nervous system may stimulate the heart to produce stronger contractions and to increase the heart rate. And during periods of physical inactivity, such as sleep, it may decrease the heart rate.

Actually, the interplay between the two branches of the autonomic nervous system—the sympathetic and parasympathetic nervous systems—causes the heart rate to change. Stimulation of the sympathetic nervous system with simultaneous inhibition of the parasympathetic nervous system commonly accelerates the heart rate. And stimulation of the parasympathetic nervous system with simultaneous inhibition of the sympathetic nervous system commonly slows the heart rate.

Parasympathetic stimulation

The parasympathetic nervous system is made up of vagal nerve fibers. The vagal fibers for myocardial stimulation start in the medulla and terminate in the SA and AV nodes of the heart.

Normally, stimulation of the parasympathetic nervous system causes the vagal fibers to release acetylcholine, which alters potassium conduction in cardiac cells. However, excessive parasympathetic stimulation causes the release of greater amounts of acetylcholine, and more potassium than normal may move out of the cells. This alteration in potassium conduction causes the membrane potential of the cells to become more negative than usual, a condition called hyperpolarization.

With hyperpolarization, the usual resting potential of cells in the SA node may change from about −60 mV to about −75 mV. Thus, reaching the threshold takes much longer, and the cells may generate impulses less frequently. Or the membrane potential may never rise high enough to reach the threshold, and the SA node loses its ability to achieve automaticity.

In the same way, parasympathetic stimulation can decrease or stop automaticity in the fibers of the AV junction. It can also decrease or stop the excitability of the cells in the AV node.

With strong vagal stimulation, the discharge of the SA node, conduction through the AV node, and excitability of the AV junctional fibers can all stop completely. If this cessation occurs, no electrical stimulation is produced to initiate ventricular contractions.

When the ventricles receive no electrical stimulation for 5 to 20 seconds, the Purkinje fibers generally initiate a rhythm, called a ventricular escape rhythm. This rhythm has a slow rate of about 15 to 40 bpm.

Sympathetic stimulation

The sympathetic nervous system is made up of sympathetic nerve fibers. Like the vagal fibers, the sympathetic fibers originate in the medulla and terminate in the SA and AV nodes of the heart.

Normally, stimulation of the sympathetic nervous system causes the sympathetic nerve fibers to release epinephrine, which may alter calcium conduction in cardiac cells. However, excessive sympathetic stimulation causes the release of greater amounts of epinephrine, and the increased movement of calcium into the cardiac cells may make them much more positive than normal.

With a more positive charge, the cardiac cells are able to reach the threshold much more quickly, which increases the automaticity of the SA node's cells and the excitability of the AV node's cells. With impulses being generated more quickly in the SA node and moving more rapidly through the AV node, the atrial and ventricular muscles have greater contractility. Such stimulation by the sympathetic nervous system can triple the heart rate and double the strength of a cardiac contraction.

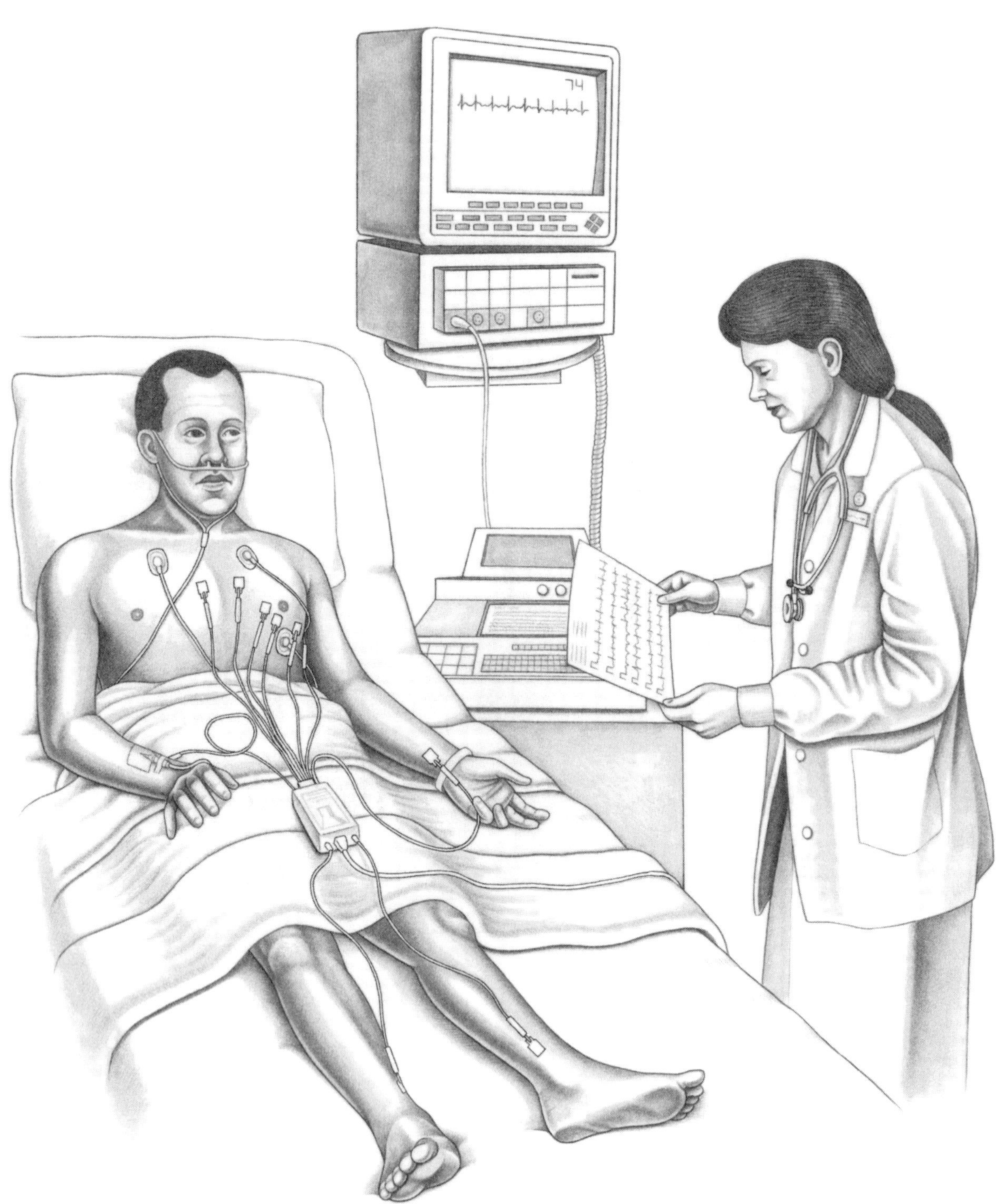
74

2

Understanding the Electrocardiogram

To give expert care to your patient with an arrhythmia, you need to read and interpret his electrocardiogram (ECG) so that you can detect subtle—perhaps dangerous—changes in his condition. In this chapter, you'll find a concise review that will refresh your memory on key ECG facts and help you hone your ECG skills.

First, you'll find a quick review of essential information about the heart's electrical currents and the ECG's electrical leads. Then comes a short section on obtaining an ECG, followed by a section on the components of an ECG. Finally, you'll find a discussion on interpreting ECGs, followed by a short section on troubleshooting the ECG tracing.

Fundamentals of electrocardiography

As you know, an ECG gives you a graphic representation of the electrical activity that stimulates the myocardium to contract during diastole and to relax during systole. But before reading about the actual components of the ECG waveforms and their interpretation, briefly review two important concepts: the electrical axis and electrical leads.

Electrical axis

Normally, the cells of the sinoatrial (SA) node produce the heart's electrical impulses. During systole, these impulses move in electrical currents from cell to cell down through the heart. The combination of all the currents during electrical systole produces the heart's electrical axis—the direction in which electrical impulses flow through the heart.

As you'd expect, a normal electrical axis runs from top right (the SA node) to bottom left (the left ventricle). You can use a hexaxial reference figure to help visualize this electrical axis. This figure shows a circle superimposed on a heart, with the circle divided into 30-degree increments. The top of the circle is designated as −90 degrees; the bottom, as +90 degrees. The point 90 degrees clockwise from the top is designated as 0 degrees; 90 degrees counterclockwise from the top, ±180 degrees. Thus, a normal electrical axis runs from about −120 degrees to about +30 degrees (see *Normal electrical axis,* page 14).

Electrical leads

The various leads you can use to assess your patient produce views of his heart's electrical activ-

Normal electrical axis

This hexaxial reference figure shows the normal directional flow of electrical impulses through the heart. This flow, called the electrical axis, runs from the sinoatrial node at about −120 degrees to the left ventricle near the apex at about +30 degrees.

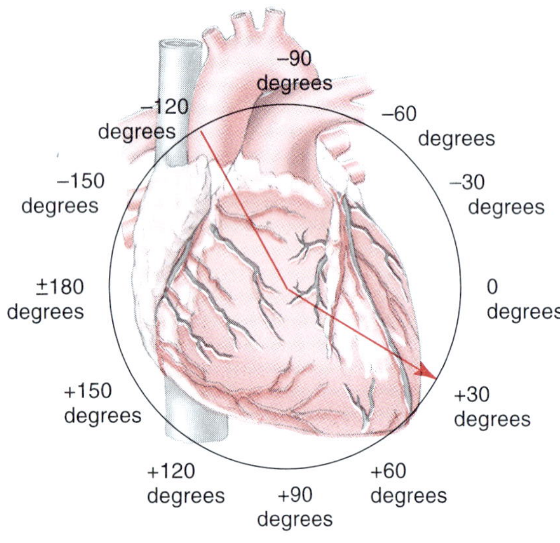

ity taken from different angles. These electrical views are created by a negative pole and a positive pole. The electrical currents running between these poles and through the heart give you the electrical views.

Deflections, the upward and downward tracings on the ECG, represent the direction and magnitude of electrical currents in the heart. When the heart's electrical axis runs parallel to a lead, the deflections may be either positive (upward) or negative (downward). When the electrical axis moves in the same direction as the lead, you'll see a positive deflection. When the electrical axis moves in the opposite direction from the lead, you'll see a negative deflection. When the electrical axis is perpendicular to a lead, the ECG produces a biphasic deflection, which is made up of a positive deflection and a negative deflection. The size of the deflection on the ECG represents the magnitude of the current.

Standard limb leads

The standard limb leads—leads I, II, and III—are called bipolar leads because you actually place a positive and a negative electrode on the patient. These three limb leads record the flow of electrical current in the frontal plane of the heart.

In lead I, the negative electrode is on the patient's right arm and the positive electrode on his left arm. This lead provides a horizontal view of the heart.

In lead II, the negative electrode is on the right arm and the positive electrode on the left leg. This lead runs parallel to the electrical axis of the heart. Usually, lead II records the highest positive deflection of all the leads.

In lead III, the negative electrode is on the left arm and the positive electrode on the left leg. Lead III records a view through the inferior wall of the left ventricle that typically is perpendicular to the normal axis of the heart (see *A look at the standard and augmented limb leads*).

Augmented unipolar limb leads

The augmented voltage leads are called unipolar leads because they use only a positive electrode applied to one of three designated limbs—the right arm, left arm, or left leg. The ECG machine computes the designated augmented voltage lead in relation to a negative pole, which is the center of the heart. Thus, augmented voltage leads provide information about electrical activity flowing to the right, to the left, and downward in relation to the center of the heart. Because the tracings formed by the augmented leads would ordinarily be quite small, the ECG machine enlarges or augments them with extra voltage.

The augmented voltage right (aV_R) lead uses the right arm as the positive electrode. The tracing that this lead produces is almost a mirror image of the tracing that lead II produces because the direction of the aV_R lead is the opposite of lead II.

The augmented voltage left (aV_L) lead uses the left arm as the positive electrode. The tracing that lead aV_L produces records the electrical current flowing through the lateral wall of the left ventricle.

The augmented voltage foot (aV_F) lead uses the left leg as the positive electrode. The tracing that lead aV_F produces records the electrical current flowing through the center of the heart.

Left precordial leads

The left precordial leads, V_1 through V_6, are unipolar leads; each requires only a positive electrode. The ECG machine uses information from the standard limb leads to determine the path of the precordial leads. These leads view the heart's electrical activity on a horizontal plane from anterior to posterior.

Lead V_1 shows a view of the right ventricle. Lead V_2 focuses on the ventricular septal wall. Lead V_3 views the anterior septal wall. Lead V_4, also called the apical lead, focuses on the anterior wall of the left ventricle. Lead V_5 focuses on the anterior wall of the heart near the lateral wall of the left ventricle. Lead V_6 shows a view of the lateral wall of the left ventricle (see *Where to place the left precordial electrodes,* page 16).

Right precordial leads

The right precordial leads, which are used to assess the right side of the heart, aren't part of a standard 12-lead ECG. If your patient has right ventricular heart failure or a right ventricular infarction, you may use these leads, which follow the pattern of leads V_4 through V_6 but are located to the right of the sternum.

Leads for continuous monitoring

Usually, you'll perform continuous cardiac monitoring using either lead II or a modified chest lead (MCL_1), a bipolar lead whose tracing resembles the one produced by lead V_1. Most commonly, you'll use lead II because it runs parallel to the heart's electrical axis. However, when dressings, clothing, or an incision line limits access to your patient's chest, you may use lead I.

To use lead MCL_1 for continuous cardiac monitoring, apply the negative electrode at the left midclavicular line below the clavicle. Apply the positive electrode at the fourth intercostal space just to the right of the sternum.

A look at the standard and augmented limb leads

This schematic illustration shows you the direction of the six limb leads.

Each of the standard limb leads—leads I, II, and III—requires two electrodes. Depending on the lead, you'll place electrodes on the right arm, the left arm, and the left leg.

Each of the unipolar augmented leads—leads aV_R, aV_L, and aV_F—requires only a positive electrode, which creates an axis perpendicular to one of the standard limb leads.

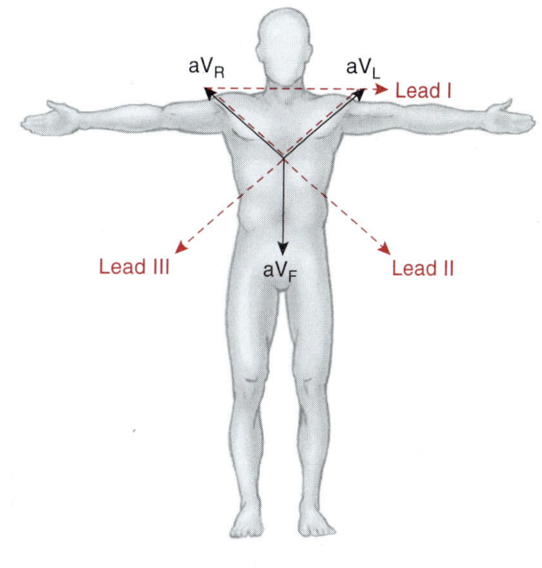

Obtaining an electrocardiogram

To obtain a useful ECG, you'll need to enlist your patient's cooperation and apply the electrodes to his skin properly. If your patient understands the procedure, he'll probably be more cooperative. Tell him that an ECG is a painless way to examine his heart function. Also, explain why he has to remain as still as possible while you obtain the tracing. Make sure that his room is warm and quiet and do what's necessary to guarantee his privacy during the procedure.

If you're using a multichannel recorder, the most common type of 12-lead ECG machine, you can apply all the leads at the same time. The machine will switch automatically from one lead view to the next. If you're using a single-channel machine, you'll have to adjust the dial manually for each limb lead. And you'll have to apply each electrode separately, in sequence, for the precordial lead tracings.

Where to place the left precordial electrodes

To obtain horizontal views of the heart's electrical activity, place the electrodes of the left precordial leads on your patient's chest in the following locations:
- V_1—fourth intercostal space at the right sternal border
- V_2—fourth intercostal space at the left sternal border
- V_3—midway between leads V_2 and V_4
- V_4—fifth intercostal space on the left midclavicular line
- V_5—fifth intercostal space on the left anterior axillary line
- V_6—fifth intercostal space on the left midaxillary line.

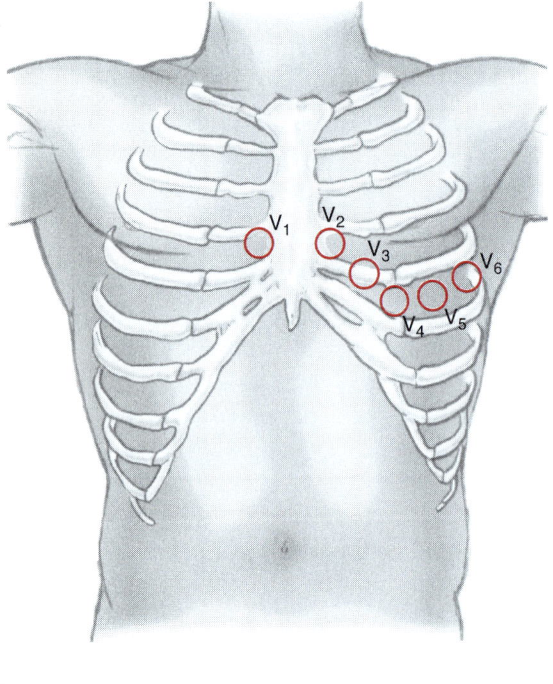

Continuous cardiac monitoring requires the use of adhesive, pre-gelled electrodes. At a minimum, this form of monitoring requires three electrodes: one positive, one negative, and one ground.

If you're using a multichannel recorder that allows you to view two leads simultaneously, you may use as many as five electrodes. The electrode placement depends on manufacturer's specifications.

Telemetry (ambulatory) monitoring commonly uses three electrodes in an MCL_1 configuration. The placement of these electrodes also may vary, depending on manufacturer's specifications.

Applying the electrodes

The electrodes for continuous cardiac monitoring and the silver oxide tabs used by the ECG machine for conducting electrical current must be applied to clean, dry skin surfaces. Good skin contact is essential for proper ECG tracings, so use an alcohol wipe to clean the areas where electrodes will be placed. If your patient's chest is particularly hairy, shave the electrode sites.

Before applying electrodes and silver oxide tabs, check that the sites are completely dry. Also, check that the electrodes or tabs are moist with electrode gel or paste.

Avoid placing electrodes against bony prominences such as your patient's clavicle, radius, and tibia. Doing so could cause the ECG to pick up electrical noise (artifact), thus decreasing the readability of your tracing.

Elements of an electrocardiogram

All ECG machines record waveforms on graph paper that has a standardized grid containing both large and small squares. The large squares, which have a darker border, contain 25 small squares. Each small square is 1 mm wide and 1 mm high (see *Electrocardiogram grid: Measuring time and amplitude*).

Five large squares roll out of the ECG machine every second. Thus, each large square on the horizontal axis represents 0.2 second. Each small square represents 0.04 second. At the top of the ECG grid, you'll see markers at intervals of 15 large squares, representing 3-second increments. When you're reading an ECG, these squares and markers allow you to pinpoint your patient's

Electrocardiogram grid: Measuring time and amplitude

The increments of the electrocardiogram grid are standardized for measuring time along the horizontal axis and amplitude along the vertical axis.

Horizontally, one small square represents 0.04 second. One large square (the equivalent of five small squares) represents 0.2 second.

Vertically, one small square represents 0.1 millivolt (mV). One large square (the equivalent of five small squares) represents 0.5 mV.

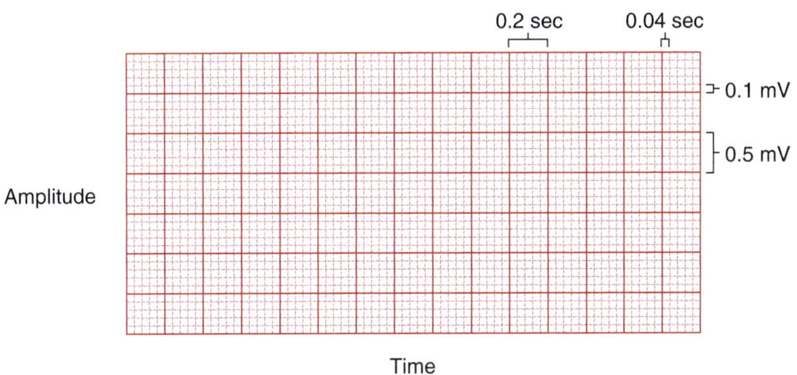

heart rate as well as the duration of each component of the cardiac cycle.

The squares on the vertical axis indicate the amplitude, or force, of the electrical current. A vertical deflection, either upward or downward, measures amplitude. Each small square indicates 0.1 millivolt (mV). Each large square represents 0.5 mV.

Waves

On the ECG tracing, each wave represents a key component of the cardiac cycle. These waves include the P wave, QRS complex, T wave, and U wave (see *Identifying the components of the cardiac cycle,* page 18).

P wave

The P wave depicts the simultaneous depolarization of the atria. Normally, a P wave is gently rounded. Because the atria are small and generate less electrical force than the ventricles, the P wave is smaller than the other components of the cardiac cycle.

Usually, P waves have positive deflections in leads I, II, aV_F, and V_1 through V_4. Because the vector of the P wave is opposite that of the heart's electrical axis, the P wave should always have a negative deflection in lead aV_R.

The P wave can be biphasic, exhibiting both positive and negative deflections in leads III, aV_L, and V_1 through V_4. Normally, the P wave is less than 3 mm high and less than 0.11 second wide. P waves initiated by the SA node have a uniform appearance.

QRS complex

Normally, the QRS complex depicts the nearly simultaneous depolarization of the ventricles. The QRS complex is larger than the P wave because the ventricles have more muscle mass and, therefore, more power than the atria.

Usually, the QRS complex has a positive deflection in leads I, II, III, aV_F, aV_L, V_5, and V_6. A negative deflection can sometimes appear in lead III. But negative deflections should always appear in leads V_3 and V_4.

The first line of the QRS complex to leave the

Identifying the components of the cardiac cycle

Normally, on an electrocardiogram (ECG), one cardiac cycle consists of a P wave, a QRS complex, and a T wave. Usually, a U wave isn't discernible on an ECG.

The ECG tracing also depicts segments (a measure of time from the end of one wave to the beginning of another) and intervals (a measure of time from one component of the cardiac cycle to another).

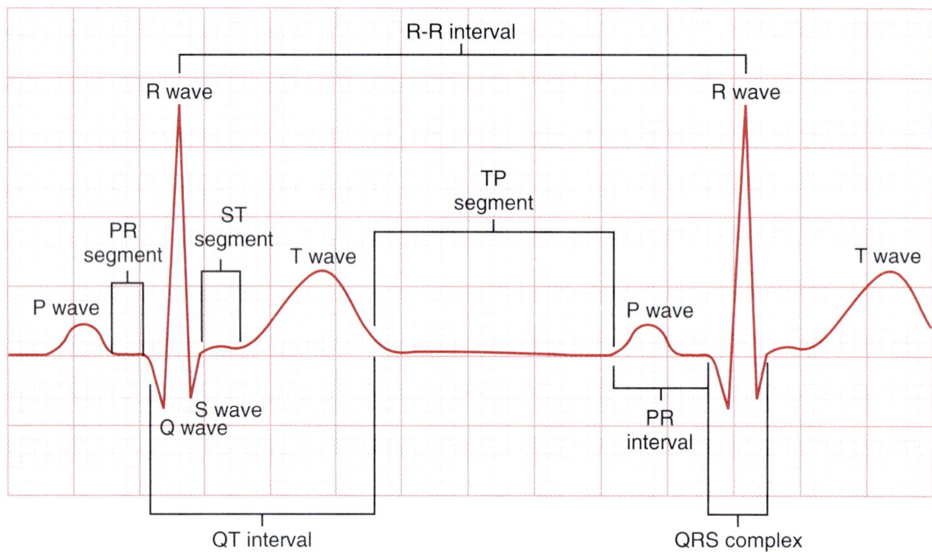

baseline in a negative deflection is the Q wave. The first line to redirect in a positive deflection is the R wave. The negative deflection that follows the R wave is the S wave.

Normally, the QRS complex is less than 25 mm high and lasts for 0.1 second or less.

T wave

After the ventricles have contracted, the heart mechanically relaxes and fills with blood. Meanwhile, the cardiac cells repolarize. This period is depicted on the ECG tracing as the T wave.

The T wave represents the refractory period, a vulnerable time for the cardiac cells. The beginning of the T wave represents the absolute refractory period, during which no impulse can depolarize the cells. The remainder of the T wave represents the relative refractory period, during which only some cells have been repolarized.

T waves vary in shape and size. These waves aren't used to determine rate and rhythm. However, they may indicate ischemia, injury to the heart muscle, hypertrophy, or a metabolic abnormality.

U wave

The U wave is a small deflection that has no significance in determining rate and rhythm. However, you'll need to be able to identify it correctly so that you don't confuse it with the P wave. The significance of the U wave isn't known, but the wave may represent further repolarization of the ventricles.

The U wave isn't always visible on the ECG tracing. When it is, you'll see it best in leads V_4 through V_6. The U wave may appear as a positive deflection in patients with hypokalemia. Or it may appear as a negative deflection in patients with either ischemia or left ventricular hypertrophy.

Intervals and segments

To achieve expertise in reading ECG tracings, familiarize yourself with intervals and segments. The three intervals—PR, R-R, and QT—are the time between sections of waves. The three segments—PR, ST, and TP—are the time from the end of one wave to the beginning of another.

PR interval

The PR interval is the time from the point at which the P wave leaves the baseline to the beginning of the QRS complex. This interval represents the movement of an electrical impulse from the SA node (depolarization of the atria) to the AV junction, then through the AV junction (up to the point of ventricular depolarization).

The PR interval normally occurs in 0.12 to 0.2 second. The interval can change depending on the heart rate. Usually, it's shorter in patients with tachycardia. A shortened PR interval may also result from steroid use and an accessory conduction path that skips the AV junction.

Usually, the PR interval is longer in patients with bradycardia. A longer interval may result from atrial hypertrophy and atrial dilation. Drug therapy given to slow impulse transmission through the AV junction, such as digitalis glycosides, beta-blockers, and calcium channel blockers, can lengthen the PR interval. And longer PR intervals are common in patients who are recovering from a myocardial infarction or sick sinus syndrome.

R-R interval

The R-R interval is the time from one R wave to the next—the time between ventricular contractions, which is determined by the heart rate. If the lengths of the R-R intervals are uniform, the heart rate is regular. If the lengths of the R-R intervals vary, the rate is irregular.

QT interval

The QT interval starts at the beginning of the QRS complex and lasts to the end of the T wave. This interval represents the time of ventricular depolarization and repolarization. Normally, the QT interval lasts 0.35 to 0.45 second.

Age, sex, and heart rate affect the length of the QT interval. Usually, the length of the interval increases slightly with age. Women commonly have longer QT intervals than men. And as the heart rate increases, the QT interval decreases. However, a slowed heart rate lengthens the QT interval.

A prolonged QT interval, which can lead to serious arrhythmias, may result from electrolyte abnormalities. It may also result from antiarrhythmic drug use.

PR segment

The PR segment is the time from the end of the P wave to the beginning of the QRS complex. And it represents the delay of an electrical impulse at the AV node. Usually, the PR segment is an isoelectric line. It's used as a baseline for comparing ST-segment depression or elevation.

ST segment

The ST segment is the time from the end of the QRS complex to the beginning of the T wave. This segment represents the time when ventricular contraction is complete and the cells begin to repolarize.

Normally, the ST segment is isoelectric, appearing flat on the baseline. A positive elevation or negative depression of less than 1 mm also is considered normal. However, an elevation or depression of more than 1 mm may result from ischemia, injury to the heart, drugs, or metabolic abnormalities.

TP segment

The TP segment is the time from the end of the T wave to the beginning of the P wave. During the TP segment, the heart muscle is completely relaxed, and the cardiac cells are able to respond to the next electrical impulse. Usually, TP segments are isoelectric, unless a U wave is discernible.

Analyzing the electrocardiogram

To analyze an ECG tracing, you need to calculate the heart rate, determine the heart rhythm, and recognize whether the tracing represents a normal sinus rhythm or an arrhythmia.

Calculating heart rate

You can calculate the heart rate from an ECG tracing using several methods: two that can be used only if the heart's rhythm is regular and one that can be used if the heart's rhythm is irregular.

If the rhythm is regular, count the number of large squares between two consecutive QRS complexes and divide the result into 300. For example, if you count three squares between the two QRS complexes, divide 300 by 3 for a heart rate of 100 beats per minute (bpm).

If the rhythm is regular, you can also use the more precise 1,500 method. Because each small square represents 0.04 second, 1,500 squares represent 1 minute. So for this method, count the number of small squares between two QRS complexes. Divide the result into 1,500. For example, if you count 15 small squares, divide 1,500 by 15 for a heart rate of 100 bpm.

If the heart rate is irregular, you can use the less precise 6-second method to calculate the heart rate. Above the ECG graph, a dash separates every 3 seconds. Count the number of QRS complexes that occur within 6 seconds—that is, the number that occur between two 3-second markers. Multiply the result by 10 to calculate the heart rate. For example, if you count seven QRS complexes in a 6-second strip, multiply 7 by 10 for a total of 70 bpm. If a QRS complex falls on the line of a 6-second strip, you also count this portion of the QRS complex. For example, if you count 7.5 QRS complexes in a 6-second strip, multiply this number by 10 for a total of 75 bpm.

Determining heart rhythm

On an ECG tracing, the rhythm consists of an atrial rhythm and a ventricular rhythm. To calculate the atrial rhythm, measure the distance from P wave to P wave. To measure the ventricular rhythm, measure the distance from R wave to R wave. You can use either calipers or pencil and paper.

If you're using calipers to determine the atrial rhythm, place the tips of the calipers at the points where two consecutive P waves start. Holding the calipers at that span, place them on successive intervals of P waves. If they match, the atrial rhythm is regular. If the distances between P waves differ, the atrial rhythm is irregular.

To determine the ventricular rhythm using calipers, place the tips of the calipers at the points where two consecutive R waves start. Holding the calipers at that span, place them on successive intervals of R waves. If the intervals are the same, the ventricular rhythm is regular. If the distances between R waves differ, the ventricular rhythm is irregular.

To determine rhythm without calipers, use pencil and paper. At the edge of the paper, mark the beginning of a P or R wave. Make another mark at the next P or R wave. Use this distance to map out successive P-to-P wave or R-to-R wave intervals. Follow the same precepts as described for using calipers.

Recognizing normal sinus rhythm

After determining rate and rhythm, you'll have to determine whether the tracing represents normal sinus rhythm or an arrhythmia. The normal sinus rhythm consists of a P wave, a QRS complex, and a T wave with equal distance between successive P waves and between successive R waves. The heart rate is 60 to 100 bpm (see *Characteristics of normal sinus rhythm*). If any of these components is missing, the tracing represents an arrhythmia.

Look closely at the P wave for shape and duration. If the impulse originated in the SA node, the PR interval should be 0.12 to 0.2 second. A QRS complex measuring 0.1 second or less should follow each P wave. In lead II, the QRS complex should be upright.

A T wave should follow each QRS complex. Examine the shape and size of the T waves. They should have smooth upward slopes from the ST segments, rounded peaks, and then downward slopes to the isoelectric line.

Troubleshooting

Sometimes you may have difficulty obtaining a clear and accurate ECG tracing. An ECG tracing may appear entirely wrong or dangerously abnormal. Electrical interference may make it difficult to distinguish normal from abnormal ECG waveforms. If your patient has such a waveform abnormality, always check him before proceeding. Assess him for physiologic signs and symp-

Characteristics of normal sinus rhythm

Rate: 60 to 100 beats per minute
Rhythm: regular
P wave: normal
PR interval: 0.12 to 0.2 second
QRS complex: ≤ 0.1 second

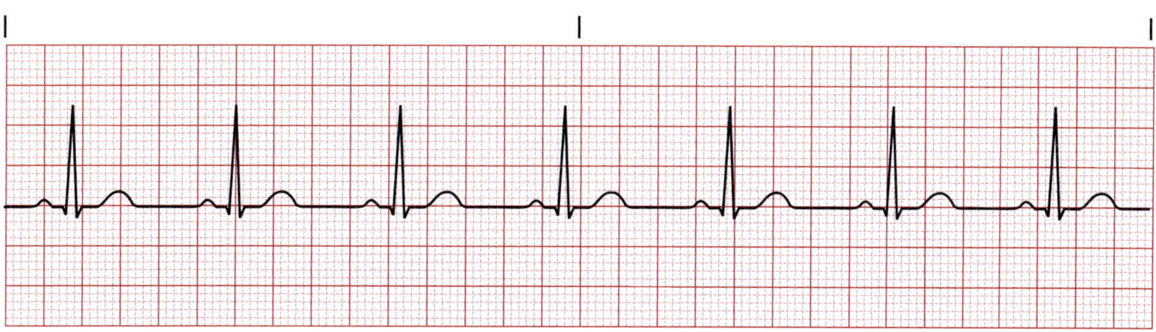

toms that would confirm any abnormality in the ECG tracing. If your patient is asymptomatic, determine whether he may have moved too much during the procedure, causing an abnormal reading.

The ECG commonly detects skeletal muscle activity and interprets it as electrical impulses. You can resolve this artifact or signal noise by repositioning the electrodes, changing the monitoring lead, or asking your patient to lie still while you reexamine the tracing.

Another possible cause of electrical interference or artifact is using old or dried-out electrodes. Be sure there's plenty of conduction gel on the electrodes to ensure a good tracing. Check each electrode for the amount of gel and the extent of skin contact. If you can't find anything wrong with the electrodes or their attachment to the patient, you may have to use a different lead to achieve a good tracing.

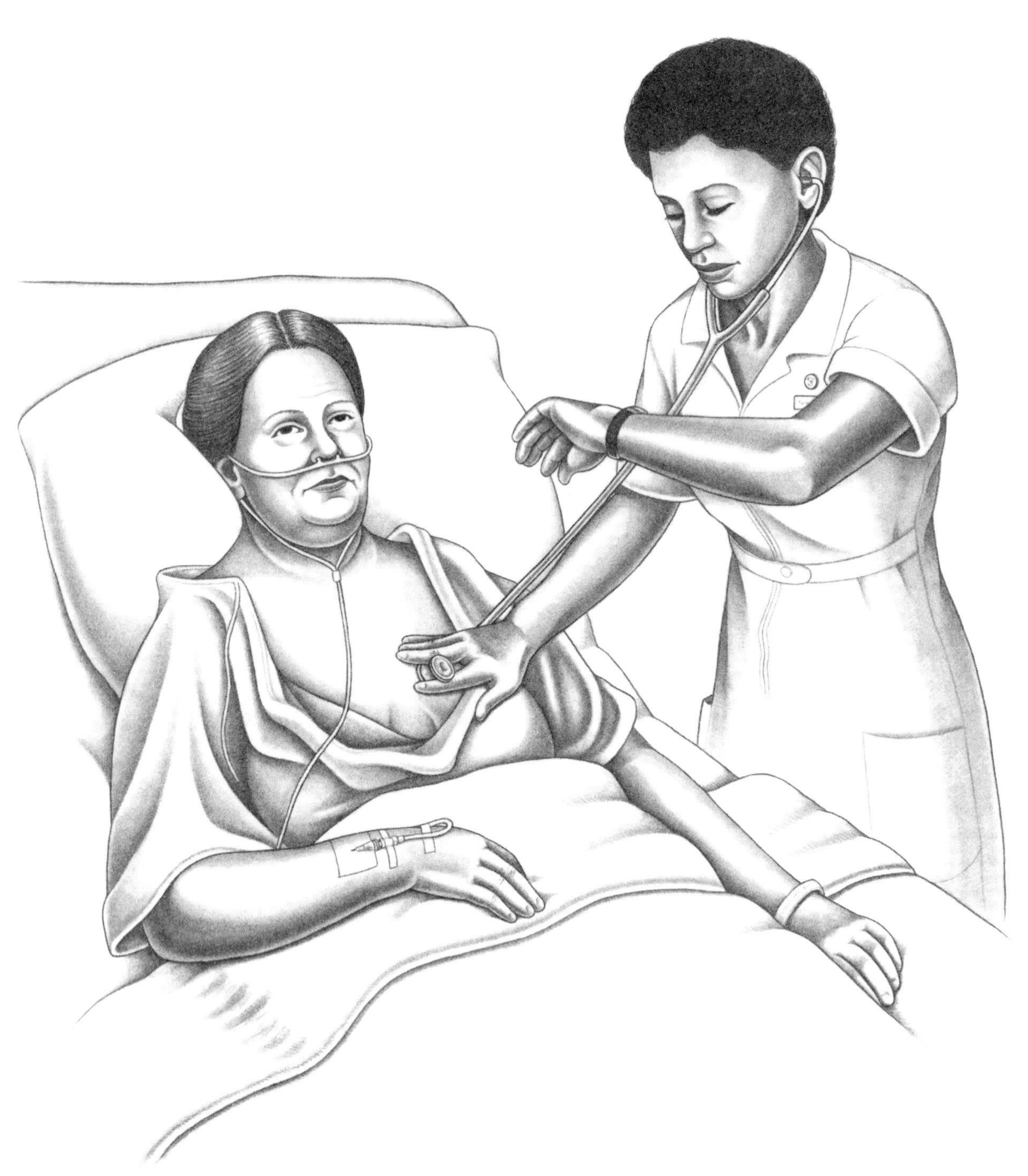

3

Sinoatrial Node Arrhythmias

When electrical impulses travel too quickly, too slowly, or irregularly from the heart's sinoatrial (SA) node, your patient has an SA node arrhythmia. Some SA node arrhythmias may be so mild that a patient has no signs or symptoms and needs no treatment; however, others may require immediate treatment to save a patient's life.

In this chapter, you'll find a comprehensive review of how to respond to the most common SA node arrhythmias—sinus arrhythmia, sinus bradycardia, sinus tachycardia, sinus arrest and SA exit block, and sick sinus syndrome.

Sinus arrhythmia

Sinus arrhythmia, which may be a normal variation in cardiac rhythm, usually doesn't produce any signs or symptoms. It commonly appears in young and elderly patients with slower heart rates. Sinus arrhythmia occurs in two forms: respiratory and nonrespiratory.

In the respiratory form, when the patient inhales, decreased intrathoracic pressure increases venous flow to the right atrium. Increased atrial pressure inhibits the parasympathetic nervous system, increasing the patient's heart rate. When the patient exhales, intrathoracic pressure increases, causing decreased venous flow and decreased pressure in the right atrium. This decreased atrial pressure stimulates the parasympathetic nervous system, thus slowing the patient's heart rate.

The nonrespiratory form of sinus arrhythmia usually occurs in older patients. It may result from or be worsened by carotid sinus massage and drugs such as digoxin, morphine, and neostigmine.

Signs and symptoms

Your patient probably won't notice the subtle signs and symptoms of sinus arrhythmia unless she knows that she has an underlying cardiovascular disease. When signs and symptoms do occur, they usually result from slow rather than fast heart rates. The lengthened atrial cycle, which has long pauses between beats, may cause dizziness, faintness, and palpitations. If your patient's heart rate drops below 30 beats per minute (bpm) and she has no escape beats, she may develop syncope. In fact, syncope is the main reason many patients with sinus arrhythmia seek medical attention.

Some patients with sinus arrhythmia develop signs and symptoms from an accelerated heart rate. If your patient's heart rate increases, the shortened atrial cycle may lead to palpitations, dyspnea, and chest discomfort.

On the electrocardiogram (ECG) of a patient with sinus arrhythmia, you'll see a variation in

Characteristics of sinus arrhythmia

Rate: 60 to 100 beats per minute
Rhythm: irregular
P wave: smooth, rounded, upright
PR interval: 0.12 to 0.2 second
QRS complex: < 0.12 second

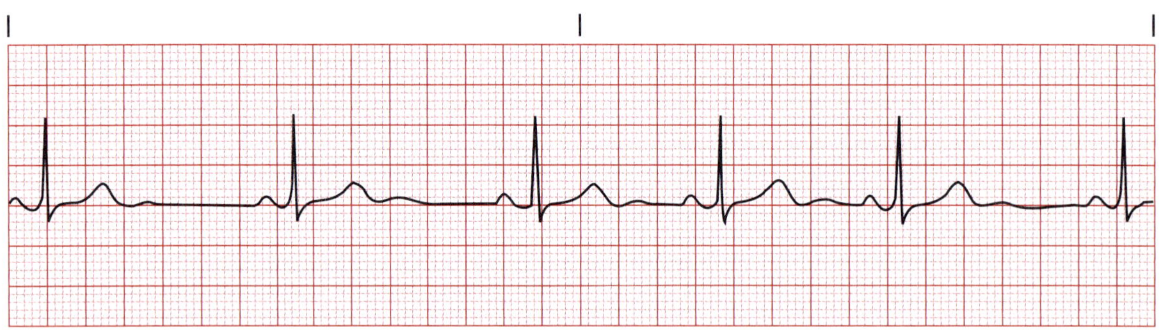

rhythm: her PR interval and R-R interval will vary by more than 0.16 second. However, other ECG characteristics will remain relatively normal (see *Characteristics of sinus arrhythmia*).

Look for a rate that remains within the normal range for the patient's age despite the alternating faster and slower rhythm. In an elderly patient, a normal range can be from 55 to 83 bpm.

The patient's P waves may differ slightly in contour but won't be inverted. Her QRS complexes will appear normal. And each QRS complex will have a P wave.

With the respiratory form of sinus arrhythmia, the P-P interval shortens during inspiration and lengthens during expiration. With the nonrespiratory form, the fluctuations in the P-P interval don't correspond to the respiratory cycle. To confirm the respiratory form of sinus arrhythmia, ask your patient to hold her breath while you observe the cardiac monitor. If the irregular cardiac cycle disappears, your patient has respiratory sinus arrhythmia.

Treatment

Most patients with sinus arrhythmia lead productive lives without ever noticing the mild variations in their cardiac rhythm. Your patient won't need treatment unless she develops significant signs and symptoms. If she does, treatment may include atropine, epinephrine, and isoproterenol (see *Drug therapy for sinus arrhythmia*). In some cases, a physician may also decide to insert an artificial permanent pacemaker.

Atropine

If your patient needs treatment for a slow heart rate caused by sinus arrhythmia, give her atropine, as prescribed. Atropine blocks the action of acetylcholine in the smooth muscle of the SA node, thus blocking vagal effects on the SA node and increasing the heart rate. Typically, you should give 0.5 to 1 mg of atropine by injection and repeat the dose every 5 minutes, as needed. The maximum total dose is 2 mg.

Monitor your patient's heart rate for tachycardia while you administer atropine. Also, be aware that low doses may actually slow her heart rate. And they may cause urinary hesitancy, urine retention, dry mucous membranes and skin, and decreased bronchial secretions.

Atropine is contraindicated in patients with acute glaucoma or a history of chronic glaucoma. Because atropine dilates the pupils, it may cause blurred vision and eye pain. Use it with extra cau-

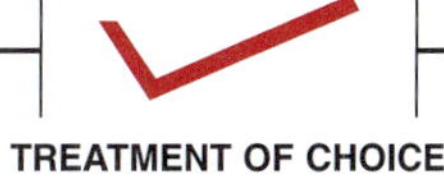

TREATMENT OF CHOICE

Drug therapy for sinus arrhythmia

Drug and action	Adverse effects	Interactions	Nursing considerations
Atropine • blocks action of acetylcholine on postganglionic receptors in cardiac muscle and on sinoatrial and atrioventricular nodes	• drowsiness, palpitations, tachycardia, dry mouth, constipation, urinary hesitancy	• May have additive effect when used with other anticholinergic drugs, including antihistamines, tricyclic antidepressants, quinidine, and disopyramide. • May alter absorption of other drugs by slowing gastrointestinal motility.	• Monitor patient's vital signs and electrocardiogram (ECG) frequently. • Observe patient for tachycardia, angina, and increased ectopia. • Monitor patient's fluid intake and output. • Increase patient's dietary fiber and fluid intake to avoid constipation.
Epinephrine • stimulates $beta_1$ and $beta_2$ receptors, which results in cardiac stimulation, bronchodilation, and vasoconstriction	• anxiety, insomnia, hypertension, arrhythmias, angina, hypoglycemia, urinary hesitancy	• May have additive effect when used with other adrenergic drugs, including decongestants. • When used with monoamine oxidase (MAO) inhibitors, may lead to hypertensive crisis. • Beta-blockers, such as propranolol, may block effects of epinephrine.	• Monitor patient's blood pressure, pulse, and ECG every 5 minutes during therapy. • Maintain peaceful environment. • Report increased restlessness, chest pain, or ectopia.
Isoproterenol • stimulates $beta_1$ and $beta_2$ receptors, which results in cardiac stimulation, bronchodilation, and vasoconstriction	• restlessness, tremors, hypertension, arrhythmias, angina, hyperglycemia	• May have additive effect when used with other adrenergic drugs. • When used with MAO inhibitors, may cause hypertensive crisis. • Beta-blockers, such as propranolol, may block effects of isoproterenol.	• Monitor patient's blood pressure, pulse, hemodynamic status, and ECG every 5 minutes during therapy. • Monitor patient's fluid intake and output. • Assess patient for chest pain, arrhythmias, and hypertension.

tion in very young and elderly patients; both groups are especially sensitive to its adverse effects.

If atropine is contraindicated or ineffective, epinephrine may be prescribed instead.

Epinephrine

Epinephrine, a natural hormone produced by the adrenal medulla, stimulates beta receptors in the heart, thus increasing the firing rate of the SA node and conductivity through the atrioventricular (AV) node and Purkinje fibers. For a patient with sinus arrhythmia, give 0.1 to 1 mg of epinephrine I.V., using a 1:10,000 solution. Repeat this dose every 5 minutes, as indicated, until you reach a maximum of 4 mg/minute.

When giving epinephrine, observe your patient for the following adverse reactions:

- changes in respiratory rate
- urinary hesitancy
- tachycardia
- increased ventricular arrhythmias
- headache
- hypertension
- tremors, facial flushing, fear, anxiety, and insomnia
- hypotension from peripheral vasodilation that results from a $beta_2$-receptor response. (You're most likely to detect hypotension 10 to 20 minutes after the initial injection.)

Epinephrine is contraindicated in patients who have tachycardia resulting from an arrhythmia or tachycardia and heart block resulting from a toxic

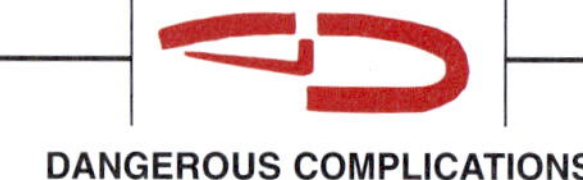

DANGEROUS COMPLICATIONS

Responding to syncope

Syncope, a frightening complication, is a temporary loss of consciousness caused by cerebral hypoxia. The hypoxia may result from problems as varied as a harmless vasovagal episode to a life-threatening cardiac arrhythmia. In fact, syncope may be an early sign of such cardiac problems as sick sinus syndrome, valvular heart disease, bradyarrhythmias, tachyarrhythmias, and pacemaker failure.

Signs and symptoms

Usually, a patient with syncope loses consciousness abruptly. She may experience dizziness, pallor, and diaphoresis shortly before syncope occurs, or she may have no warning. In most cases, syncope lasts only a few seconds, and the patient recovers quickly, although she may be pale and diaphoretic.

Your patient's skin may offer clues to the cause of her syncope. If she has vasovagal syncope, her skin may appear pale and feel moist, and then gradually return to normal. Sudden pain, acute grief, anger, and even the sight of blood may cause such syncope. It also may result from hot environments, crowds, extreme fatigue, and straining to have a bowel movement. Many patients with vasovagal syncope report several minutes of warning symptoms, such as palpitations and dizziness, before they lose consciousness.

In contrast, a patient with cardiac syncope may have a gray, cyanotic appearance that rapidly changes to a flushed appearance when cardiac output resumes. The patient may complain of a hot or cold sensation just before losing consciousness. Cardiac syncope usually occurs within 15 seconds—and sometimes as quickly as 3 seconds—after the patient experiences these symptoms.

Nursing interventions

Immediately verify that your patient has a patent airway, adequate respirations, and a pulse. If she has no respirations or pulse, call for help and begin performing cardiopulmonary resuscitation. If she's breathing and has a pulse, lower her head, maintain a patent airway, and observe her for seizure activity. If necessary, have someone bring emergency equipment to her room. Establish cardiac monitoring and observe her heart rate and rhythm.

Address your patient's immediate signs and symptoms, which may include a slow and weak pulse, urinary incontinence, and apprehension. She may complain of nausea and the need to have a bowel movement. Provide emotional support and a quiet environment while you assess her vital signs and document her signs and symptoms. Document her appearance, any seizure activity, incontinence, the duration of her unconsciousness, and the vital signs you obtained during and after the episode.

Pay special attention to any important events that preceded or followed the syncope. For example, if your patient fell when she fainted, note her posture, activity, and signs and symptoms before the episode. Also, explore your patient's history for previous episodes of syncope, arrhythmias, heart disease, and neurologic disorders.

Follow-up care

A young, vigorous patient who has a single episode of syncope probably won't require follow-up. However, if your patient is elderly and has a history of cardiac problems, she may need cardiovascular tests, Holter monitoring, and laboratory studies.

Treatment for cardiac syncope may include drugs, corrective surgery, and permanent pacemaker insertion.

reaction to a digitalis glycoside. Use epinephrine with caution in patients who have coronary artery insufficiency, ischemic heart disease, heart failure, or hypertension.

Isoproterenol

Isoproterenol, which is used to treat symptomatic bradycardia caused by sinus arrhythmia, has actions similar to those of epinephrine. Isoproterenol stimulates $beta_1$ and $beta_2$ receptors to increase the heart rate and contractility by enhancing the pacemaker function of the SA node and improving AV conduction.

Administer isoproterenol I.V. at 5 μg/minute using a solution prepared by diluting 10 ml of 1:5,000 solution in 500 ml of 5% dextrose in water (D_5W). As you administer the drug, monitor your patient's ECG for changes in heart rate and rhythm. Isoproterenol may quickly cause the following adverse effects:

- rapid heart rates
- ectopic arrhythmias and ischemic changes resulting from increased myocardial oxygen consumption
- ventricular ectopic beats
- vasoconstrictor effects, including angina, headache, dizziness, skin flushing, nausea, diaphoresis, and generalized weakness.

Pacemaker

In extreme cases of symptomatic sinus arrhythmia, your patient may need long-term management of the arrhythmia with an implanted permanent pacemaker. This device has a power source, usually a battery; a pulse generator, which contains electronic circuitry for generating an appropriately timed stimulus; and electrodes or wires to complete the electrical connection between the pulse generator and the myocardium. The pulse generator is inserted permanently under the patient's skin.

The physician's decision to use permanent pacing depends on the cause of your patient's signs and symptoms. If her sinus arrhythmia results from an acute myocardial infarction (MI) or a toxic reaction to digoxin, the arrhythmia is probably reversible, and she'll most likely need only a temporary pacemaker. Patients with symptomatic bradycardia typically require permanent pacing.

Complications

Altered cardiac output (CO), the most serious acute complication of sinus arrhythmia, usually stems from bradycardia. If your patient's heart rate drops below 40 bpm and the AV node doesn't initiate impulses, she may experience syncope—a transient loss of consciousness caused by temporarily reduced blood flow to the brain. Dizziness, pallor, and diaphoresis are warning signs and symptoms of impending syncope. Most patients recover spontaneously after several moments and suffer no lasting effects. However, patients with sinus arrhythmia who commonly experience syncope need a permanent pacemaker (see *Responding to syncope*).

Chronic complications usually occur in patients whose sinus arrhythmia is accompanied by other cardiac arrhythmias. Because low CO decreases peripheral vascular circulation, venous stasis may result. If drug therapy doesn't help control the arrhythmia and increase CO, the patient may need permanent pacing.

Nursing considerations

Appropriate interventions for sinus arrhythmia depend on its cause and its signs and symptoms. Assess your patient for specific evidence of cardiac disease, including chest pain, palpitations, dyspnea, syncope, cough, fatigue, and edema. Also, monitor her ECG and document her response to treatment. Changes in blood pressure, mental status, and urine output may reflect altered CO. Remember, elderly patients who've had an acute MI are the most likely to develop complications from this arrhythmia.

During epinephrine administration, explain to your patient that she may experience feelings of anxiety because epinephrine mimics the body's response to stress.

Teach your patient and her family how to check her radial pulse, especially if she takes digoxin. Also, teach them the signs and symptoms of bradycardia and decreased CO. Review the names, dosages, actions, and adverse effects of any prescribed drugs.

Make sure that she knows when to contact her physician and that she understands the importance of keeping follow-up appointments with her physician, cardiologist, or other health care professional.

Sinus bradycardia

If your patient's SA node consistently conducts less than 60 bpm, she has sinus bradycardia. In some people, such a slowed heart rate occurs normally. For example, in athletes and other physically fit people who have a highly efficient cardiovascular system, the heart can pump more blood with each contraction, thus maintaining a normal CO with a slower heart rate.

However, in other people, sinus bradycardia isn't normal. And if the arrhythmia causes them to experience the signs and symptoms of reduced CO, they may require drug therapy or a pacemaker.

Pathophysiology

Sinus bradycardia is caused by decreased impulse formation in the pacemaker cells of the SA node. This decreased impulse formation may result from problems in the pacemaker cells themselves or from extracardiac problems, including underlying diseases, drug effects, and electrolyte abnormalities.

Conditions that can contribute to sinus bradycardia include a previous MI, underlying heart disease, obstructive jaundice, hypopituitarism, myxedema, and intracranial tumors and bleeding. In patients with obstructive jaundice, bile salts that have accumulated in the body's tissues have a depressant effect on the SA node. Hypopituitarism and myxedema can reduce sympathetic stimulation by decreasing metabolism. Elevated intracranial pressure from tumors and bleeding may reduce the heart rate by stimulating the parasympathetic nervous system.

Other causes of sinus bradycardia include increased vagal tone and decreased sympathetic stimulation resulting from prolonged vomiting, pharyngeal suctioning, vasovagal syncope, and Valsalva's maneuver during forced voiding or straining at stool.

When assessing the underlying causes of sinus bradycardia, always consider adverse drug effects. Your patient may be taking a drug intended to slow an abnormally fast heart rate or to prevent more serious cardiac arrhythmias—for example, a beta-blocker or a digitalis glycoside. In patients with sinus bradycardia, a beta-blocker may slow the heart rate to dangerously low levels. Propranolol, one type of beta-blocker, may also slow AV conduction and decrease myocardial contractility and CO. A digitalis glycoside increases the force of myocardial contractions by slowing electrical impulses across the AV node. If your patient takes digoxin, bradycardia may be a warning sign of a toxic reaction.

Elevated blood potassium levels (hyperkalemia) may be an underlying cause of sinus bradycardia as well. The cardiac muscle is extremely sensitive to altered potassium levels. Blood potassium levels above 4.5 mEq/L can decrease the resting potential and increase the membrane excitability of cardiac cells. Repolarization of the SA node slows, resulting in bradycardia and hypotension. To assess your patient for possible hyperkalemia, ask her about noncardiac signs and symptoms of the condition, such as diarrhea, nausea, muscle cramping, and paresthesia.

Signs and symptoms

In sinus bradycardia, the slow heart rate may allow an irritable focus in the heart to take over the pacemaker function and create dangerous ventricular arrhythmias, such as ventricular tachycardia and ventricular fibrillation. In patients with heart disease or other serious health problems, sinus bradycardia can trigger the signs and symptoms of low CO. If your patient's heart rate drops below 40 bpm, she may develop hypotension, angina, dizziness, syncope, weakness, and diaphoresis. Also, she may become confused and restless and have a decreased urine output.

On your patient's ECG, you'll see a heart rate below 60 bpm. The atrial and ventricular rates are identical, and escape beats may be present. Typically, other ECG characteristics are normal. But if she also has sinus arrhythmia, her rhythm may be irregular (see *Characteristics of sinus bradycardia*).

Treatment

Begin treatment for sinus bradycardia with an accurate ECG interpretation of the arrhythmia. Collaborate with your patient's physician to isolate the cause of the arrhythmia and diagnose any underlying heart disease, and assess your patient for the signs and symptoms of decreased CO. Obtain a complete health history and perform a physical examination. Record any complaints of chest pain, palpitations, dyspnea, syncope, cough, fatigue, and edema.

As in sinus arrhythmia, atropine and isoproterenol form the first line of drug treatment for sinus bradycardia. In some cases, a physician may also prescribe theophylline or arrange for temporary or permanent pacemaker insertion.

Atropine

Patients who need drug treatment for sinus bradycardia typically receive I.V. atropine. Within minutes after administration, your patient's heart rate should increase. And this increase in heart rate should quickly alleviate all signs and symptoms related to low CO and decreased cerebral perfusion.

Characteristics of sinus bradycardia

Rate: < 60 beats per minute
Rhythm: regular
P wave: smooth, rounded, upright
PR interval: 0.12 to 0.2 second
QRS complex: < 0.12 second

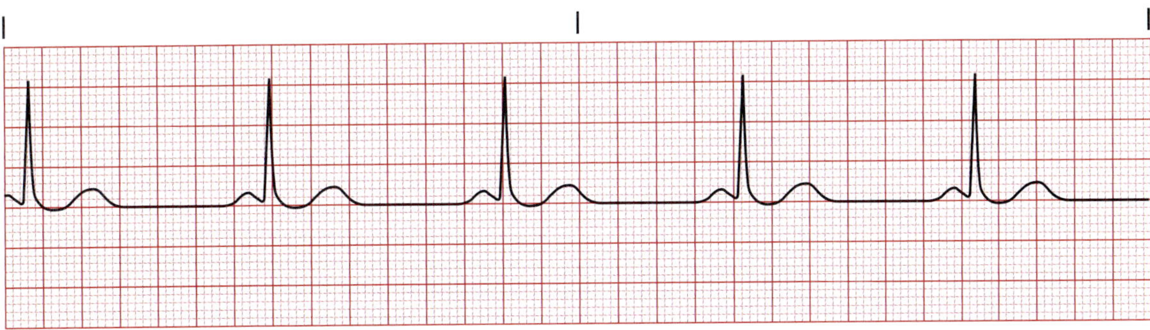

The standard dosage of atropine is 0.5 to 1 mg, repeated every 5 minutes to a total of 2 mg, as needed. Monitor your patient carefully while administering atropine because the increase in heart rate that this drug produces will increase myocardial oxygen consumption and possibly induce myocardial ischemia. Also, keep in mind that a patient who has had an MI may be at risk for ventricular ectopia. The ischemia may cause further infarction and increase irritability in the ventricles.

Be alert for other adverse effects of atropine, such as tachycardia, dry mucous membranes and skin, decreased bronchial secretions, urinary hesitancy, urine retention, and increased intraocular pressure. Remember that atropine is contraindicated in patients with acute glaucoma or a history of chronic glaucoma because it can increase intraocular pressure, leading to pain and blurred vision. Use it cautiously in very young and elderly patients.

Isoproterenol

If atropine is contraindicated or proves to be ineffective for your patient's signs and symptoms, the second drug of choice for sinus bradycardia is isoproterenol. Isoproterenol increases the heart rate and contractility by stimulating beta$_1$ and beta$_2$ receptors.

Usually, give isoproterenol at 5 µg/minute using a solution prepared by diluting 10 ml of 1:5,000 solution in 500 ml of D_5W. Monitor your patient closely because isoproterenol increases myocardial oxygen consumption. Ventricular ectopic beats are common during administration of this potent drug. Other effects include an excessive heart rate, ectopic arrhythmias, and ischemic changes. Your patient may also experience headache, skin flushing, angina, nausea, dizziness, diaphoresis, and generalized weakness.

Theophylline

If your patient can't tolerate atropine or isoproterenol or fails to respond to them, the physician may prescribe theophylline. Although not the most common or desirable treatment for this arrhythmia, theophylline stimulates the pacemaker cells of the SA node.

Pacemaker

Patients with symptomatic sinus bradycardia who can't tolerate drug therapy will probably need temporary or permanent pacing for long-term management of the arrhythmia.

If your patient has sinus bradycardia accompanied by other health problems, she may not be able to attain an acceptable heart rate or tolerate

Investigating your patient's palpitations

A patient with palpitations commonly describes—with some alarm—a sensation of fluttering, butterflies, or pounding in her chest. Although frightening, the episodes usually subside before the symptoms can be recorded or the patient reaches a medical facility.

What to do

Begin investigating possible causes for your patient's palpitations by obtaining a thorough health history. Be sure to ask about possible physiologic causes, such as mitral valve prolapse, hyperthyroidism, and cardiac conduction defects.

Keep in mind that palpitations occur normally with exercise. They also may result from caffeine or nicotine intake, lack of sleep, hyperventilation, antihistamines, a heavy meal, or stress.

In many cases, the electrocardiogram reveals a normal sinus rhythm when palpitations occur. However, if your patient's cardiac rhythm becomes irregular during palpitations, she may be having premature beats or short bursts of an arrhythmia. Significant bradycardia (less than 50 beats per minute) may indicate atrioventricular block or sinoatrial node dysfunction.

What to teach your patient

If your patient has palpitations, teach her to take these measures:

- stop what she's doing and rest until the symptoms subside
- count her radial pulse during episodes
- note whether her heartbeat is regular, irregular, rapid, normal, or slow
- seek immediate medical attention if the palpitations occur with other signs and symptoms, such as chest pain, dizziness, or fainting.

Commonly, palpitations result from anxiety and a stressful lifestyle. You may need to help your patient explore lifestyle changes, adopt relaxation techniques, and eliminate caffeine and nicotine.

the hemodynamic effects of the arrhythmia. For such a patient, the physician may insert a permanent cardiac pacemaker. Such health problems include an extensive anterior-wall infarction and a chronic heart disease, such as heart failure.

If your patient is recovering from open-heart surgery or a small area of MI, temporary transvenous or transcutaneous pacing may be more appropriate. In some cases, a physician may use a temporary pacemaker until a permanent one can be inserted.

Complications

Acute complications from sinus bradycardia include an altered hemodynamic status and the onset of more dangerous arrhythmias, such as premature ventricular contractions (PVCs). The PVCs that arise from sinus bradycardia result from the body's compensatory response to a decreased CO. Consequently, you most likely won't administer lidocaine I.V., the standard treatment for PVCs, to a patient who also has sinus bradycardia because the drug would further decrease her heart rate. Instead, treat ectopic beats by resolving the underlying bradycardia. This can be done either with drugs or with a pacemaker.

Your patient with chronic sinus bradycardia may develop dependent edema, especially if she also has underlying heart disease or a previous MI. For those patients with a history of decreased ejection fraction, long-term management may include I.V. therapy with an inotropic drug.

Remember, if your patient's heart rate drops below 40 bpm and doesn't respond to treatment, she may have sick sinus syndrome.

Nursing considerations

When you first notice sinus bradycardia, perform a baseline assessment that includes your patient's vital signs and neurologic status. Observe your patient for the signs and symptoms of decreased CO, including chest pain, dyspnea, syncope, cough, fatigue, edema, and palpitations (see *Investigating your patient's palpitations*). Be alert for changes in mental status and decreased urine output.

In uncomplicated cases of sinus bradycardia, careful monitoring and documentation of the patient's ECG usually are sufficient treatment. Assess her ECG for heart rate and rhythm and for signs of a more serious arrhythmia, such as AV block or a junctional escape rhythm. If your patient shows significant ECG changes or new signs and symptoms related to the sinus bradycardia, immediately notify the physician. Also, be prepared to implement emergency measures.

If your patient experiences hypotension from sinus bradycardia during sleep, you may need to awaken or turn her to help increase her heart rate and CO. Also, assess your patient's blood pressure, pulses, mental status, and urine output to determine if she's experiencing other signs and symptoms.

Whenever possible, include family members or your patient's primary caregiver in your teaching sessions. Make sure your teaching includes the following:

- pulse and blood pressure monitoring
- the signs and symptoms of significant bradycardia
- developments that warrant a call for medical help
- the dosages, actions, and adverse effects of her drugs
- the importance of keeping follow-up appointments with her physician or other health care professional.

Your patient's ability to monitor her own cardiac status will help her manage her condition and prevent complications.

Sinus tachycardia

The most common of all the arrhythmias, sinus tachycardia may occur in some patients as a natural result of the body's reaction to stress. When the sympathetic nervous system's fight or flight response is activated, the heart rate increases to meet the body's demands for more oxygen. In healthy patients, such a response is normal. However, in other patients, prolonged, persistent sinus tachycardia isn't normal and may require treatment.

Pathophysiology

In sinus tachycardia, the normal pacemaker of the heart fires impulses much more rapidly than usual. Causes of sinus tachycardia include physical exercise, emotional and physical stress, increased body temperature, and the use of stimulants, such as caffeine and cigarettes. Exercise stimulates the heart rate by increasing the body's oxygen demand and consumption. A sudden drop in blood pressure also results in tachycardia because the heart increases its effort to maintain peripheral perfusion. If your patient has decreased tissue perfusion because of anemia or a hypermetabolic state, such as fever, her heart rate will increase when chemoreceptor mechanisms stimulate the vasomotor center.

If your patient has prolonged sinus tachycardia, she's at risk for heart failure when sympathetic neurotransmitters or myocardial energy stores become depleted. During high rates of sinus tachycardia, cardiac stroke volume may decrease because of shortened diastolic filling time, causing a decrease in coronary perfusion and subsequent ischemia.

Certain drugs with a positive chronotropic (rate-accelerating) effect also may cause sinus tachycardia, including:

- epinephrine (a sympathetic agonist)
- atropine (an anticholinergic)
- caffeine
- nicotine
- alcohol
- methamphetamine
- cocaine.

Signs and symptoms

As discussed, sinus tachycardia may occur in some patients as a normal adaptive response. This arrhythmia develops in healthy people during activities such as running and exercising and during states of heightened anxiety. Thus, the condition is usually asymptomatic. But if the patient has limited cardiac reserves or other health problems, she may experience signs and symptoms such as palpitations, restlessness, anxiety, and diaphoresis. If your patient has coronary artery disease (CAD), rapid or sustained tachycardia may also cause her to experience signs and symptoms of ischemia and angina pectoris.

On the ECG of a patient with sinus tachycardia, the heart rate is 100 to 150 bpm. Because the conduction pathways are normal, cardiac conduction remains at a 1:1 ratio for each cycle, and other ECG characteristics remain normal. The rhythm is regular (see *Characteristics of sinus tachycardia,* page 32).

Characteristics of sinus tachycardia

Rate: 100 to 150 beats per minute
Rhythm: regular
P wave: uniform, upright
PR interval: 0.12 to 0.2 second
QRS complex: < 0.12 second

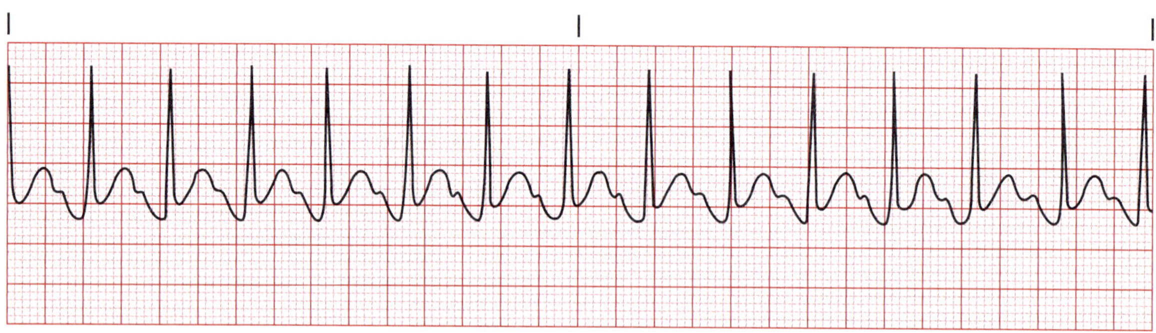

Treatment

When treating sinus tachycardia, you'll need to identify the underlying cause. If it's a prescribed drug, you may need to adjust the dosage, as ordered, to eliminate a positive chronotropic effect. Also, advise your patient to avoid stimulants such as caffeine and nicotine.

A physician may coach the patient through Valsalva's maneuver or use carotid sinus massage or other vagal maneuvers to help slow the heart rate. However, it probably will accelerate again unless the underlying cause is corrected.

A patient with symptomatic sinus tachycardia usually requires drug therapy. Typically, a physician may prescribe propranolol, a calcium channel blocker, or digoxin.

Propranolol

If your patient has persistent, symptomatic sinus tachycardia unrelated to a manageable cause, the arrhythmia may be treated with propranolol, a beta-blocker that decreases AV conduction and slows the heart rate by blocking stimulation of beta$_1$ and beta$_2$ receptors. Propranolol also has a direct membrane-stabilizing action on cardiac cells. The normal dosage is 10 to 60 mg orally four times daily.

Propranolol isn't recommended for arrhythmias related to thyrotoxicosis, mitral valve prolapse, or anxiety. If your patient's pulse is less than 50 bpm, consult with the physician before giving the drug.

When giving propranolol, monitor your patient's blood pressure and pulse frequently. Assess her for adverse reactions to the drug, such as bradycardia, worsening heart failure, hypotension, pulmonary edema, fatigue, drowsiness, depression, mental changes (such as memory loss or confusion), bronchospasm, wheezing, diarrhea, and nausea. If your patient is male, ask him about impotence and decreased libido, which also may be caused by propranolol.

Warn your patient that smoking can overstimulate the heart rate, increase myocardial oxygen demand, decrease the cardioprotective effects of propranolol, and interfere with her body's ability to clear the drug. Propranolol masks the signs and symptoms of hypoglycemia, so advise diabetic patients to monitor their blood glucose level regularly.

Calcium channel blockers

A calcium channel blocker can help decrease your patient's heart rate by blocking the movement of calcium across cardiac cell membranes. As a result, the rate of depolarization decreases. Calcium

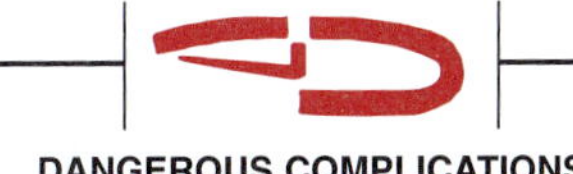

DANGEROUS COMPLICATIONS

Avoiding the adverse effects of digoxin

Digoxin, a plant alkaloid derived from the foxglove flower, is one of the oldest and most effective drugs for treating heart failure and certain cardiac tachyarrhythmias. It strengthens contractions of the heart muscle, increases stroke volume and cardiac output, and reduces preload and electrical impulse transmission across the atrioventricular (AV) node, thereby slowing the heart rate.

However, in addition to its therapeutic effects, digoxin also has some associated dangers. It has a narrow therapeutic range, and toxic blood levels can cause the following adverse effects:

- arrhythmias, including sinus bradycardia, sinoatrial arrest, second-degree and third-degree AV block, atrial fibrillation with a slowed ventricular response, junctional escape rhythm, and ventricular arrhythmias
- gastrointestinal (GI) disturbances, including anorexia, vomiting, and nausea, which may be the first warning sign of toxic blood digoxin levels
- visual disturbances, such as yellow or green halos around objects
- central nervous system effects, such as disorientation, delirium, headache, and drowsiness
- hypokalemia, which can lead to cardiac arrhythmias, hypotension, muscle weakness, and respiratory distress.

Nursing considerations

To ensure safe digoxin therapy, take the following measures:

- Before administering digoxin, check your patient's heart rate. If it's below 60 beats per minute, confirm the dosage with the patient's physician before giving the drug.
- Before admininstering digoxin, also check your patient's blood potassium level. If it's below 3.5 mEq/L, you must correct it before giving the drug.
- Avoid giving digoxin to a patient with hypertrophic obstructive cardiomyopathy. Digoxin may increase ventricular contractility, which can worsen obstruction of the left ventricular outflow.
- Give digoxin with food to decrease the adverse GI effects. However, be aware that high-fiber foods may interact with the drug.
- If your patient takes quinidine, cut the digoxin dose in half, as ordered. Remember that quinidine and amiodarone can raise blood digoxin levels, as can protein-bound drugs such as verapamil, warfarin, erythromycin, tetracycline, and phenytoin.
- Watch your patient carefully for signs of a toxic reaction. Remember that patients with low albumin levels and decreased muscle mass have a greater risk of a toxic reaction because of a decreased ability to bind the drug.
- Monitor the patient's blood digoxin level, as ordered.
- Teach your patient about the drug's intended actions, dosage, and adverse effects. If she develops adverse effects, make sure she knows when to contact the physician.

channel blockers decrease SA and AV node conduction and prolong AV node refractory periods in cardiac conduction tissue, resulting in a slower heart rate. Such drugs include verapamil, nifedipine, diltiazem, nicardipine, felodipine, and amlodipine.

Calcium channel blockers are contraindicated in patients with advanced heart block, severe heart failure, or episodes of sinus bradycardia. When giving a calcium channel blocker, monitor your patient for adverse reactions such as dizziness, headache, fatigue, bradycardia, hypotension, edema, heart block, and heart failure. Your patient also may develop sinus arrest or asystole, constipation, nausea, abdominal discomfort, or pulmonary edema.

Digoxin

You may administer digoxin to prolong the AV node's refractory period and to decrease conduction through the SA and AV nodes, effects that result from increased parasympathetic tone and decreased sympathetic tone. The usual maintenance dose is 0.125 to 0.5 mg/day, administered orally.

Digoxin can cause adverse reactions (see *Avoiding the adverse effects of digoxin*). Also, it interacts with several other drugs. Amiodarone and antibiotics may increase the absorption of digoxin, leading to a toxic reaction. Antidiarrheal medications, antacids, and anion exchange resins such as cholestyramine can impair the absorption of digoxin, diminishing its therapeutic effects. Calcium salts and thyroid medications used with digoxin increase the risk of cardiac arrhythmias.

Because digoxin slows the heart rate and increases CO, it's contraindicated in patients with AV block and ventricular arrhythmias. When administering digoxin, observe your patient for such signs and symptoms as fatigue, weakness, headache, blurred vision, yellow vision, nausea, vomiting, anorexia, and diarrhea. Document the development of arrhythmias, bradycardia, and ECG abnormalities and notify the physician immediately.

As ordered, check your patient's blood electrolyte levels and blood digoxin level periodically during therapy. If her heart rate is less than 60 bpm, withhold digoxin, as indicated.

Nursing considerations

Although sinus tachycardia isn't a life-threatening arrhythmia, your patient's increased heart rate may indicate a serious underlying problem. Perform a baseline assessment of her vital signs, peripheral pulses, skin color, capillary refill, and urine output. Monitor her ECG and stay alert for signs and symptoms of heart failure, such as dyspnea, cough, crackles, peripheral edema, and distended neck veins.

Sinus tachycardia may reduce your patient's CO and worsen other medical problems. As you know, decreased CO can reduce oxygen exchange in the lungs, leading to changes in her level of consciousness, such as agitation or confusion. Your patient also may become anxious from feeling short of breath.

Keep in mind that external stimulation can increase your patient's oxygen consumption. Maintain a quiet, comfortable environment and regulate her visiting hours, if necessary. Anxiety and pain stimulate the sympathetic nervous system, worsening sinus tachycardia. Offer analgesics, as needed, and take measures to decrease your patient's anxiety.

Encourage your patient to participate in her treatment by checking her own pulse and blood pressure; using relaxation techniques at home, such as biofeedback, meditation, and guided imagery; and avoiding cardiostimulants such as caffeine, alcohol, nicotine, and antihistamines. Also, advise her not to smoke.

Take time to review your patient's drug regimen with her. Make sure she knows the names, dosages, actions, and adverse effects of her prescribed drugs. If she is diabetic and taking propranolol, tell her to monitor her blood glucose level regularly.

If your patient is taking digoxin, tell her to check her pulse before taking the drug. And tell her that if her heart rate is less than 60 bpm, she should call the physician before she takes it.

Sinus arrest and sinoatrial exit block

If your patient's SA node fails to initiate an impulse at the expected time in the cardiac cycle, one of two problems has occurred: the SA node didn't generate an electrical impulse (sinus arrest), or the SA node generated an impulse that failed to exit the node (SA exit block).

Sinus arrest and SA exit block are difficult to tell apart because SA node depolarization isn't recorded on the ECG. What's more, these two arrhythmias produce the same clinical result: the sinus mechanism fails to deliver its current into the surrounding tissue.

Pathophysiology

During sinus arrest, SA node automaticity is depressed and impulses aren't formed as expected. When only one sinus impulse fails to form, the rhythm is called a sinus pause. If more than one impulse fails to form, the rhythm is called sinus arrest.

Fortunately, the heart has pacemaker cells scattered throughout the myocardium to supplement the main pacemaker cells found in the SA node. When sinus arrest occurs, these lower pacemakers fire escape beats from the junctional or ventricular pacemaker cells. However, if the SA node stops firing and no escape beats occur, your patient will experience sudden cardiac death.

During SA exit block, impulse conduction is either slowed or blocked from leaving the SA node.

Characteristics of sinus arrest

Rate: 60 to 100 beats per minute
Rhythm: irregular
P wave: smooth, rounded, upright
PR interval: > 0.2 second; absent during arrest
QRS complex: < 0.12 second

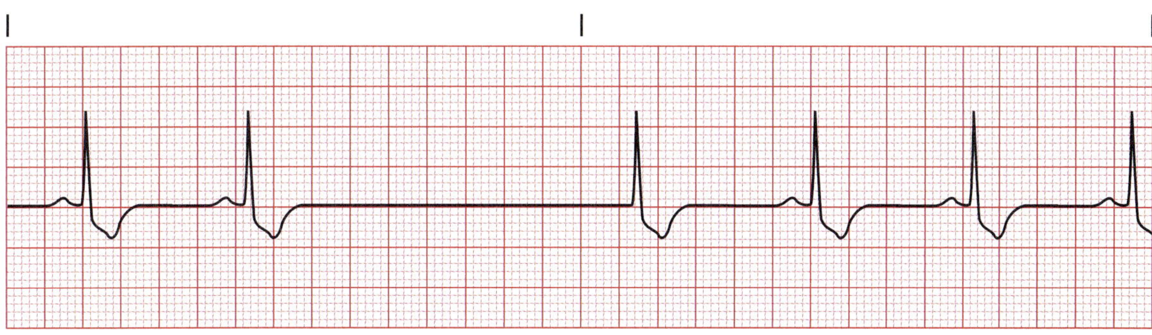

This arrhythmia is divided into three types based on the length of delay: first-degree, second-degree, and third-degree block.

If your patient has first-degree SA exit block, conduction time is prolonged from the SA node to the surrounding atrial tissue. You can't see this abnormality on a standard ECG. Typically, the AV node takes over, and your patient may develop a second-degree AV block type I arrhythmia.

Second-degree SA exit block results from an intermittent failure in the conduction of sinus impulses to the surrounding atrial tissue. Third-degree SA block results from a complete failure in impulse conduction between the SA node and the atria. On a standard ECG, this latter form of SA exit block looks the same as sinus arrest. However, with third-degree SA block, another pacemaker usually takes over, and the patient's rhythm changes.

Several underlying problems can lead to sinus arrest or SA exit block, such as the following:

- an occlusion of the SA node artery resulting from an MI
- stretched myocardial fibers during volume overload, which can inhibit SA node activity
- an adverse reaction to a beta-blocker, a calcium channel blocker, or digoxin
- degenerative heart disease
- myocarditis
- trauma to the conduction system after heart surgery
- vagal stimulation.

Signs and symptoms

Usually, sinus arrest and SA exit block are transient arrhythmias. During episodes of the arrhythmia, the patient typically has a slow, irregular pulse. She may experience only mild symptoms or none at all. However, if escape beats fail to occur, your patient may experience the signs and symptoms of decreased CO and cerebral insufficiency, including hypotension, vertigo, confusion, dizziness, and syncope.

On the ECG of a patient with sinus arrest or SA exit block, the atrial rate is normal, except when several sinus impulses fail to form or fail to exit the SA node. In the latter case, the patient will have bradycardia. The ventricular rate also is normal except in the absence of sinus impulses or escape beats (see *Characteristics of sinus arrest*).

You should see P waves when the SA node fires, but not during sinus arrest, second-degree exit block, or third-degree exit block. When P waves are present, the PR interval usually is normal. However, if the P wave accompanies a junctional

QRS complex, the PR interval may be shortened.

The R-R interval may be normal when P waves are present, but it won't be measurable when P waves are absent. Expect to see normal QRS complexes with normal SA node function, wide QRS complexes with ventricular escape beats, and no QRS complexes during periods of sinus arrest.

Treatment

Your patient won't need treatment for sinus arrest or SA exit block unless she has signs and symptoms of hemodynamic compromise. If she has these signs and symptoms, treatment typically includes atropine, isoproterenol, and pacemaker insertion.

Atropine

Administer atropine to help restore the normal formation or conduction of SA node impulses. As ordered, give the standard dosage: 0.5 to 1 mg repeated every 5 minutes, as needed, to a total of 2 mg.

Watch your patient for adverse reactions to atropine, such as urinary hesitancy, urine retention, dry mucous membranes and skin, and decreased bronchial secretions. Monitor your patient's heart rate for tachycardia during atropine injection. And remember that low doses of this drug may actually slow her heart rate.

As in the treatment of other SA node arrhythmias, use atropine cautiously in young and elderly patients, who are especially sensitive to its effects. Also, avoid giving atropine to a patient with acute glaucoma or a history of chronic glaucoma.

Isoproterenol

Give isoproterenol to increase your patient's heart rate and contractility, enhance the pacemaker function of the SA node, and improve AV conduction. As with other SA node arrhythmias, administer the drug at 5 μg/minute using a solution prepared by diluting 10 ml of 1:5,000 solution in 500 ml of D_5W.

Isoproterenol may quickly cause excessive heart rates and other adverse effects. Also, because the drug increases myocardial oxygen consumption, it may cause ectopic arrhythmias and ischemic changes. Ventricular ectopic beats are common. The patient also may develop a headache, flushed skin, angina, nausea, dizziness, and diaphoresis.

Pacemaker

If your patient's symptomatic sinus arrest or SA exit block doesn't respond to drug therapy, the physician may insert a pacemaker to maintain your patient's CO and heart rate at acceptable levels.

Complications

For many patients, sinus arrest and SA exit block are harmless, asymptomatic arrhythmias. However, if your patient with sinus arrest or SA exit block also has another cardiac condition—such as an MI, heart failure, or CAD—she may require treatment for the arrhythmia. Also, in some patients, extended periods of bradycardia often decrease CO and may lead to hypotension, decreased cerebral perfusion, and syncope, which may require treatment.

The pauses caused by sinus arrest or SA exit block may decrease oxygen supply to the coronary arteries, causing myocardial ischemia. This situation is critical for patients who've had an MI because the myocardium is already damaged by decreased blood flow.

If your patient has heart failure or CAD, sinus arrest or SA exit block may contribute to chronic complications. If your patient has heart failure, assess her for weakness, fatigue, cough, crackles, dyspnea, dependent edema, and distended neck veins. If she has CAD or has had an MI, watch for ischemic changes. If your patient has had an inferior-wall MI, expect to see chronic arrhythmias because this type of an MI damages the right coronary artery, which in turn affects the SA node and causes conduction disturbances.

Complete sinus arrest without escape beats results in cardiac standstill and sudden death. If your patient has episodes of asystole, be prepared to take emergency measures.

Nursing considerations

Observe your patient for early signs and symptoms of hemodynamic compromise. Assess her peripheral and apical pulses, and report changes in her cardiac rhythm. Be alert for signs and symptoms of decreased CO, heart failure, and inadequate cerebral perfusion.

If you need to suction your patient, watch her ECG carefully. To prevent vagal stimulation and hypoxia, which may trigger an increased heart rate and ectopic escape beats, don't suction for more than 10 to 15 seconds.

If your patient takes a drug that decreases the heart rate, such as a beta-blocker, a calcium channel blocker, digoxin, or quinidine, observe her carefully for adverse reactions. Also, if she's taking digoxin, check her blood digoxin level frequently.

As with other sinus arrhythmias, tell your patient to take her pulse regularly, especially if she takes digoxin. Teach your patient, her family members, and any caregivers to recognize the signs and symptoms of bradycardia and decreased CO. And carefully review her drug regimen with her, including the names, dosages, actions, and adverse effects of all her drugs.

Explain when she should contact her physician. Stress the importance of keeping follow-up appointments with her physician, cardiologist, or other health care professional. Teach her how to avoid vagal stimulation caused by gagging, straining, coughing, and other activities that could cause Valsalva's maneuver.

Sick sinus syndrome

In sick sinus syndrome, also called SA node dysfunction, the SA node fails to initiate impulses normally. And because of anatomic or physiologic abnormalities, the SA node conducts impulses at a slow rate or fails to conduct them at all, producing sinus pauses or sinus block. In sick sinus syndrome, the SA node also may fire erratically, producing rapid heart rates.

Usually, sick sinus syndrome begins with sinus bradycardia and progresses to sinus arrest or sinus block. In bradycardia-tachycardia syndrome, which is one type of sick sinus syndrome, the heartbeat alternates between rapid and slow rates.

Pathophysiology

Sick sinus syndrome may result from problems in the SA node itself or from problems outside the SA node. Such problems may include altered SA automaticity, abnormal SA conduction, and altered function of the autonomic nervous system or endocrine system.

Although sick sinus syndrome appears in patients of all ages, this arrhythmia most commonly occurs in the elderly. Also, it may accompany other cardiovascular abnormalities, such as hypertension, CAD, and cerebrovascular disease.

A patient with a history of cardiomyopathy or an MI may develop sick sinus syndrome from a decreased blood supply to the SA node or from atrial muscle that is compromised by amyloidosis, diffuse fibrosis, collagen vascular disease, infection, pericardial disease, or degenerative retinopathy. This arrhythmia also occurs after cardiac surgery and in young adults with a history of congenital heart defects. Also, drugs such as digoxin, propranolol, and quinidine commonly cause reversible dysfunction of the SA node.

Signs and symptoms

With sick sinus syndrome, your patient's signs and symptoms may range from mild to life threatening. Your patient's ability to tolerate this arrhythmia depends on the extent of damage to the SA node and the functional capacity of the lower pacemaker sites. Myocardial contractility and the level of perfusion in other primary organs, including the brain and kidneys, also affect her tolerance for the arrhythmia.

Signs and symptoms of sick sinus syndrome may develop quickly, but the onset usually is insidious and progressive. Your patient may experience weakness, dizziness, altered mental status, syncope, and chest pressure and pain. Persistent, severe, and unexplained sinus bradycardia commonly results from sick sinus syndrome. And periodic cessation of the sinus rhythm may result in sinus pauses, sinus arrest, and SA block, which may be accompanied by the failure of other pacemaker sites in the heart.

Long pauses in the heart rate or periods of sinus arrest can cause syncope and seizures. If your patient has bradycardia-tachycardia syndrome, she also may experience the signs and symptoms of tachycardia, such as weakness, recurrent uncompensated episodes of heart failure, changes in mental status, and palpitations.

Unlike other cardiac arrhythmias that are diagnosed from a single ECG, sick sinus syndrome is diagnosed from a series of ECGs made after ruling out alternative diagnoses. Patients with sick sinus syndrome tend to have a slow heart rate except during the tachycardia phase of bradycardia-tachycardia syndrome. If your patient has this type of sick sinus syndrome, her heart rate may al-

Characteristics of sick sinus syndrome

Rate: 60 to 100 beats per minute
Rhythm: periods of irregularity
P wave: usually smooth, rounded, upright; shape depends on pacemaker site
PR interval: 0.12 to 0.2 second
QRS complex: < 0.12 second

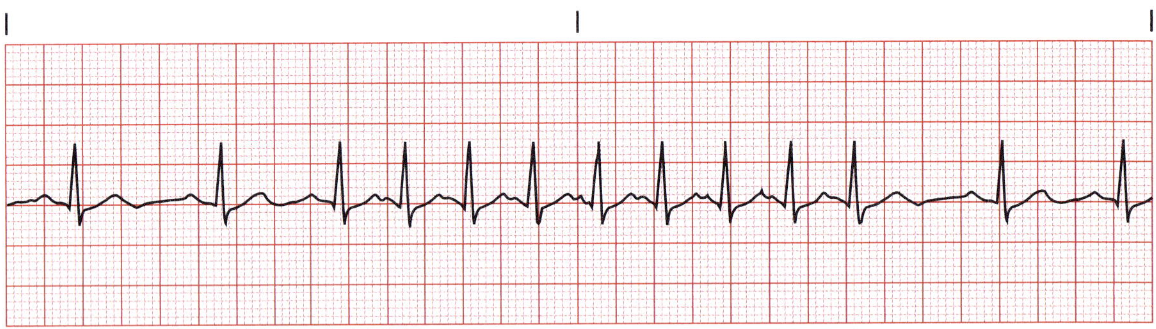

ternate between 30 and 180 bpm (see *Characteristics of sick sinus syndrome*).

Your patient's rhythm may be regular, irregular, or a combination of the two. Rhythm disturbances that accompany sick sinus syndrome include persistent and severe sinus bradycardia, sinus pauses, sinus arrest, sinus arrhythmia, SA block, and deviations from the normal SA node pacemaker site, such as a wandering pacemaker. Other rhythm disturbances include junctional-ventricular escape beats, tachyarrhythmias, and AV block.

With sick sinus syndrome, the pacemaker function originates in the SA node. However, because of the abnormal conduction, other ectopic sites pace the heart from time to time. The heart's lower pacemakers commonly are impaired in patients with SA conduction defect, and they tend to produce long pauses in systole.

The shape of the P wave depends on which pacemaker site controls the cardiac cycle when you observe the arrhythmia. You may see normal or abnormal P waves with positive or negative deflections on the ECG. At a normal heart rate, the P wave is normal in shape and size because conduction comes from the SA node. But if the heart rate drops below 60 bpm, the P wave may be notched and won't necessarily appear with each QRS complex. If the heart rate rises above 100 bpm, the P wave may become small and peaked. And it may seem to ride the downward slope of the preceding T wave.

The PR interval may be prolonged or at the upper limit of normal (0.2 second). In some patients, the rate of conduction through the atrium drops, and you'll observe a short PR interval of less than 0.12 second.

Your patient's R-R interval may be regular or irregular depending on the severity of the arrhythmia. And the QRS complex probably will be normal unless your patient has underlying cardiac disease. In that case, her QRS complex may be widened to more than 0.1 second.

Treatment

In the early stages of sick sinus syndrome, your patient's symptoms may be limited to mild palpitations and dizziness, which don't require treatment. However, when signs and symptoms become significant, look for underlying problems that may contribute to the arrhythmia. Obtain a detailed history and perform a physical examination. Also, obtain ECGs to document your patient's response to treatment.

Drugs may help to control sick sinus syndrome, but drug treatment alone usually either fails or worsens the arrhythmia. For example, if your patient has bradycardia-tachycardia syndrome, a drug used to decrease the tachyarrhythmia may depress an already failing SA node and worsen your patient's bradyarrhythmia. If you administer atropine or isoproterenol for your patient's bradycardia, her tachyarrhythmia may increase. Electrical cardioversion can also worsen your patient's arrhythmia. Subsequently, permanent pacing typically is the treatment of choice for patients with sick sinus syndrome. Also, in conjunction with pacing, a physician may prescribe a drug to control the arrhythmia.

Pacemaker

For a patient with sick sinus syndrome, especially one with bradycardia-tachycardia syndrome, a pacemaker has two benefits: it protects the patient during bradyarrhythmia, and it allows her to safely use drugs to control tachycardia. For example, with a pacemaker in place, you can give a calcium channel blocker to lower your patient's heart rate without the fear of decreasing her heart rate below the settings of the pacemaker.

Quinidine

Quinidine, a broad-spectrum drug that's used to control both atrial and ventricular arrhythmias, blocks sodium channels in the heart, which slows impulse conduction in the atria, ventricles, and His-Purkinje fibers. Quinidine delays repolarization at these sites. And it blocks vagal input to the heart, increasing SA node automaticity and AV conduction.

To prevent quinidine from overstimulating the ventricles, physicians usually pretreat patients with digoxin, verapamil, or a beta-blocker, all of which suppress AV conduction. Quinidine is usually prescribed as quinidine sulfate, and the typical dose in adults is 200 to 400 mg every 4 to 6 hours. Quinidine sulfate is also available in 300-mg extended-release tablets. The usual dose of these tablets is 300 to 600 mg every 8 to 12 hours, adjusted as necessary to maintain a quinidine blood level between 2 and 5 µg/ml.

Quinidine may also be given I.V. at a rate of 16 mg/minute. During I.V. administration, observe the patient carefully for adverse ECG changes, including lengthened PR and QT intervals and widened QRS complexes. If your patient's PR interval lengthens or if her QRS complexes widen by 50% or more, notify the physician immediately.

The most common adverse effects of quinidine include abdominal pain and cramping, nausea, vomiting, and diarrhea. Nausea may be both immediate and intense.

Procainamide

Procainamide is a second drug of choice for treating tachyarrhythmias that result from sick sinus syndrome. Like quinidine, this drug blocks sodium channels in the heart, decreasing conduction in the atria, ventricles, and His-Purkinje system. Procainamide also delays repolarization. Effects on the ECG include lengthened QT intervals and widened QRS complexes.

Procainamide may be administered I.V. at an initial rate of 20 mg/minute, increased to a maximum loading dose of 600 mg. After the loading dose is attained, an infusion rate of 2 to 6 mg/minute should be used.

When the arrhythmia is controlled, the patient should be started on oral doses of procainamide. The standard oral dose is 50 mg/kg/day in divided doses. The drug is available in both sustained and nonsustained forms and is administered every 4 to 6 hours, adjusted as necessary to maintain a plasma procainamide level of 4 to 10 µg/ml.

Adverse effects of procainamide include nausea, vomiting, abdominal cramping, and diarrhea. Occasionally, patients may experience giddiness and weakness. Patients should be supine during the administration of I.V. procainamide. During I.V. administration, observe the patient closely for hypotension.

Propranolol

Propranolol, a nonselective beta-blocker, is sometimes used to treat tachyarrhythmias that result from sick sinus syndrome. By blocking $beta_1$ receptors, propranolol decreases SA node automaticity, AV node conduction, and myocardial contractility. The reduction in AV conduction appears on the ECG as a prolonged PR interval.

Propranolol may be administered either I.V. or orally. The standard I.V. dose is 1 to 3 mg injected at the rate of 1 mg/minute. Oral doses of 10 to 80 mg may be given every 6 to 8 hours, as prescribed.

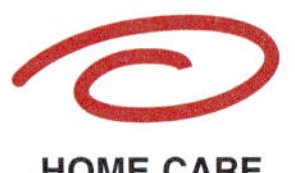

HOME CARE

Using ambulatory electrocardiographic monitoring

If your patient has fleeting arrhythmias, syncope, angina, or palpitations, or if she has a newly implanted pacemaker or just started taking a new cardiac drug, she may benefit from ambulatory electrocardiographic (ECG) monitoring.

In this procedure, the patient's ECG is recorded continuously as she goes about her normal activities. For most patients, the recording period lasts 24 hours.

The patient wears a Holter monitor, which is a small recording box carried in a pouch on a shoulder strap, as shown. Electrodes from the recording box are attached to her chest. The monitor keeps a continuous, timed record of the patient's cardiac activity for the time that she wears it.

During the recording period, the patient keeps a diary of her physical activities and any cardiac signs and symptoms that she experiences. Also, if she develops such signs and symptoms as chest pain, palpitations, or dyspnea, she can push the appropriate button on the Holter monitor to mark the time.

When the recording period ends, the patient turns in the monitor and her diary. Special equipment is used to quickly scan the 24-hour ECG tape. This equipment produces a 24-hour ECG tracing, which the physician can review for abnormal cardiac activity.

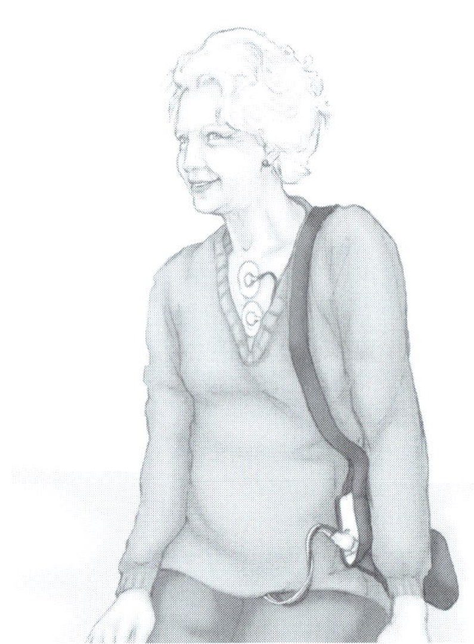

Adverse effects, although rare, include bradycardia, peripheral vascular insufficiency, dizziness, and fatigue.

Warfarin

Because periods of atrial inactivity promote clot formation, your patient with sick sinus syndrome faces an increased risk of transient ischemic attack and cerebrovascular accident (CVA). Consequently, a physician may prescribe warfarin—an oral anticoagulant—to help prevent clots that could turn into emboli after being dislodged by an episode of tachyarrhythmia.

Warfarin inhibits clot formation by interfering with hepatic synthesis of vitamin K–dependent clotting factors. The standard dosage is 5 to 15 mg/day for 2 to 5 days. The dose is then adjusted to achieve a desired prothrombin time and an international normalized ratio. Usually, an adult patient takes 2 to 10 mg/day as a maintenance dose.

Bleeding is the major adverse effect of warfarin. Because complications of anticoagulant therapy can be serious and usually result from noncompliance, you should teach your patient how to safely take this high-risk drug.

Nursing considerations

Because an ECG doesn't directly measure SA node activity, a single ECG of a patient with sick sinus syndrome may show a normal sinus rhythm. Therefore, your patient needs continual assessment and documentation of ECG changes and related signs and symptoms. Ambulatory ECG monitoring is a useful diagnostic tool for a patient with sick sinus syndrome. It allows continuous recording of myocardial activity while your patient performs her normal daily activities (see *Using ambulatory electrocardiographic monitoring*).

If your patient undergoes ambulatory ECG monitoring, emphasize the importance of keeping an accurate diary during the recording period. Tell her which activities to document, including eating, toileting, receiving visitors, and watching television. Also, make sure she knows how to push the marking button on the Holter monitor.

If you are monitoring the patient during the recording period, watch for any signs of activity intolerance. Document any signs and symptoms that may arise and the administration times of drugs. Keep in mind that analgesics, inotropic drugs, and anxiolytic drugs can alter cardiac conduction.

If an unexplained cardiac event occurs, your documentation and your patient's diary will provide essential information to help the physician correlate these signs and symptoms of hemodynamic compromise with ECG recordings of the patient's cardiac arrhythmias. Ultimately, this detailed information may yield an effective treatment for a complex cardiac disorder.

Besides Holter monitoring, other procedures can help you evaluate sick sinus syndrome. Assess the patient's vital signs, apical and radial pulses, and neurologic status frequently. Combine these data with the patient's ECG to document her arrhythmias. Also, a physician may perform complete neurologic and thyroid function studies before arriving at a diagnosis of sick sinus syndrome.

Observe your patient for signs of syncope, renal failure, and decreased CO. Look for signs and symptoms of impaired cerebral arterial blood flow resulting from variations in cardiac rhythm. Monitor your patient for fatigue, muscle aches, and slight personality changes. Document her mental status, including emotional lability, memory lapses, irritability, apathy, nocturnal wakefulness, confusion, and impaired judgment. You may need input from family members to accurately assess such signs and symptoms.

In elderly patients, the cerebral effects of sick sinus syndrome can easily be misinterpreted as senility. Carefully watch for evidence of emboli or a CVA, especially if your patient has atrial fibrillation. Also, assess your patient for signs of heart failure: jugular vein distention, peripheral edema, crackles, dyspnea, and orthopnea.

Know which of your patient's drugs may affect SA node conduction, and observe the cardiac monitor for signs of myocardial ischemia or irritability after administering these drugs. Stay alert for changes in heart rate or rhythm, which may be early signs of progression of sick sinus syndrome. Observe your patient's ECG for changes in the ST segment, such as abnormal depression or elevation. Look for the development of premature atrial contractions—a sign that SA node function may be impaired.

If your patient with sick sinus syndrome also has hypertension, make sure she doesn't take an antihypertensive drug that depresses the SA node, such as propranolol, metoprolol, labetalol, verapamil, or diltiazem. Beta-blockers that inhibit the cardiac response to sympathetic stimulation can reduce your patient's heart rate. But a diuretic combined with a drug such as hydralazine, a direct-acting vasodilator, can effectively control blood pressure without inhibiting the patient's SA function.

Finally, teach your patient and her caregivers the following:

- how to check her pulse and blood pressure
- how to identify bradycardia and tachycardia
- when to call for help and what to do until it arrives
- the importance of keeping all follow-up medical appointments
- how to recognize signs and symptoms of decreased cerebral blood flow, such as personality changes, memory loss, or confusion
- the names, actions, dosages, and possible adverse effects of her prescribed drugs
- why compliance with warfarin is particularly important.

Taking warfarin for sick sinus syndrome can lead to serious complications, usually because of patient noncompliance. For best results, teach your patient over several sessions and provide written material for her to review.

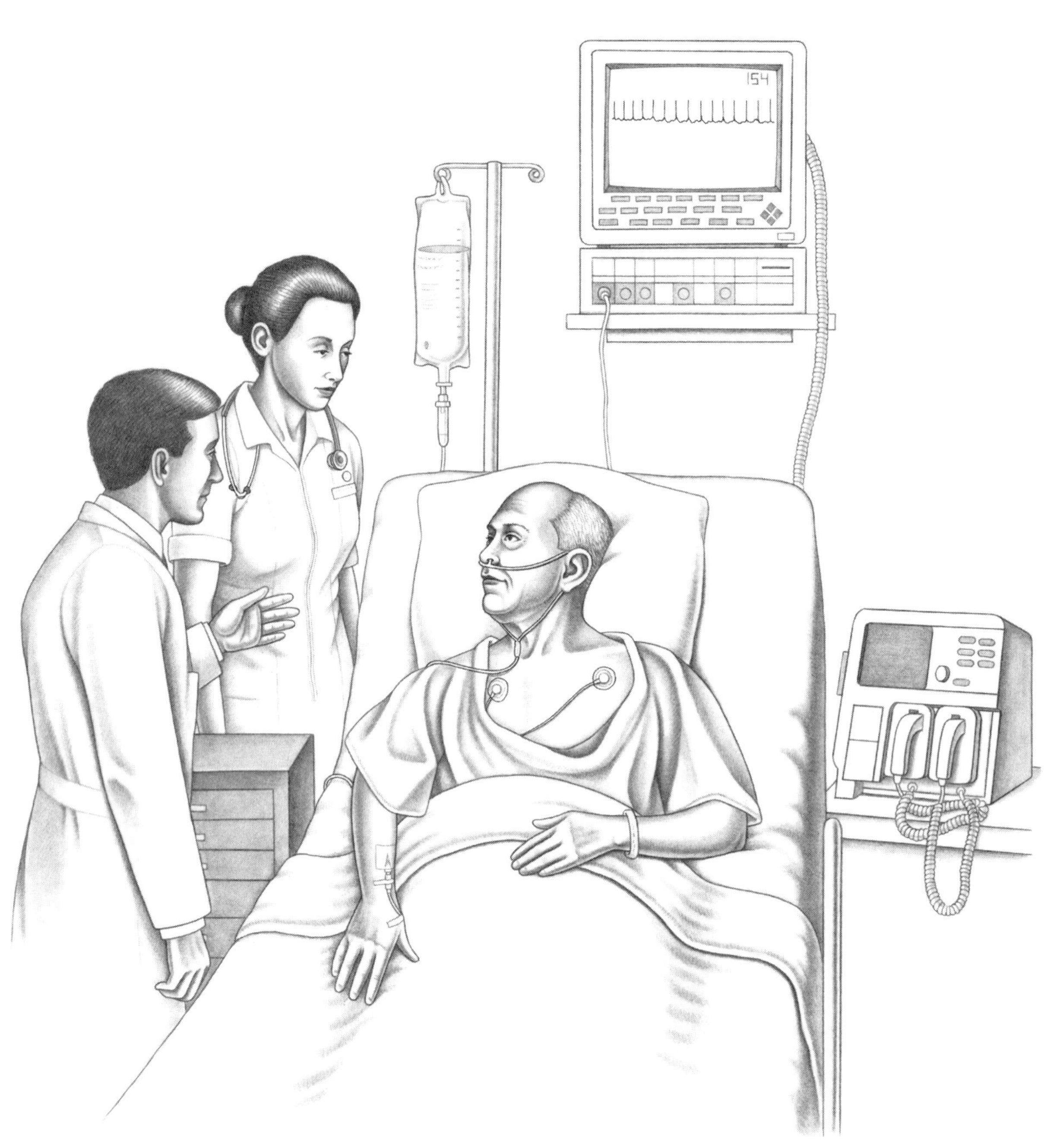
154

4

Atrial Arrhythmias

The most common type of cardiac arrhythmia, atrial arrhythmias typically result from altered automaticity in cardiac cells, reentry phenomenon, or partial depolarization that leads to repetitive ectopic firing and afterdepolarization. In many cases, the focus of irritable atrial automaticity lies where the atrial conductive pathways converge near the cardiac sulcus between the left atrium and ventricle. From this location, the focus can short-circuit the heart's normal pacemaker, the sinoatrial (SA) node.

In this chapter, you'll find a review of the most common atrial arrhythmias—atrial fibrillation, atrial flutter, premature atrial contractions, atrial tachycardia, and wandering atrial pacemaker—as well as important information on caring for and teaching patients who have them.

Atrial fibrillation

Among Americans, especially those over age 75, atrial fibrillation is the most common sustained arrhythmia. It's also the arrhythmia most likely to require hospitalization.

In atrial fibrillation, the atria quiver ineffectively, allowing blood to pool and possibly form clots inside the atria. And if the patient's ventricular rate exceeds 100 beats per minute (bpm), he may experience hemodynamic compromise.

Pathophysiology

Atrial fibrillation that lasts for only a short time can be a normal response in a healthy person. Usually, this intermittent form of atrial fibrillation results from increased catecholamine release caused by emotional stress, postoperative stress, exercise, and acute alcohol intoxication. The condition is called lone atrial fibrillation because it develops in people who have no evidence of structural heart disease. Other causes of lone atrial fibrillation include excessive tobacco smoking or chewing, caffeine consumption, and use of recreational drugs.

Patients with thyrotoxicosis or pheochromocytoma also experience increased catecholamine release. Consequently, they also may develop atrial fibrillation. In thyrotoxicosis, the myocytes have an increased sensitivity to epinephrine and norepinephrine. Thus, they're more irritable, which increases the automaticity of the atria. A pheochromocytoma is a catecholamine-producing tumor that can cause your patient to excrete excessively high levels of catecholamines in his urine.

Chronic atrial fibrillation, in contrast, typically results from structural heart disease. Essentially, any structural abnormality that can lead to atrial enlargement also can lead to atrial fibrillation. In many cases, the abnormality involves a valve. For example, a person with rheumatic heart disease may develop structural problems in the mitral valve that cause mitral regurgitation, mitral stenosis, or both. Rheumatic fever sometimes affects the aortic valve as well, resulting in stenosis with or without regurgitation.

In mitral stenosis, the left atrium must increase its contractile force to propel blood into the left ventricle. Eventually, the left atrium enlarges as a result of this effort, and the atrial myocardium stretches, disrupting normal atrial conduction. Diseases of connective-tissue infiltration, such as amyloidosis and sarcoidosis, also interrupt the conductive pathways and may cause atrial fibrillation.

Aortic insufficiency and aortic stenosis can cause atrial fibrillation when volume overload from the left ventricle progresses to left ventricular heart failure. The volume overload backs up into the left atrium, resulting in left atrial enlargement. Left ventricular heart failure and the resulting atrial overload also can result from a myocardial infarction (MI), dilated cardiomyopathy, or ventricular hypertrophy caused by uncontrolled hypertension.

Atrial septal defect is another structural abnormality that can lead to atrial fibrillation when volume overload stretches and enlarges the atria. Volume overload, atrial stretching, and atrial enlargement also can result from decreased contractility. Chronic alcohol ingestion, right ventricular heart failure, and dilated cardiomyopathy may ultimately lead to decreased myocardial contractility and interruption of the conduction system. Other causes of decreased or impaired myocardial contractility include ischemic cardiomyopathy, hypertrophic cardiomyopathy, and cardiomyopathies of viral or parasitic origin.

Signs and symptoms

In all likelihood, a patient with atrial fibrillation will have a predictable set of signs and symptoms along with the signs you can see on his ECG because, normally, atrial contractions contribute up to 20% of the total cardiac output (CO). But in atrial fibrillation, loss of the atrial kick and decreased ventricular filling time result in diminished CO.

Patients with atrial fibrillation commonly experience palpitations from the rapid ventricular rate. Loss of atrial function and decreased ventricular filling time also can cause myocardial ischemia, pulmonary edema, and decreased cerebral blood flow. And patients may experience angina, dyspnea, light-headedness, and syncope. If your patient's CO declines significantly, he may be hypotensive. Also, you may hear crackles from heart failure when you auscultate his posterior lung fields.

Your physical examination also will reveal an irregular pulse that, in untreated atrial fibrillation, usually exceeds 100 bpm. Palpation of the arterial pulse reveals varying amplitudes of pulsatile sensation. Cardiac auscultation confirms a first heart sound (S_1) that varies in intensity. If your patient has decreased left ventricular compliance from diastolic dysfunction or left ventricular heart failure from volume overload caused by the reduced CO, you may hear a third heart sound (called an S_3 gallop).

When assessing jugular vein distention, you'll note an absence of the *a*-wave portion of your patient's jugular venous pulse. Also, you'll detect a radial pulse deficit when assessing the apical-radial pulse. This deficit occurs because some of the impulses conducted from the atria to the ventricles aren't strong enough to produce a palpable ventricular contraction.

In atrial fibrillation, the atrial rate usually is 350 to 600 bpm—too fast to count. Atrial activity is chaotic and disorganized, with several foci depolarizing simultaneously. On the patient's ECG, you'll see fine fibrillatory waves called f waves between QRS complexes, instead of the usual P waves. These fine f waves tend to accompany atherosclerotic cardiovascular and hypertensive disease (see *Characteristics of atrial fibrillation*).

The patient will have an irregular rhythm because the pacemakers of atrial fibrillation alternate between multiple atrial areas of reentry and multiple, simultaneously depolarizing, ectopic foci. Multiple atrial impulses reach the atrioventricular (AV) node during its refractory period and aren't conducted. This effect can only be seen on the next conducted beat when analyzing the ECG.

The ventricular response rate is relatively slow compared with the atrial rate. This slow response rate results from concealed conduction, in which an atrial impulse only partially penetrates the AV node and doesn't proceed to the ventricles.

If the patient develops atrial fibrillation after having an MI, he may have experienced an atrial infarction. If so, you'll see changes in his ECG that suggest an atrial infarction, including PR segment elevation in the left chest leads and lead I, with reciprocal depression in the right chest leads and lead III.

Treatment

Treatment for atrial fibrillation depends on several variables: the patient's hemodynamic stability, the duration and cause of atrial fibrillation, and the

Characteristics of atrial fibrillation

Atrial rate: 350 to 600 beats per minute (bpm)
Ventricular rate: 60 to 100 bpm
Atrial rhythm: can't be determined
Ventricular rhythm: irregular

P wave: replaced by f waves
PR interval: can't be determined
QRS complex: < 0.12 second

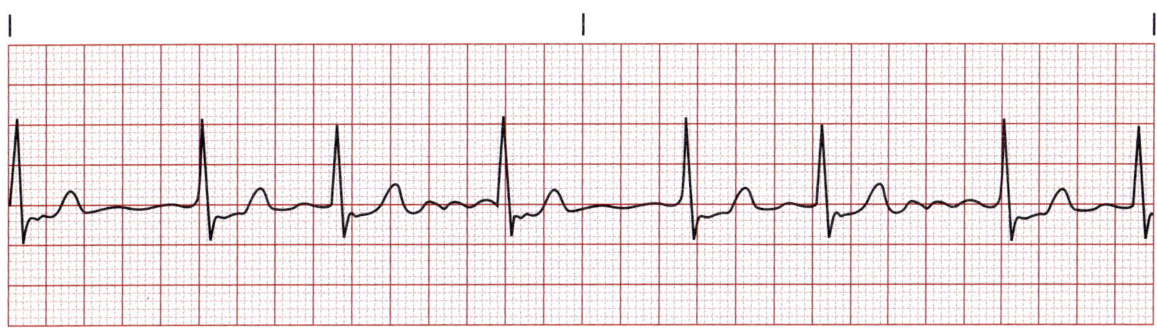

probability of converting to and maintaining sinus rhythm. Of these variables, maintaining your patient's hemodynamic stability is always the first priority.

Most patients with atrial fibrillation receive therapy with anticoagulant or antiarrhythmic drugs. Those who can't tolerate the arrhythmia or the drug therapy may undergo electrical cardioversion, ablation therapy, or surgical correction (see *Caring for a patient with atrial fibrillation,* pages 46 and 47).

Anticoagulant drugs

If your patient has had atrial fibrillation for more than 48 hours, a physician most likely will start him on anticoagulation therapy to reduce the risk of systemic thromboembolism when he converts to a normal sinus rhythm. If your patient will undergo chemical or electrical cardioversion, he'll probably receive anticoagulants for at least 3 weeks before and 3 weeks after the cardioversion.

The principal anticoagulants used to treat atrial fibrillation are heparin and warfarin. Most patients start anticoagulation therapy on heparin rather than warfarin because of the possible risk of a hypercoagulable state when therapy starts with warfarin. Heparin helps to establish anticoagulation more quickly. For long-term, outpatient use, however, warfarin remains the anticoagulant of choice.

Heparin

Patients receiving heparin for anticoagulation should be hospitalized for frequent monitoring of the activated partial thromboplastin time (APTT), adjustment of the drug dose, and observation for heparin-related complications. Heparin potentiates the action of antithrombin III, thereby inactivating thrombin, certain activated coagulation factors (IX, X, XI, and XII), and plasmin. Heparin also prevents conversion of fibrinogen to fibrin.

Regimens for heparin therapy vary. Typically, start by giving the patient an I.V. bolus of 5,000 units, immediately followed by a continuous heparin infusion starting at 1,000 units/hour, as ordered. Check your patient's blood APTT 4 hours after starting the heparin therapy, as ordered, and 4 hours after each adjustment of the heparin dose.

Your goal during therapeutic anticoagulation with heparin is an APTT of 1.5 to 2 times normal, or 1.5 to 2 times the patient's APTT baseline before anticoagulation. Once you've achieved a stable APTT, the patient can start warfarin therapy, as or-

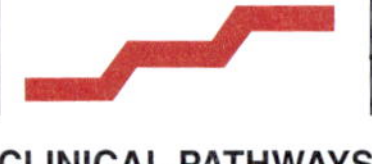

CLINICAL PATHWAYS

Caring for a patient with atrial fibrillation

	History and physical examination	Diagnostic tests	Discharge planning
Day 1	• signs and symptoms and chief complaint on admission • physical assessment on admission • cardiac history and precipitating factors • duration of arrhythmia • vital signs (every 15 minutes for 4 hours if patient has ibutilide infusion; every 30 minutes if he has diltiazem drip, then every 4 hours as needed) • baseline QT interval	• continuous cardiac monitoring • 12-lead electrocardiogram (ECG) • oxygen saturation • chest X-ray, as indicated • laboratory tests, including complete blood count, hematocrit, and hemoglobin level • arterial blood gas measurement, as needed • drug levels, as indicated • prothrombin time (PT) or activated partial thromboplastin time (APTT), as indicated	• Determine cause of arrhythmia. • Identify patient's support systems.
Day 2	• vital signs every 4 hours, as needed • systems review each shift • cardiac rhythm and QT interval	• continuous cardiac monitoring • 12-lead ECG • oxygen saturation each shift, as needed • laboratory tests, as ordered • PT or APTT	• Assess patient's understanding of disorder. • Initiate review of arrhythmia management.
Day 3	• vital signs every 4 to 8 hours, as needed • systems review each shift	• continuous cardiac monitoring • 12-lead ECG • oxygen saturation and laboratory tests, as ordered • PT or APTT	• Obtain dietary consultation for food and drug interactions. • Participate in interdisciplinary review of patient's anticipated home care needs.
Day 4	• vital signs every 4 to 8 hours, as needed • systems review each shift	• continuous cardiac monitoring • 12-lead ECG • oxygen saturation and laboratory tests, as ordered • PT or APTT	• Provide resource options for continued needs. • Schedule follow-up care.

dered. Heparin and warfarin therapy may overlap for 3 to 5 days.

Adverse effects of heparin therapy include a mild decrease in the platelet count and, in 10% of patients, thrombocytopenia. If your patient's platelet count falls below 100,000/mm^3, discontinue heparin therapy, as ordered. If your patient develops heparin-related thrombocytopenia, low-molecular-

Drugs	Interventions	Patient teaching
• antiarrhythmic therapy: diltiazem I.V. drip or ibutilide infusion if atrial fibrillation lasted less than 90 days, systolic blood pressure is above 90 mm Hg, and baseline QT interval is less than 0.44 second; alternatively, digoxin • anticoagulant therapy: continuous heparin infusion • I.V. fluid and potassium replacement, as needed • antianxiety drugs, as needed • sedation for electrical cardioversion, as needed	• Continuously monitor cardiac rhythm. • Measure QT interval each shift, as needed. • Ensure that emergency equipment is available. • Use bleeding precautions. • Assess PT or APTT, as indicated, and adjust anticoagulant dose, as needed. • Apply antiembolism stockings. • Maintain bed rest. • Monitor fluid intake and output. • Administer oxygen, as needed.	• Orient patient to unit. • Explain all procedures and treatments to allay anxiety. • Include family, as appropriate.
• oral antiarrhythmics, as prescribed • anticoagulant therapy, as ordered • oral potassium, as needed	• Continuously monitor cardiac rhythm. • Measure QT interval each shift, as needed. • Use bleeding precautions. • Assess PT or APTT and adjust anticoagulant dose, as needed. • Apply antiembolism stockings. • Monitor fluid intake and output. • Encourage ambulation, as tolerated. • Administer oxygen, as needed.	• Review basic cardiac anatomy and physiology. • Teach patient and family about causes and early signs and symptoms of atrial fibrillation. • Teach patient to take his pulse.
• antiarrhythmics, as ordered • anticoagulant therapy, as ordered	• Continuously monitor cardiac rhythm. • Measure QT interval each shift, as needed. • Use bleeding precautions. • Assess PT or APTT and adjust anticoagulant dose, as needed. • Apply antiembolism stockings. • Monitor fluid intake and output. • Increase patient's activity level, as tolerated. • Administer oxygen, as needed.	• Review purpose and desired results of PT or APTT tests. • Review possible food and drug interactions and dietary restrictions. • Explain bleeding precautions.
• antiarrhythmics, as ordered • anticoagulant therapy, as ordered	• Continuously monitor cardiac rhythm. • Measure QT interval each shift, as needed. • Use bleeding precautions. • Assess PT or APTT and adjust anticoagulant dose, as needed. • Apply antiembolism stockings. • Monitor fluid intake and output. • Increase patient's activity level, as tolerated. • Administer oxygen, as needed.	• Review patient's diet, exercise, and stress level. • Reinforce importance of follow-up, including tests of clotting time.

weight heparin may provide another therapeutic option for anticoagulation.

Another risk raised by heparin therapy is uncontrolled bleeding. If your patient develops excessive anticoagulation, give protamine sulfate—a heparin antagonist—to reverse heparin's effects. Protamine sulfate neutralizes heparin by binding to the heparin molecule and rendering it ineffective until excretion. The protamine dose is determined by the dose of heparin the patient is receiving; 1 mg of protamine sulfate neutralizes about 100 units of heparin. The maximum dose of protamine is 250 mg; usually, give 50 mg over 10 minutes by I.V. infusion. Allergic reactions to protamine can occur because the drug is synthesized from fish.

Warfarin

Although appropriate warfarin therapy widely varies from patient to patient, typically you should start by giving 10 mg orally for 2 days. Then measure the patient's prothrombin time (PT) and international normalized ratio (INR) before establishing a continued dose. The therapeutic goal for warfarin anticoagulation in atrial fibrillation is a PT of 15 to 17 seconds with an INR of 2 to 3. Once the PT and INR are stabilized, maintenance doses of warfarin can be determined; they usually range from 2 to 10 mg.

Antiarrhythmic drugs

Conversion of atrial fibrillation to sinus rhythm is desirable only when the patient will benefit hemodynamically. In patients who would not benefit from cardioversion or who have hemodynamically stable atrial fibrillation, the goal of treatment is to slow the ventricular response rate while trying to identify the cause of the fibrillation. The target ventricular rate for controlling atrial fibrillation is 60 to 100 bpm, which is achieved most rapidly with beta-blockers or calcium channel blockers. A physician also may prescribe digoxin, a sodium channel blocker, or a potassium channel blocker.

Beta-blockers

A physician prescribes a beta-blocker to slow the patient's ventricular response rate to less than 100 bpm while maintaining the patient's blood pressure in a normal range. If your patient has ischemic heart disease, you should decrease the ventricular rate to 60 to 70 bpm.

Usually, a selective beta-blocker is preferable to a nonselective beta-blocker because it's less likely to cause bronchospasm. Beta-blockers commonly used to treat atrial fibrillation include metoprolol, atenolol, and propranolol.

Metoprolol: As ordered, give 5 mg of metoprolol I.V. every 5 minutes until you reach a total dose of 15 mg. Then switch to the oral form of the drug, giving a maintenance dose of 50 to 225 mg twice daily, preferably 8 to 12 hours apart.

Atenolol: Typically prescribed for a patient who needs only maintenance therapy, atenolol allows once-daily dosing. As ordered, instruct the patient to take 50 to 200 mg/day.

Propranolol: A nonselective beta-blocker used to control atrial tachycardia, propranolol also possesses membrane-stabilizing potential, a class Ib antiarrhythmic property. This drug is available for both oral and I.V. administration. Give 1 mg of the drug I.V. slowly, over 1 minute. If this dose fails to control the patient's ventricular response, give repeated 1-mg doses, as indicated, up to a total of 5 mg. Then give 10 to 80 mg of the oral form every 6 to 8 hours. Propranolol is contraindicated in uncompensated heart failure, chronic bronchitis, emphysema, and asthma.

Calcium channel blockers

As a group, calcium channel blockers block the slow influx of calcium into myocytes. Calcium channel blockers used to control the ventricular rate in atrial tachycardia include diltiazem and verapamil. Both are available in I.V. and oral forms.

Diltiazem: Give 0.25 mg/kg of diltiazem I.V. over 2 minutes. If your patient's ventricular rate remains above 100 bpm, give a second bolus of 0.35 mg/kg over 2 minutes, as prescribed. For maintenance, infuse 5 to 15 mg/hour.

To convert the I.V. dose to an oral maintenance dose, calculate 150% of the cumulative 24-hour I.V. dose to determine the 24-hour oral dose. Maintenance oral doses are available as regular-release, sustained-release, and once-daily forms.

Contraindications to diltiazem include sick sinus syndrome, hypotension, and cardiogenic shock. It also is contraindicated in atrial flutter when the patient may have an accessory bypass tract, as in Wolff-Parkinson-White (WPW) syndrome and short PR-interval syndrome (see *Understanding reentry phenomenon*). Giving diltiazem or verapamil for these preexcitation syndromes can cause a 1:1 conduction of atrial impulses, which in turn can produce ventricular rates of up to 350 bpm.

Verapamil: Give 2.5 to 5 mg of verapamil I.V. over 2 minutes. If the patient's ventricular rate doesn't respond well enough, repeat the dose once after 5 minutes. Regular-release and sustained-release forms are available for maintenance therapy; usually, instruct the patient to take an oral dose of 120 to 480 mg every 24 hours.

Understanding reentry phenomenon

In reentrant tachycardias, a process called reentry phenomenon perpetuates a rapid rhythm. Usually, reentry phenomenon occurs when a premature atrial contraction prompts an impulse to travel to the bundle of Kent because the normal pathway is still refractory.

The bundle of Kent directly connects the atria to the ventricles, bypassing the atrioventricular (AV) node and the bundle of His. Electrical impulses conducted through this accessory pathway cause abnormally fast ventricular depolarization. Also, the bundle of Kent conducts impulses in both antegrade (forward) and retrograde (backward) directions. So an impulse that moves into the ventricles through the AV node can also travel back to the atria through the bundle of Kent. The impulse then circles back to the ventricles through the AV node, perpetuating the tachycardia.

Normal conduction

Sinoatrial node

Atrioventricular node

Purkinje fibers

Reentry phenomenon

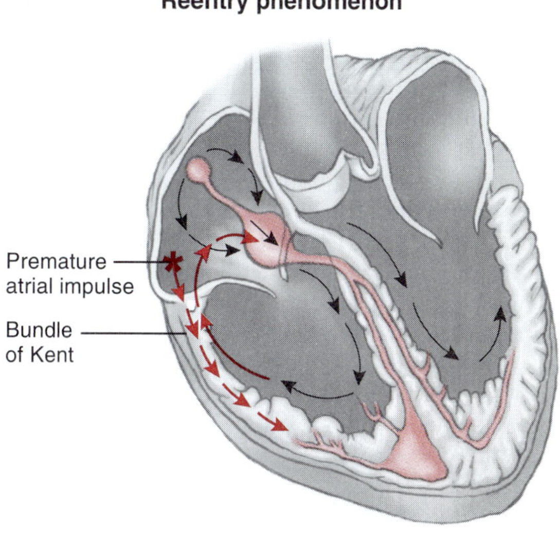

Keep in mind that most patients develop hypotension during I.V. administration of verapamil. If your patient has an ejection fraction less than 30%, hypotension, sick sinus syndrome, atrial fibrillation, or atrial flutter with WPW syndrome, don't give the drug. Remember that verapamil can increase blood digoxin levels by 50% to 75%.

Digoxin

Digoxin is classified as both an antiarrhythmic and a digitalis glycoside. This drug is ideal for slowing the ventricular response rate of patients who have atrial fibrillation with severe left ventricular dysfunction, supraventricular arrhythmias, or heart failure. The patient also receives the added benefit of positive inotropy. Digoxin's positive inotropic effect improves ventricular contractility in patients whose ejection fractions have decreased to less than 55%.

As ordered, give 0.25 to 0.5 mg of digoxin I.V. as an initial bolus. Follow that with 0.25 mg every 6 to 8 hours until the patient's ventricular rate is controlled or you've given a total of 1 mg. Then the patient will continue to take 0.125 to 0.5 mg of oral digoxin once daily, as ordered.

Keep in mind that the negative chronotropic effect of digoxin takes several hours to reduce the patient's ventricular response rate. For a quicker response, use a calcium channel blocker or beta-blocker.

Digoxin has a narrow therapeutic range, so you must monitor the patient carefully. Therapeutic blood levels of digoxin are 1 to 2 ng/ml. And a toxic reaction usually occurs with blood levels greater than 2 ng/ml and can cause atrial and ventricular arrhythmias, fatigue, anorexia, nausea, visual disturbances (such as yellow halos or scotomas), and dizziness.

Many drugs—such as verapamil, warfarin, erythromycin, tetracycline, and phenytoin—raise blood digoxin levels because digoxin is highly bound to protein. These drugs also readily bind to proteins. If your patient receiving digoxin also receives one of these drugs, the drugs will compete for protein-binding sites, causing increased blood digoxin levels and a potential toxic reaction. Giving quinidine with digoxin can double blood digoxin levels, so cut your patient's digoxin level in half as you start giving quinidine. Also, reduce the digoxin dose for patients with decreased creatinine clearance. Low creatinine clearance may indicate decreased muscle mass. In such patients, digoxin is less able to bind to protein and more of the drug is available in the circulation.

When giving digoxin, watch your patient's electrolyte levels closely because hypokalemia, hypomagnesemia, and hypercalcemia can prompt digoxin-related arrhythmias.

Sodium channel blockers

When your patient's ventricular rate is controlled, you can start giving class Ia antiarrhythmic drugs to try to convert his atrial fibrillation to a sinus rhythm. Class I drugs, including subclasses Ia, Ib, and Ic, are called sodium channel blockers because they exert their effects by inhibiting the influx of sodium into the cell by binding to the sodium channels.

Class Ia drugs prolong the refractory period of the ventricles as well as the QT interval. These drugs include quinidine, procainamide, and disopyramide. They're used to treat atrial tachycardias, to prevent recurrence of atrial fibrillation and flutter, and to suppress ventricular ectopia. Class Ib drugs shorten the action potential and refractory threshold at high tissue concentrations. Examples of such drugs include lidocaine, mexiletine, tocainide, and phenytoin. Class Ic includes the most potent sodium channel–blocking drugs. They profoundly slow conduction and have minor effects on repolarization.

Keep in mind, however, that successful cardioversion, whether chemical or electrical, depends on the duration of atrial fibrillation, atrial size, underlying causes of the arrhythmia, and blood levels of antiarrhythmic drugs.

Patients with chronic atrial fibrillation are less likely to achieve or maintain a sinus rhythm than those with atrial fibrillation of new onset. Patients with left atrial diameters larger than 4.5 cm also are less likely to convert or remain converted. Patients with endogenous or exogenous catecholamine excess should have these anomalies corrected before attempting cardioversion; however, the ventricular response rate should still be controlled with a beta-blocker, a calcium channel blocker, or digoxin.

Quinidine: Give 200 to 400 mg of regular-release quinidine every 6 hours, as ordered, even if your patient has decreased renal function. Give Quinaglute, a longer-acting form of quinidine gluconate, at 324 to 648 mg every 8 to 12 hours. Therapeutic blood levels are 1.3 to 5 µg/ml.

Quinidine is highly protein bound and increases blood digoxin levels by up to 100%. It also prolongs the PT in patients taking warfarin. The blood half-life of quinidine significantly increases with the patient's age and with liver dysfunction.

The most common adverse effects are nausea, vomiting, and diarrhea, especially at higher doses. Sometimes these effects are intolerable and require the patient to discontinue the drug. Quinidine also can produce fever and flulike symptoms, and it decreases counts of white blood cells (WBCs), red blood cells (RBCs), and platelets. Cinchonism, a toxic reaction of the central nervous system, produces tinnitus, hearing loss, visual disturbances, confusion, delirium, and psychosis.

Quinidine increases the conduction of atrial impulses through the AV node, and 1:1 conduction can result in detrimental ventricular rates. Before using quinidine to treat atrial fibrillation, the ventricular rate must be controlled with a beta-blocker, a calcium channel blocker, or digoxin.

Procainamide: Give a 100-mg loading dose of procainamide I.V. every 3 to 5 minutes until you've given a total of 1 to 1.5 g, as ordered. If your patient develops hypotension—a common reaction—you may need to adopt longer dosing intervals. After the loading dose, give a maintenance infusion at 2 to 4 mg/minute. Oral forms are available as regular-release doses (500 to 1,000 mg every 4 to 6 hours) and sustained-release doses (500 to 1,000 mg every 8 hours).

During administration, you need to monitor and control several indicators. Watch your patient's ventricular rate carefully. Also, before and during administration, measure his QT interval corrected for heart rate (QTc). A normal QT interval is measured from the beginning of the Q wave to the end of the T wave. But because the interval varies with the ventricular rate, you must calculate your patient's QTc interval using the following formula:

$$QTc = \frac{\text{QT interval}}{\sqrt{\text{R-R interval}}}$$

A significantly prolonged QTc interval is more than 500 milliseconds or greater than 25% of the original QTc interval before antiarrhythmic therapy began. Recall that hypokalemia, hypomagnesemia, and severe left ventricular dysfunction also prolong the QT interval.

To detect a toxic reaction, monitor your patient's blood levels of procainamide and its active metabolite, *N*-acetylprocainamide. If your patient has combined procainamide and metabolite levels above 30 µg/ml, he faces a risk of adverse reactions and arrhythmias because the metabolite acts as a potassium channel blocker.

Procainamide produces a lupus-like syndrome in up to one-third of patients receiving long-term therapy. Signs and symptoms include fever, arthralgias, pleuropericarditis, and hepatomegaly. And antinuclear antibodies develop in 75% of patients receiving long-term therapy. Procainamide should be discontinued in patients who are symptomatic. Lupus-like effects resolve with discontinuation of the drug.

Sensitivity reactions to procainamide include agranulocytosis, fever, rash, and cardiovascular signs and symptoms of hypotension, ventricular escape rhythms, and conduction abnormalities (widened QRS complexes and prolonged QT intervals). These adverse effects also require prompt cessation of therapy. Also, if the patient's atrial fibrillation is suppressed, the QRS complex has widened by more than 50% of baseline, or you've given a total dose of 15 mg/kg, stop giving procainamide.

Disopyramide: Oral disopyramide is available as regular-release doses, given at 100 to 200 mg every 6 to 8 hours, and sustained-release doses, given at 100 to 300 mg twice daily. Dosing should be adjusted for patients with renal insufficiency. If creatinine clearance is more than 15 ml/minute, instruct your patient to take 100 mg every 12 hours. If his creatinine clearance is 15 ml/minute or less, tell him to take 100 mg/day.

Adverse effects of disopyramide include anticholinergic signs and symptoms and myasthenic crisis. Also, the drug's negative inotropic effects may prompt heart failure. As with other class Ia drugs, you must control your patient's ventricular rate before administration, and you should monitor his QTc intervals.

Potassium channel blockers

If your patient's atrial fibrillation fails to respond to conventional therapies, the physician may prescribe a potassium channel blocker. Potassium channel blockers prolong the duration of action potential and repolarization. They also prolong the sinus rate, recovery time, and conduction through the AV node. And they decrease systemic vascular resistance and mean arterial pressure (MAP) without depressing left ventricular function, thereby reducing afterload. Drugs used to convert or suppress atrial fibrillation include amiodarone and ibutilide.

Amiodarone: Amiodarone blocks conversion of thyroxine (T_4) to triiodothyronine, blocks noncompetitive alpha-blockers and beta-blockers, and prevents angina. Give 600 mg/day orally for 1 week, followed by 400 mg/day for 2 weeks. If the atrial fibrillation converts to a sinus rhythm, switch to maintenance dosing at 200 mg/day. Keep in mind, however, that the drug may not convert or suppress the arrhythmia for 4 to 6 weeks.

Pulmonary infiltrates and fibrosis occurs in about 15% of patients who receive amiodarone, but these effects are unlikely among patients who receive less than 300 mg/day. Pulmonary function tests and chest X-rays should be performed every 3 to 6 months. If undetected, amiodarone-induced pulmonary fibrosis is fatal in about 10% of patients.

Because of amiodarone's effect on the thyroid gland, about 3% of patients develop thyroid dysfunction. Encourage your patient to have thyroid function tests at least once a year. Remember that T_4 is always elevated in patients who receive long-term amiodarone therapy. *Amiodarone-induced hyperthyroidism* is defined as a thyroid-stimulating hormone (TSH) level of less than 0.1 μg/ml together with an elevated T_4.

Ibutilide: The proper dose of ibutilide depends on your patient's weight. If he weighs more than 80 kg, infuse 1 mg of the drug I.V. over 10 minutes; if he weighs less than 80 kg, give him 0.01 mg/kg. If the atrial fibrillation persists, repeat the initial dose 20 minutes after the first infusion. The physician may prescribe long-term suppressive therapy with a potassium channel blocker or a calcium channel blocker after the patient converts to a sinus rhythm.

During cardioversion with ibutilide, continuously monitor your patient's ECG, blood pressure, and QTc interval for polymorphic ventricular tachycardia (VT) and hypotension. A QTc interval greater than 0.44 second can potentiate torsades de pointes. Also, hypokalemia and hypomagnesemia can prompt lethal polymorphic VT and torsades de pointes.

Electrical cardioversion

As you know, electrical cardioversion involves the delivery of electrical impulses across the thoracic wall to halt a sustained arrhythmia. If drug therapy fails to convert your patient to a sinus rhythm and he's hemodynamically unstable, the physician may order electrical cardioversion after the patient's antiarrhythmic drugs reach their proper therapeutic levels. Also, if your patient has unstable atrial fibrillation accompanied by myocardial ischemia, an MI, hypotension, or worsening heart failure, the physician may order electrical cardioversion.

During treatment with electrical cardioversion, the operator usually can use a toggle switch to choose between synchronous or asynchronous cardioversion. In the synchronous mode, which is used for electrical cardioversion, the current is delivered during ventricular depolarization. R waves highlighted on the cardioversion monitor indicate synchronous mode. Synchronous mode must be reset after each discharge. It's contraindicated in patients who've had a toxic reaction to a digitalis glycoside.

Typically, direct-current synchronized cardioversion is administered with a starting current of 100 joules. Additional shocks of up to 360 joules may be necessary to convert atrial fibrillation to a sinus rhythm. Cardioversion pads should be strategically placed for the most effective delivery of current. For atrial fibrillation, place the anterior pad at the left sternal border between the third and fourth intercostal space. Place the posterior pad slightly below the left scapula.

Keep both pads at least 6 cm away from permanent pacers or automatic implantable cardioverter-defibrillators. You can minimize transthoracic current impedance by applying the paddles firmly to the patient's chest wall and discharging the selected current at the end of expiration.

Cardioversion can provoke transient nodal, atrial, and ventricular escape beats during and after the procedure. Rhythms other than atrial fibrillation can result from the release of catecholamines, acetylcholine, and potassium after the delivery of electrical current. Monitor your patient's laboratory results because blood levels of lactate dehydrogenase (LD), aspartate aminotransferase (AST), and creatine kinase (CK) rise when electrical current traverses the skeletal muscle. The isoenzyme CK-MB also may rise after a cumulative discharge of 425 joules has been administered.

Pretreating atrial fibrillation with quinidine before electrical cardioversion improves the chances of maintaining normal sinus rhythm after cardioversion. It also reduces the number of shocks needed and the energy required to convert to a sinus rhythm. In about 90% of such pretreated patients, electrical cardioversion successfully converts the rhythm.

Ablation therapy

If antiarrhythmic drugs fail to control the ventricular rate or the patient can't tolerate medical therapy, the physician may use radiofrequency catheter-induced ablation of the AV node to control the arrhythmia. Ablation is performed by delivering localized thermal energy to the AV node via radio frequency. Afterward, the patient will require permanent dual-chamber pacing because ablation of the AV node terminates communication between the atria and ventricles through the accessory pathways.

Ablation treatment for atrial fibrillation doesn't alter the patient's risk of cerebrovascular accident (CVA) caused by thromboembolism, so he'll continue to need anticoagulation therapy.

Surgical treatment

If your patient with atrial fibrillation needs open-heart surgery to treat some other cardiac condition, the physician may also decide to perform a maze

Maze procedure: Organizing atrial impulses

In atrial fibrillation, the atria produce chaotic electrical impulses. These impulses originate in several locations, and they don't proceed along normal pathways to the ventricles.

In the maze procedure, a surgeon creates a maze of incisions that channel ectopic impulses in a single direction through the atrial myocardium and into the normal conduction system, thus restoring normal sinus rhythm.

During the open-heart procedure, the surgeon makes several incisions in strategic locations around the right and left atria. He then uses small sutures to reassemble the atrial walls. The healed incisions act as circuit breakers because electrical impulses can't travel across the resulting scar tissue.

Thus, appropriately placed incisions interrupt the ectopic conduction routes and help organize the atrial impulses.

Anterior view

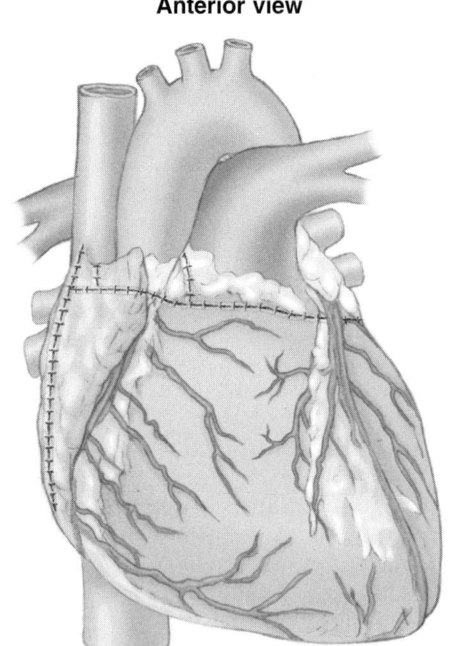

Posterior view

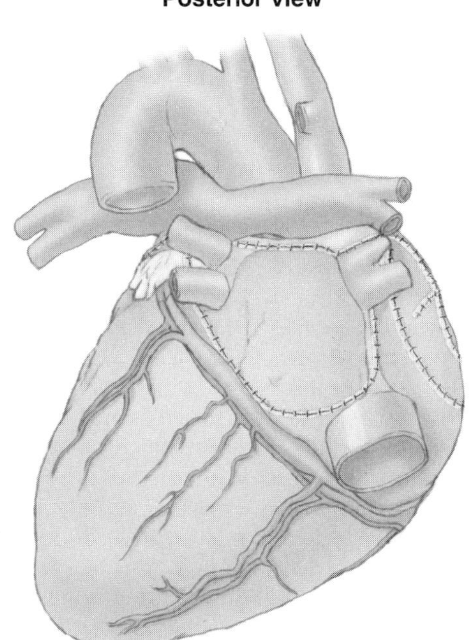

procedure to control the arrhythmia. This surgical procedure interrupts ectopic conduction with strategically placed atrial incisions (see *Maze procedure: Organizing atrial impulses*).

Complications

About 3 in 10 patients with atrial fibrillation develop systemic or pulmonary emboli—a potentially catastrophic complication. In fact, patients with atrial fibrillation have 5 times the risk of CVA as those without it, and patients with both rheumatic heart disease and atrial fibrillation have 17 times the risk.

Also, uncontrolled ventricular rates and the loss of atrial kick can culminate in diminished CO. In a diseased heart, myocardial ischemia and heart failure may result. A patient with decreased CO may try to avoid experiencing the signs and symptoms of angina, dyspnea, and syncope by limiting his activities, which decreases his quality of life. Also, orthopnea and palpitations may interfere with his sleep.

Chronic atrial fibrillation can lead to cardiac dilation and hypertrophy. Combined with the decreased CO, these changes decrease his activity tolerance.

Even when chronic atrial fibrillation is controlled, patients may experience complications from anticoagulant and antiarrhythmic therapy. For example, the risk of bleeding events is about 4% per year of treatment with warfarin. Intracranial bleeding occurs at a rate of 1% to 2% per treatment year. On average, patients with atrial fibrillation have a shorter life span than those without it because of these and other complications.

Nursing considerations

Keep in mind that various antiarrhythmic drugs are contraindicated in certain medical conditions. For example, propranolol is contraindicated in uncompensated heart failure, chronic bronchitis, and emphysema. If your patient has hypotension, cardiogenic shock, or sick sinus syndrome, don't administer diltiazem or verapamil. These drugs are also contraindicated when the patient may have an accessory bypass tract, as in WPW syndrome and short PR-interval syndrome. Also, if your patient has an ejection fraction of less than 30%, don't administer verapamil. Avoid digoxin in patients with hypertrophic, obstructive cardiomyopathy because the increase in contractility may worsen obstruction of the left ventricular outflow tract.

When administering digoxin, monitor your patient's electrolyte levels closely. Keep his blood potassium levels in the high-normal range. Also, keep in mind that patients with low albumin levels and decreased muscle mass, particularly elderly patients, have a higher risk of a toxic reaction to a digitalis glycoside because of their decreased ability to bind the drug. Monitor your patient's blood digoxin levels, ECGs, and adverse effects, as ordered. However, avoid drawing blood to check digoxin levels within 6 hours of an I.V. dose or 8 hours after oral dosing because blood concentrations are highest at this time.

Remember that hypotension is common during I.V. administration of procainamide; if it develops, adopt a longer dosing interval, as ordered. When giving procainamide or quinidine, monitor the patient's ventricular rates and QTc intervals before and during administration. Check blood levels of procainamide and *N*-acetylprocainamide for signs and symptoms of a toxic reaction.

If your patient takes high doses of amiodarone, tell him that he'll need to have pulmonary function tests and chest X-rays every 3 to 6 months because infiltrates may be reversible if detected early. Stress the importance of thyroid function tests, especially TSH levels.

Before starting ibutilide therapy, monitor your patient's blood electrolyte levels, especially his potassium and magnesium levels, and correct any abnormalities. If your patient's atrial fibrillation has lasted more than 48 hours, he'll also need anticoagulation before starting ibutilide. During therapy, continuously monitor the patient's ECG, blood pressure, and QTc interval for potential polymorphic VT, hypotension, and torsades de pointes. Because of the potential for VT, keep resuscitative equipment available at your patient's bedside.

If your patient receives anticoagulation therapy, assess him regularly for occult bleeding. If he receives heparin, watch his APTT, observe him for thrombocytopenia, and adjust the drug dose, as necessary. If he takes warfarin, have him take it in the evening. Laboratory testing is usually done in the morning, and results of his PT and INR tests will reflect a warfarin dose taken 24 to 48 hours before the blood is drawn.

If you administer protamine, monitor your patient's vital signs during and at least 3 hours after administration. Allergic reactions can occur, especially in patients allergic to fish. If large doses are administered, observe your patient for signs and symptoms of bleeding because protamine is a weak anticoagulant.

For electrical cardioversion, always keep resuscitative equipment nearby so that the patient can be intubated and given supplemental oxygen immediately, if needed. Establish reliable I.V. access with a large-bore catheter before cardioversion. The patient probably will be given 1 to 2 mg of midazolam I.V. every 2 minutes, up to a maximum of 5 mg. Any health care provider involved with administering electrical cardioversion must avoid direct contact with the patient and his bed while electrical current is delivered.

If ablation therapy is the chosen treatment, assess your patient for the development of systemic emboli by observing his mental status, respiratory rate, cardiac status, peripheral circulation, and urine output.

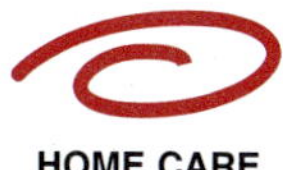

HOME CARE

Teaching your patient about anticoagulant therapy

If your patient will be taking warfarin at home, you'll need to teach him how to detect problems promptly before they become dangerous. Start by reminding him that he'll need to have his clotting time checked regularly to make sure he's taking the correct dose.

Tell your patient to immediately report the following signs and symptoms because they may warn of internal bleeding:

- abdominal pain or swelling
- back pain or backaches
- bloody or black, tarry stools
- cloudy or bloody urine
- blood visible in sputum
- dizziness
- severe or continual headaches
- blood visible in vomitus
- blurred vision.

Also, urge your patient to avoid all contact sports and activities in which he may fall or receive a blow to his body. Tell him not to take over-the-counter products containing aspirin without first checking with his physician.

Evidence of overdose

Teach your patient the signs and symptoms that may warn of an anticoagulant overdose:

- bleeding from his gums when brushing his teeth
- excessive bleeding or oozing from wounds
- unexplained bruising
- unexplained nosebleeds
- unexpected, heavy menstrual bleeding.

Vitamin K reminders

Tell your patient that wide variations in his intake of foods containing vitamin K can interfere with his anticoagulant therapy. Explain that, in general, most fruits and grains are low in vitamin K, as are many meats and the fish abalone, mackerel, and tuna. And tell him to maintain a consistent intake of foods high in vitamin K, such as the following:

- broccoli
- brussels sprouts
- cabbage
- collard greens
- cucumbers
- endives
- green scallions
- kale
- lettuce
- mustard greens
- parsley
- turnip greens
- watercress.

Patient teaching

Teach your patient about the therapeutic and adverse effects of his drugs to help him better comply with his therapy. (see *Teaching your patient about anticoagulant therapy*). Reinforce the need for strict adherence to the prescribed regimen, especially if he has an underlying condition such as heart disease. Make sure he understands the danger of stopping his drugs prematurely. Urge him to keep his follow-up appointments.

Show your patient how to check his pulse, and explain which changes he should report to his physician, such as dizziness, chest pain, palpitations, and shortness of breath. If your patient's drug is known to cause hypotension, caution him to sit up and stand up slowly, especially when getting out of bed in the morning.

If your patient takes amiodarone, warn him that his skin may turn a bluish color and that he needs sunscreen and protective clothing outdoors. If he also takes digoxin, teach him the signs and symptoms of a toxic reaction to digoxin. If he receives heparin, tell him why his APTT and platelet count must be monitored. If he takes warfarin, teach him how to monitor himself for occult bleeding.

Finally, encourage your patient to reduce stress in his life, to perform exercises for relaxation, and to eat a low-fat, low-sodium diet. Urge him to stop smoking and to avoid caffeine and alcohol.

Atrial flutter

Atrial flutter, which is usually transient, results from conditions similar to those that cause atrial fibrillation. In fact, if untreated, atrial flutter usually deteriorates into atrial fibrillation.

Atrial flutter is most common in people over age 40 who have ischemic heart disease. It's also common during the first week after cardiothoracic surgery. Typically, the mechanism of atrial flutter is a single ectopic atrial focus recurring through a reentrant pathway within the atria.

The ventricular rate is difficult to control in atrial flutter because of a mechanism called concealed conduction. In concealed conduction, some atrial impulses penetrate the AV node only partially and aren't transmitted to the ventricles. As a result, the ventricular rate remains slower than the atrial rate.

Pathophysiology

Occasionally, atrial flutter may occur in healthy people who ingest stimulants or develop acute alcohol intoxication. Both stimulants and alcohol lead to atrial irritability, which predisposes the heart to increased automaticity. Also, with alcohol intoxication, catecholamine rebound occurs after the depressant effects of the alcohol wear off.

Usually, however, atrial flutter results from organic heart disease. Like atrial flutter, atrial fibrillation can result from any condition that increases left atrial mass and diameter. When the atria are enlarged, atrial conduction is delayed, which alters the excitability of myocytes and, therefore, the automaticity of cardiac tissues.

Commonly, atrial enlargement results from reduced left ventricular function caused by aortic regurgitation, aortic insufficiency, aortic stenosis, an MI, or dilated cardiomyopathy. Patients with uncontrolled hypertension can develop left ventricular hypertrophy and stiffness, which impede left ventricular emptying. Pericarditis also impedes emptying, causing volume overload in all the chambers and abnormal atrial stretch, resulting in atrial flutter.

Increases in endogenous catecholamines from such endocrine disorders as hyperthyroidism, the overtreatment of hypothyroidism with thyroid replacement hormone, and pheochromocytoma also increase atrial excitability and can cause atrial flutter. And thyrotoxicosis increases sensitivity of the cardiac myocytes to circulating epinephrine and norepinephrine, resulting in atrial irritability.

Structural disease of the mitral valve is another common cause of atrial enlargement that can result in atrial flutter. Mitral stenosis is a common outcome of rheumatic heart disease that can occur 2 to 3 decades after the original infection. In mitral stenosis, the left atrium enlarges because of its inability to empty completely into the left ventricle. In mitral regurgitation, the loose AV valve allows backflow of blood from the left ventricle to the left atrium, resulting in volume overload and stretching of the left atrium. Atrial flutter related to AV block may result from the effects of digoxin, beta-blockers, or calcium channel blockers.

Signs and symptoms

If your patient has atrial flutter, his signs and symptoms will relate largely to his ventricular response rate. If he has a normal ventricular rate of 60 to 100 bpm, he may have no signs or symptoms. However, he may report palpitations. And when you check his jugular vein distention, you may notice cannon *a* waves, which are accentuated *a* waves of the jugular venous pulse. These waves can be observed in the neck veins as the atria contract against a closed AV valve.

If the patient has a ventricular rate above 100 bpm, he may complain of light-headedness, shortness of breath, or chest pain. These symptoms stem from reduced CO caused by a decrease in ventricular filling time. Some patients may also experience presyncope or syncope.

The atrial rate in atrial flutter is about 250 to 350 bpm. It results from a unifocal ectopic atrial focus in the caudal region of the atrium. Because the intrinsic rate of the ectopic focus exceeds that of the SA node, the ectopic focus outpaces or overdrives the SA node. Not all the atrial impulses reach the ventricles, however, so the ventricular rate is slower (see *Characteristics of atrial flutter*).

Sometimes the atria conduct impulses to the ventricles in a steady ratio, resulting in a regular ventricular rhythm. For example, one atrial impulse may reach the ventricles for every three atrial impulses, creating a ratio of 3:1 and a ventricular rate of 83 to 113 bpm. If one of every two atrial impulses moves through to the ventricles, it creates a 2:1 ratio and a ventricular rate of 125 to 177 bpm.

Conduction of atrial impulses through the AV node can also be variable, which is known as atrial flutter with varying block. This results in an irregular ventricular rhythm.

The hallmark of atrial flutter is characteristic sawtooth-edged F waves on the patient's ECG.

Characteristics of atrial flutter

Atrial rate: 250 to 350 beats per minute
Ventricular rate: varies
Atrial rhythm: regular
Ventricular rhythm: regular or irregular

P wave: replaced by sawtooth F waves, usually in multiples of 2, 3, or 4
PR interval: can't be determined
QRS complex: < 0.12 second

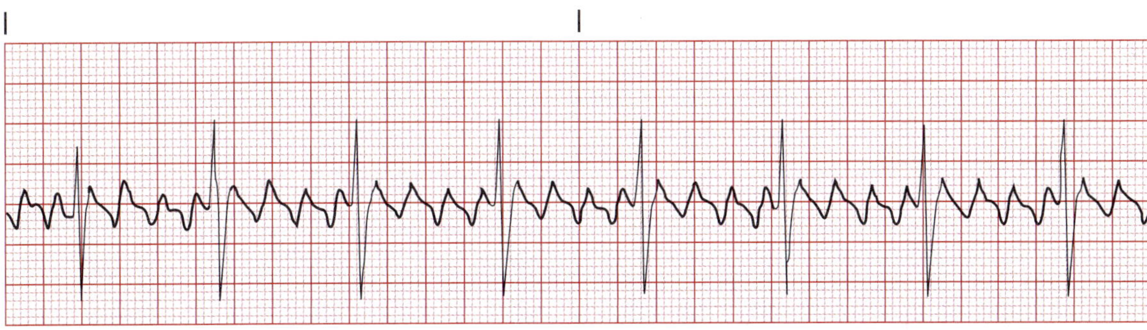

These waves are best seen in leads II, III, aV_F, and V_1. T waves blur into the F waves, making them difficult or impossible to discern. The isoelectric baseline in atrial flutter disappears at higher atrial rates.

The PR interval (more accurately called the FR interval) is usually prolonged at 0.26 to 0.46 second and can be fixed or variable. At rapid rates, such as in 2:1 conduction, some of the flutter waves are obscured because they are buried in the QRS complex. PR intervals may be undetectable. The R-R interval is fixed when the patient has a regular rhythm and variable when the patient has atrial flutter with varying block.

Atrial impulses become blocked because atrial depolarizations conduct through to the AV node during its refractory period. Therefore, the QRS complex appears normal. However, if your patient has an intraventricular conduction defect, such as a right bundle-branch block, the QRS complex may be prolonged.

Treatment

When treating a patient with atrial flutter, your goal is to determine and treat the cause. The ventricular response rate should be controlled with a beta-blocker, a calcium channel blocker, or digoxin until the patient converts to a more stable or manageable rhythm—such as a sinus rhythm or atrial fibrillation. The physician may order chemical cardioversion using a sodium channel blocker or a potassium channel blocker. If drug therapy fails to convert the rhythm, the patient may undergo electrical cardioversion, rapid atrial pacing, or ablation therapy.

Antiarrhythmic drugs

A physician may prescribe a beta-blocker, a calcium channel blocker, or digoxin to slow the ventricular response rate in atrial flutter. The I.V. route is preferred. The goal is to maintain a ventricular rate of less than 100 bpm while avoiding hypotension.

Beta-blockers

If your patient has excessive circulating catecholamines, whether endogenous or exogenous, treat that problem before giving him drugs or other treatment for atrial flutter, as ordered. Although primarily used to treat hypertension, beta-blockers also are the treatment of choice for atrial flutter caused by increased catecholamines.

As a group, beta-blockers decrease the receptiveness of myocytes to epinephrine and norepinephrine, which in turn diminishes atrial myocyte irritability. The result is a decrease in the ventricular response rate to atrial depolarization.

Beta-blockers provide an excellent option for treating atrial flutter related to an MI because slower atrial and ventricular rates minimize myocardial oxygen demand, thereby reducing ischemia and irritability. However, the negative inotropic and chronotropic effects of beta-blockers can be undesirable when treating certain patients. For example, negative inotropic properties can worsen heart failure in patients with depressed left ventricular function. Also, toxic levels of beta-blockers can produce symptomatic bradycardia when heart rates dip below 60 bpm. If bradycardia occurs, your patient may complain of light-headedness or fainting.

Beta-blockers can cause many other effects as well. For example, they mask the adrenergic response to hypoglycemia, which includes an increased heart rate, increased blood pressure, shakiness, and sweating. This masking effect can make it difficult for you and your patient to recognize the usual warning signs and symptoms of hypoglycemia. Indeed, a diabetic patient having a hypoglycemic reaction may have no signs or symptoms other than a depressed level of consciousness.

Other adverse effects of beta-blockers may include hypotension, heart failure, bronchospasm, lethargy, confusion, reduced concentration, depression, erectile dysfunction, nightmares, and insomnia.

Explain to your patient the necessity of taking beta-blockers as prescribed. Stress the need to avoid stopping the drug abruptly because of the risk of rebound tachycardias and adrenergic surges. Keep in mind that your patient may experience arrhythmias or angina as a result of withdrawal. The best way to discontinue beta-blocker therapy is by weaning the patient over several days. Remember that your patient with severely decreased ejection fraction or obstructive airway disease has an increased risk of heart failure and bronchospasm when beta-blockers are used to treat atrial flutter. When administering a beta-blocker, observe your patient for shortness of breath, orthopnea, and edema. Also, assess him for crackles and expiratory wheezing.

Calcium channel blockers

Calcium channel blockers used to control the ventricular rate include diltiazem and verapamil. Both are available in I.V. and oral forms.

Diltiazem: Give 0.25 mg/kg of diltiazem I.V. over 2 minutes. If the patient's ventricular rate stays above 100 bpm, give a second bolus of 0.35 mg/kg over 2 minutes. Then switch to a maintenance infusion at 5 to 15 mg/hour, as ordered. To determine the oral maintenance dose, multiply the cumulative 24-hour I.V. dose by 150%. The total oral dose can be given as divided doses or as a once-daily dose, depending on whether the physician prescribes a regular-release or sustained-release form.

Contraindications to diltiazem include sick sinus syndrome, hypotension, cardiogenic shock, and atrial flutter accompanied by WPW syndrome or short PR-interval syndrome.

Verapamil: Give 2.5 to 5 mg of verapamil I.V. over 2 minutes. If the patient's ventricular rate doesn't respond quickly enough, repeat the dose once after 5 minutes. Regular-release and sustained-release preparations are available for maintenance oral dosing. Typically, the starting dose is 120 mg every 24 hours. The maximum dose is 480 mg every 24 hours, divided or given as a single dose, depending on the preparation.

Verapamil is contraindicated in patients with an ejection fraction under 30%, hypotension, sick sinus syndrome, and atrial flutter or atrial fibrillation accompanied by WPW syndrome or short PR-interval syndrome. Remember that verapamil can increase blood digoxin levels by 50% to 75% because it's highly protein bound. Therefore, monitor your patient's blood digoxin levels and ECG closely when giving verapamil. Hypotension is common during I.V. administration.

Digoxin

As ordered, give 0.25 to 0.5 mg of digoxin I.V. as an initial bolus, followed by 0.25 mg every 6 to 8 hours until the patient's ventricular rate is controlled or you've given a total of 1 mg. Tell the patient to take 0.125 to 0.5 mg of oral digoxin once daily, as ordered.

Keep in mind that the negative chronotropic effect of digoxin takes several hours to reduce the patient's ventricular response rate. For a quicker response, use a calcium channel blocker or a beta-blocker, as ordered.

Therapeutic blood levels of digoxin are 1 to 2 ng/ml. A toxic reaction usually occurs with blood levels greater than 2 ng/ml and can cause atrial and ventricular arrhythmias, fatigue, anorexia, nausea,

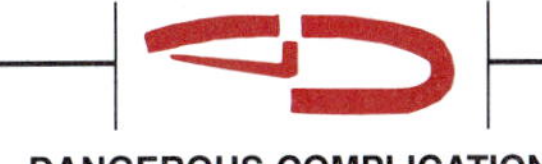

DANGEROUS COMPLICATIONS

Treating a toxic reaction to digoxin

To control ventricular response rates in supraventricular arrhythmias, a physician may prescribe digoxin. For maintenance therapy, the patient probably will take 0.125 to 0.5 mg once daily—less if he has decreased creatinine clearance.

Therapeutic blood levels are 1 to 2 ng/ml. Because of the narrow therapeutic range, the patient taking digoxin requires special care. Here's how to minimize the dangers of digoxin.

What to do immediately

If you suspect a toxic reaction to digoxin, check your patient's blood electrolyte levels right away. Hypokalemia, hypomagnesemia, and hypercalcemia worsen arrhythmias caused by digoxin. Keep your patient's blood potassium levels in the high-normal range.

Monitor your patient closely for changes in his heart rate and rhythm. If tachycardia persists even after you correct his blood electrolyte levels, discontinue digoxin temporarily or indefinitely, as ordered.

If the patient develops a life-threatening toxic reaction, give him digoxin immune FAB, as ordered. Typically, you'll administer it as an 800-mg I.V. push.The FAB antibody binds to digoxin, and the complex is then excreted. The appropriate dose depends on the patient's current blood digoxin level and goal blood digoxin level. Each 40-mg vial neutralizes 0.6 mg of blood digoxin.

visual disturbances (such as yellow halos or scotomas), and dizziness. Many drugs—such as verapamil, warfarin, erythromycin, tetracycline, and phenytoin—raise blood digoxin levels because digoxin is highly bound to protein (see *Treating a toxic reaction to digoxin*). Giving quinidine with digoxin can double blood digoxin levels, so cut your patient's digoxin level in half as you start giving quinidine. Also, if your patient has decreased creatinine clearance, reduce the dose of digoxin. Monitor your patient's electrolyte levels closely because hypokalemia, hypomagnesemia, and hypercalcemia can cause digoxin-related arrhythmias.

Sodium channel blockers

Sodium channel blockers used to convert and suppress atrial flutter include quinidine, procainamide, and disopyramide. Once the mainstay of treatment for supraventricular arrhythmias, sodium channel blockers now have limited use because of their proarrhythmic effects, significant toxicity, and marked adverse effects.

Quinidine: As with atrial fibrillation, patients with atrial flutter can receive 200 to 400 mg of regular-release quinidine every 6 hours, even if renal function is decreased. The longer-acting form of quinidine gluconate, called Quinaglute, is given at 324 to 648 mg every 8 to 12 hours. Therapeutic blood levels are 1.3 to 5 µg/ml.

Because quinidine is highly protein bound, it can double blood digoxin levels, and it prolongs the PT in patients taking warfarin. The half-life of quinidine in the blood significantly increases with age and liver dysfunction.

The most common adverse effects are nausea, vomiting, and diarrhea, and these may require discontinuation of the drug. Quinidine also can produce fever and flulike signs and symptoms, and it decreases counts of WBCs, RBCs, and platelets. Patients with cinchonism, a toxic reaction of the central nervous system, may experience tinnitus, hearing loss, visual disturbances, confusion, delirium, and psychosis.

As with atrial fibrillation, a patient with atrial flutter must receive digoxin, a beta-blocker, or a calcium channel blocker to control his ventricular rate before treatment with quinidine. Pretreatment prevents 1:1 conduction and detrimental increases in the ventricular rate due to quinidine.

Procainamide: The dosage of procainamide for atrial flutter is the same as that for atrial fibrillation: a 100-mg loading dose I.V. every 3 to 5 minutes, up to a total of 1 to 1.5 g. If hypotension develops, use a longer dosing interval. After the loading dose, the maintenance infusion is 2 to 4 mg/minute. Give the oral forms at 500 to 1,000 mg every 4 to 6 hours for regular release and 500 to 1,000 mg every 8 hours for sustained release.

Adverse reactions and arrhythmias may occur with excessive blood levels of procainamide and *N*-acetylprocainamide. So monitor your patient's blood levels to ensure that his combined procainamide and *N*-acetylprocainamide levels aren't above 30 µg/ml.

Procainamide produces a lupus-like syndrome in up to one-third of recipients of long-term therapy, with signs and symptoms of fever, arthralgias, pleuropericarditis, and hepatomegaly. Lupus-like effects resolve with discontinuation of the drug. Also, antinuclear antibodies develop in three-quarters of patients receiving long-term treatment. If your patient becomes symptomatic, you may need to discontinue procainamide.

Also, if your patient develops sensitivity reactions such as agranulocytosis, fever, rash, and cardiovascular signs and symptoms; if his atrial flutter is suppressed; if the QRS complex has widened by more than 50% of baseline; or if you've given a total dose of 15 mg/kg, stop therapy with procainamide.

Disopyramide: As with atrial fibrillation, give oral disopyramide at one of two dosages: 100 to 200 mg every 6 to 8 hours for regular release or 100 to 300 mg twice daily for sustained release. If your patient has renal insufficiency, adjust the dose, as necessary. If his creatinine clearance is 15 to 40 ml/minute or greater, give 100 mg every 12 hours. If his creatinine clearance is 15 ml/minute or less, give him 100 mg/day.

Adverse effects of disopyramide may include anticholinergic signs and symptoms, myasthenic crisis, and heart failure. As with other sodium channel blockers, control your patient's ventricular rate before administering disopyramide. Also, monitor his QTc interval during administration.

Potassium channel blockers

If your patient has refractory atrial flutter, the next choice of therapy may be a potassium channel blocker. The mechanism of action for a potassium channel blocker is the same as that described for the treatment of atrial fibrillation. Potassium channel blockers prolong action potential and repolarization as well as sinus rate, recovery time, and conduction through the AV node. And they reduce afterload by decreasing systemic vascular resistance and MAP without depressing left ventricular function.

The most common potassium channel blockers prescribed for atrial flutter are amiodarone and ibutilide. Patients who have had atrial flutter for more than 48 hours should receive anticoagulation therapy before chemical cardioversion with these drugs.

Amiodarone: Amiodarone is the most commonly used potassium channel blocker for atrial flutter. As prescribed, give 600 mg/day orally for 1 week, followed by 400 mg/day for 2 weeks. If the atrial flutter converts to a sinus rhythm, switch to maintenance dosing at 200 mg/day. Keep in mind that conversion or suppression of the arrhythmia may take 4 to 6 weeks.

About 3% of patients taking amiodarone develop thyroid dysfunction, so urge your patient to have thyroid function tests at least once a year. Remember that T_4 is always elevated in patients who receive long-term amiodarone therapy. As described, amiodarone-induced hyperthyroidism is a TSH level of less than 0.1 mg/ml together with an elevated T_4. Other important adverse effects of amiodarone can include corneal or pulmonary infiltrates, liver dysfunction, and electrolyte abnormalities (see *Reviewing the adverse effects of amiodarone*).

Ibutilide: This short-acting potassium channel blocker is used to convert atrial flutter to sinus rhythm. The proper dose depends on your patient's weight. If he weighs more than 80 kg, infuse 1 mg of the drug I.V. over 10 minutes. If he weighs less than 80 kg, give him 0.01 mg/kg. For persistent atrial flutter, repeat the initial dose 20 minutes after the first infusion. After sinus rhythm returns, the physician may prescribe long-term suppressive therapy with potassium channel blockers or calcium channel blockers.

During ibutilide treatment, continuously monitor your patient's ECG, blood pressure, and QTc interval for polymorphic VT and hypotension. A QTc interval greater than 0.44 second can potentiate torsades de pointes. Also, monitor electrolyte levels. Hypokalemia and hypomagnesemia can cause lethal polymorphic VT and torsades de pointes.

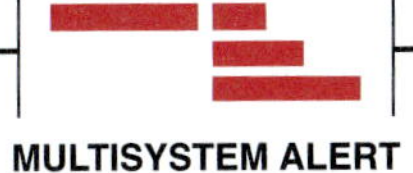

MULTISYSTEM ALERT

Reviewing the adverse effects of amiodarone

Amiodarone can have adverse effects on several body systems. Use this chart to review these effects and to help your patient make sure they're detected early.

System	Drug effects	Patient teaching
Cardiac	• Amiodarone can elevate blood digoxin levels, prolong PR intervals, widen QRS complexes, and lengthen QT intervals.	• Tell your patient to notify his physician if he develops a dry cough, numbness or loss of sensation, nausea, vomiting, constipation, or a loss of appetite.
Endocrine	• Amiodarone can block the conversion of thyroxine to triiodothyronine.	• Instruct your patient to have a thyroid function test at least once a year to detect silent thyrotoxicosis.
Hepatic	• Liver transaminase can rise to three times normal levels, even in patients who have normal liver function at the start of therapy.	• Urge your patient to have follow-up tests of liver function.
Ocular	• Most patients develop corneal infiltrates made up of amiodarone crystals.	• Encourage your patient to have periodic eye examinations.
Respiratory	• Pulmonary infiltrates and fibrosis occur in up to 15% of patients. • Infiltrates are unlikely among patients who take less than 300 mg daily.	• Instruct your patient to have chest X-rays and pulmonary function tests every 3 to 6 months, as prescribed.

Electrical cardioversion

If chemical cardioversion with antiarrhythmic drugs fails to convert your patient to a normal sinus rhythm or if he has unstable atrial flutter, the physician may prescribe electrical cardioversion after the patient has attained therapeutic blood levels of his antiarrhythmic drugs.

Atrial flutter is considered unstable when it causes angina, dyspnea, a decreased level of consciousness, hypotension, pulmonary edema, or an acute MI. A patient with unstable atrial flutter typically has a ventricular rate above 150 bpm.

Energy levels for cardioversion can start at 50 joules delivered in synchronous mode. If the atrial flutter doesn't convert to a sinus rhythm or atrial fibrillation, subsequent shocks of 100, 200, 300, and 360 joules may be necessary. Although conversion to a sinus rhythm is the best result, conversion to atrial fibrillation is also acceptable. Ventricular rates are easier to control in atrial fibrillation than in atrial flutter because of the concealed conduction in atrial flutter.

Atrial, nodal, and ventricular escape beats can occur briefly during and after cardioversion. Also, rhythms other than atrial flutter can result from the release of catecholamines, acetylcholine, and potassium caused by delivery of an electrical current. The patient's blood levels of LD, AST, and CK may rise in response to electrical current coursing through skeletal muscle. However, the isoenzyme CK-MB typically doesn't rise until the patient receives a cumulative discharge of 425 joules.

The worst adverse effect of cardioversion is the conversion of atrial flutter to VT or ventricular fibrillation (VF). This rare complication usually accompanies a toxic reaction to a digitalis glycoside. If cardioversion causes VT, the defibrillator should immediately be switched to asynchronous mode and a countershock should be administered, starting at 200 joules.

Other adverse effects of cardioversion include first-degree and second-degree burns on the chest wall and tenderness of the chest-wall muscles. Burns can be avoided by properly using electrolyte gel or pads and by maintaining firm contact between the defibrillator paddles and the patient's skin.

Successful cardioversion depends on the duration of atrial flutter, atrial size, precipitating drugs, and blood levels of antiarrhythmic drugs. The longer your patient remains in atrial flutter, the less likely he is to successfully convert to or maintain sinus rhythm. Patients with left atrial diameters of greater than 4.5 cm are also less likely to convert or remain converted.

Pretreating atrial fibrillation with quinidine before electrical cardioversion improves the chances of maintaining normal sinus rhythm after cardioversion. It also may reduce the number of shocks and the energy required to convert to a sinus rhythm. In patients who are optimal candidates for cardioversion, the success rate is 90%.

Rapid atrial pacing

If your patient develops atrial flutter after having a cardiotomy, he may benefit from rapid atrial pacing. He'll most likely have epicardial pacing wires in place until a few days before discharge.

Rapid atrial pacing involves connecting the atrial leads to a pacer generator and pacing the patient's heart at an atrial rate that is 115% to 130% of the flutter rate. In other words, an atrial rate of 250 bpm would be overdrive paced at 285 to 325 bpm.

Only pacer generators specially designed for rapid atrial pacing can be used for this procedure. Standard pacer generators can't reach a high enough rate to overdrive pace the atria. When overdrive pacing does reach a high enough rate, it can convert atrial flutter to a normal sinus rhythm by suppressing the ectopic atrial focus.

Ablation therapy

Radiofrequency catheter-induced ablation therapy is another option for a patient in whom drug therapy fails. Before ablation, electrophysiologic studies record intracardiac electrograms and locate the arrhythmic focus. Then, radio frequency is used to produce a localized thermal injury to the endocardium. The success rate of this procedure is 95%. Radiofrequency catheter-induced ablation may ultimately reduce the need for suppressive drug therapy for atrial flutter.

Complications

Acute complications of atrial flutter typically stem from an uncontrolled, rapid ventricular response rate that decreases ventricular filling time, reduces CO, and increases myocardial oxygen demand. If the patient also has coronary artery disease (CAD), he faces a heightened danger of myocardial ischemia and an MI. Myocardial ischemia and decreased CO also can cause heart failure and, in turn, hypoxia and hemodynamic compromise. Decreased CO reduces cerebral blood flow as well, possibly causing syncope.

Emboli are uncommon in atrial flutter. When they do occur, they usually affect patients whose atrial flutter has lasted longer than 3 days or who have a history of mitral stenosis from rheumatic heart disease. Thromboemboli develop in the atrial walls as blood pools in the fluttering chambers. These emboli are then ejected out of the atria, possibly causing a CVA, an MI, limb ischemia, pulmonary emboli, or other systemic emboli.

The risk of thromboembolism increases when atrial flutter converts to sinus rhythm because the atria finally contract effectively, possibly releasing the emboli. The decision to use anticoagulation therapy is made on a case-by-case basis.

Electrophysiologic complications of atrial flutter include deterioration of atrial flutter to atrial fibrillation and atrial flutter coupled with preexcitation or WPW syndrome. Conversion to atrial fibrillation is dangerous because of the loss of atrial kick and the propensity for thrombus formation. However, the ventricular rate in atrial fibrillation is easy to manage. In atrial flutter with preexcitation, administration of AV nodal blocking drugs to slow the ventricular rate can lead to the disastrous consequence of 1:1 conduction of atrial impulses through the AV node to the ventricles, resulting in VT. Such drugs include cardizem, verapamil, and digoxin.

Nursing considerations

Closely monitor your patient's ECG and clinical findings during drug treatment or electrical cardioversion for atrial flutter. Stay alert for possible drug interactions. For example, because verapamil is highly bound to protein, it can increase blood digoxin levels by 50% to 75%. Assess your patient's blood digoxin level and ECG carefully and frequently during concurrent administration.

Other nursing interventions for patients receiving digoxin include maintaining blood potassium levels in the high-normal range. Avoid obtaining blood drug levels within 6 hours after an I.V. dose or 8 hours after an oral dose, when blood concentrations are highest. Avoid giving digoxin to patients with hypertrophic, obstructive cardiomyopathy because the resulting increase in contractility could worsen obstruction of the left ventricular outflow tract. Also, keep in mind that patients with low albumin levels and decreased muscle mass—usually elderly patients—face an increased risk of a toxic reaction to a digitalis glycoside because of their decreased ability to bind the drug.

When giving a sodium channel blocker, such as quinidine or procainamide, monitor and control your patient's ventricular rates. Check blood procainamide and metabolite levels for a toxic reaction. With disopyramide, monitor your patient's blood chemistry results and adjust the dose, as ordered, if your patient has renal insufficiency. Also, monitor your patient's QTc interval.

As possible, avoid giving drugs in combination with antiarrhythmic therapy that could prolong the patient's QT interval. Such drugs include erythromycin, haloperidol, phenothiazines, quinidine, and tricyclic antidepressants.

When giving a potassium channel blocker, examine your patient for evidence of dependent edema from decreased systemic vascular resistance. If the patient takes amiodarone, watch for thyroid dysfunction.

Monitor the patient's blood electrolyte levels, especially potassium and magnesium, before giving ibutilide. Monitor his QTc interval both before and during therapy. A QTc interval greater than 0.44 second commonly accompanies torsades de pointes. Continuously check your patient's ECG and blood pressure for polymorphic VT and hypotension. Remember that hypokalemia and hypomagnesemia can provoke lethal polymorphic VT and torsades de pointes, so keep resuscitative equipment at the bedside.

Patient teaching

Tell your patient what he should expect during evaluation and treatment for his arrhythmia. Encourage him to participate in his own treatment by quitting smoking and limiting his use of alcohol, caffeine, and other stimulants. Teach him how to take his pulse and explain which signs and symptoms warrant calling his physician, including an increase in the number of irregular heartbeats, dizziness, palpitations, and chest pain. Remind him to move slowly when standing or sitting up, especially first thing in the morning, to avoid the adverse effects of postural hypotension.

Explain the mechanism of action and adverse effects specific to the drug that he's taking. For example, explain the signs and symptoms of a toxic reaction to digoxin and the gastrointestinal (GI) adverse effects of quinidine. Tell him when to expect his signs and symptoms to improve. Explain that he may not feel any improvement for 4 to 6 weeks after he starts therapy with amiodarone.

Stress the importance of taking his drug as prescribed, especially if he has an underlying condition such as an MI, hypertension, or mitral valve disease. Make sure he understands not to stop taking his drug unless his physician directs him to stop. Urge him to faithfully keep all follow-up appointments.

Premature atrial contractions

If the heart has an irritable ectopic focus anywhere in the atria except the SA node, this focus can produce a premature atrial contraction. You'll notice it as an early beat on the patient's ECG that interrupts an otherwise regular rhythm.

If the AV node and the ventricles have fully repolarized when the irritable focus produces an impulse, it will conduct through to the ventricles and produce a QRS complex on the patient's ECG. If the AV node isn't fully repolarized, however, the impulse will be blocked, producing no QRS complex on the patient's ECG.

Pathophysiology

Premature atrial contractions may occur in patients who have cardiac problems such as atherosclerotic heart disease, valvular heart disease, enlarged atria, mitral valve prolapse, and heart failure. Also, in patients who don't have heart disease, the arrhythmia may result from causes such as the following:

- emotional stress
- excessive use of caffeine, tobacco, or alcohol
- infection or inflammation
- hyperthyroidism
- emphysema or bronchitis
- hypokalemia or hypomagnesemia
- digoxin therapy.

Signs and symptoms

A patient with premature atrial contractions may experience a number of signs and symptoms, including palpitations, dizziness, and feelings of occasionally skipped or rapid heartbeats. If frequent premature contractions lead to atrial fibrillation, atrial flutter, or paroxysmal supraventricular tachycardia, your patient may develop even more signs and symptoms, such as the following:

- anxiety
- hypotension
- light-headedness
- syncope
- chest pain
- shortness of breath
- pulmonary crackles.

When assessing your patient for premature atrial contractions, look for the early P wave in the T wave of the preceding beat. If you can't see the P wave easily, it may be buried in the T wave. Look for a T wave that is abnormally high or peaked or one that has a notch or an extra hump in its downward slope (see *Characteristics of premature atrial contractions*).

When the impulse arrives after the ventricles have repolarized, it's conducted normally. Thus, the QRS complex that follows an early P wave has a normal shape and duration.

If the AV node and ventricles are in an absolute refractory period, the impulse may be blocked at the AV node and fail to produce a QRS complex. If the ventricles are in a relative refractory period, however, the result may be a wide, aberrant QRS complex similar to that seen in right bundle-branch block. In that case, the patient has what's called an aberrantly conducted premature atrial contraction.

Premature atrial contractions may be difficult to differentiate from premature ventricular contractions. However, the type of pause—compensatory or noncompensatory—reveals the difference. If a P wave precedes the premature beat, it's a premature atrial contraction. Usually, the affected patient has a normal heart rate and a regular underlying rhythm. And the QRS complexes are less than 0.12 second.

Treatment

Your patient won't need any treatment for premature atrial contractions unless his signs and symptoms warrant treatment or his premature atrial contractions become frequent enough to raise his risk of developing other arrhythmias, such as atrial fibrillation, atrial flutter, or paroxysmal supraventricular tachycardia. If he needs treatment, anticipate giving him drugs to correct the underlying cause of the premature contractions and antiarrhythmic drugs.

Treating the underlying cause

To help reduce the effects of underlying conditions on your patient's premature atrial contractions, make sure he's being fully treated with appropriate drugs. For example, if he has heart failure, check to make sure that he's faithfully following his drug regimen. Make sure his electrolyte levels remain within normal limits. Anticipate giving him supplemental oxygen, an inotropic drug, a vasodilator drug, and a diuretic. Restrict his fluid intake and provide low-sodium meals. Urge him to avoid caffeine, tobacco, and alcohol.

If your patient is receiving digoxin when premature atrial contractions begin, a toxic reaction to the drug may be causing the arrhythmia. Withhold the drug and notify the physician immediately.

Your patient may experience premature atrial contractions as a result of stress, especially if he has a history of mitral valve prolapse. Be aware that in such patients, frequent premature atrial contractions are commonly treated with anxiolytic (antianxiety) drugs such as alprazolam, oxazepam, or lorazepam. If the premature atrial con-

Characteristics of premature atrial contractions

Rate: depends on underlying rhythm
Rhythm: regular or irregular
P wave: peaked
PR interval: 0.12 to 0.2 second
QRS complex: < 0.12 second

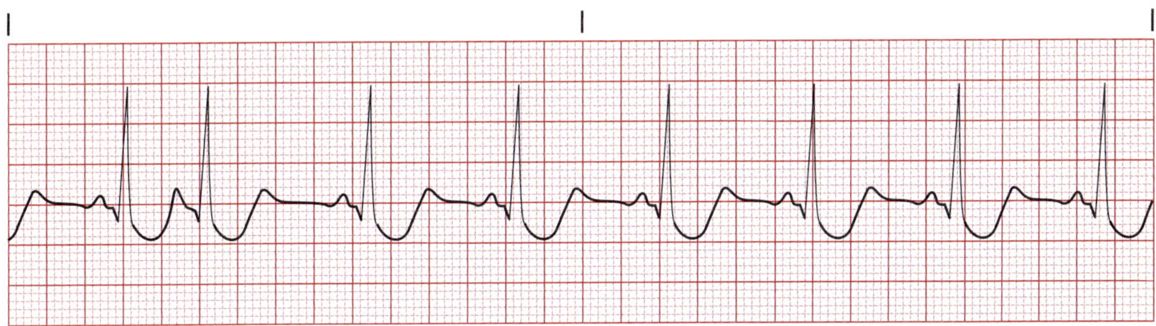

tractions are caused by stress alone, drug therapy may not be indicated. Effectively alleviating stress can decrease the incidence of premature atrial contractions. Help your patient identify possible sources of stress and teach him new coping skills, such as guided imagery, music therapy, and relaxation techniques.

Antiarrhythmic drugs

If treating the underlying cause doesn't reduce or stop the patient's premature atrial contractions, expect to give him an oral antiarrhythmic drug, such as quinidine or procainamide. If your patient is experiencing significant signs and symptoms such as palpitations or chest discomfort, he may require these drugs by the I.V. route.

Carefully monitor your patient's ECG for the development of other abnormalities when administering these drugs, such as ventricular arrhythmias and heart block. Prolongation of the QT interval increases the patient's risk of torsades de pointes. Measure his PR interval, QT interval, and QRS complex, and report lengthening intervals to the physician.

Be aware that quinidine can cause many adverse effects, such as respiratory depression, nausea, diarrhea, vomiting, dizziness, headache, hypotension, thrombocytopenia, hemolytic anemia, and anaphylaxis. If prescribed together with digoxin, quinidine also increases the risk of a toxic reaction to digoxin. Anticipate that future doses of digoxin will need to be reduced.

Also, anticipate the adverse effects of procainamide. These include hypotension, nausea, vomiting, diarrhea, rash, a lupus-like syndrome, and agranulocytosis. Keep in mind that antiarrhythmic drugs can have a proarrhythmic effect, which means that they can cause other dangerous arrhythmias (see *Proarrhythmia: Spotting early trouble,* page 66).

Complications

Even without taking antiarrhythmic drugs, a patient with premature atrial contractions has an increased risk of developing other arrhythmias, such as atrial fibrillation, atrial flutter, paroxysmal supraventricular tachycardia, and reentrant tachycardias. In a reentrant tachycardia, the irritable atria can increase the number of premature atrial contractions produced because of an accessory pathway—an area of depressed conduction between the boundaries of the atria and ventricles. If he develops a reentrant tachycardia, your patient's heart rate could reach or exceed 200 bpm.

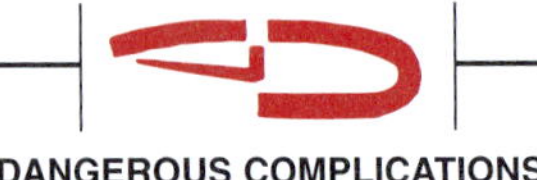

DANGEROUS COMPLICATIONS

Proarrhythmia: Spotting early trouble

The beginning of drug therapy with a sodium channel blocker can be a dangerous time for your patient, especially if he has ischemic heart disease or left ventricular dysfunction or if he receives a high dose of the drug. That's because of the risk of proarrhythmia—an arrhythmia triggered by sodium channel blockers and certain other antiarrhythmic drugs. These drugs prolong the QT interval, which raises the patient's risk of ventricular tachycardia, ventricular fibrillation, and torsades de pointes.

What you should do

Closely monitor the cardiac status of any patient receiving a sodium channel blocker—especially a patient with prolonged QT intervals, ischemic heart disease, or left ventricular dysfunction. Check your patient's electrocardiogram at least once each shift, as indicated. Measure his QT interval from the beginning of the Q wave to the end of the T wave. Although the QT interval varies with the ventricular rate, it's probably prolonged if it measures more than half as long as the R-R interval.

Combining other drugs with a sodium channel blocker can dramatically raise your patient's risk of new arrhythmias. If you must administer more than one drug, watch your patient's condition closely. In particular, monitor him for hypokalemia and hypomagnesemia, either of which can contribute to a prolonged QT interval. Whenever possible, avoid giving the following drugs in combination with a sodium channel blocker:

- astemizole
- bepridil
- droperidol
- erythromycin
- haloperidol
- indapamide
- itraconazole
- ketoconazole
- pentamidine
- quinidine
- terfenadine.

Because premature atrial contractions commonly result from chronic conditions, such as chronic bronchitis, emphysema, heart failure, valvular heart disease, and hyperthyroidism, expect your patient to have future episodes of premature atrial contractions and possibly to develop other arrhythmias, as previously discussed.

Nursing considerations

If your patient develops premature atrial contractions, obtain a baseline ECG, as ordered, so that you can tell how they change over time. Also, perform a baseline physical assessment so that you can quickly detect changes in his status—especially changes that stem from reduced CO. Assess the patient's cardiovascular status, including his vital signs, heart sounds, breath sounds, capillary refill, skin color and temperature, peripheral pulses, level of consciousness, and urine output. When assessing his pulse, count the apical beats for a full minute. Report any abnormal findings, such as hypotension, diaphoresis, or the onset of new arrhythmias, to the physician.

If your patient is receiving an antiarrhythmic drug, track his blood electrolyte levels, blood drug levels, complete blood cell count (to detect hematologic abnormalities), and liver and renal studies. Be prepared to report abnormal values to the physician and suggest follow-up laboratory tests to monitor the return to normal values or therapeutic drug levels. Anticipate electrolyte replacement therapy for abnormally low values; they occur commonly in patients who experience adverse GI effects from drug therapy.

In the acute stage of treatment, reassure your patient to reduce his anxiety. Offer simple explanations of the condition and its treatment; more detailed teaching can be done when the arrhythmia is under control. Administer anxiolytics, as prescribed.

Patient teaching

Explain measures that your patient can take to reduce the risk of recurrence. Urge him to stop smoking, as appropriate, and to cut back on caffeine and alcohol. If an underlying condition such as heart failure caused his arrhythmia, make sure he knows the importance of taking his drugs and following his treatment plan faithfully.

Teach your patient to take his pulse. Tell him to call his physician if he detects an irregular pulse or an increase in the number of irregular beats. Explain the symptoms that he should report to his physician, such as dizziness, palpitations, and chest pain. Remind your patient to rise slowly to the sitting or standing position, especially first thing in the morning, to avoid the effects of postural hypotension.

Explain the purpose of all the drugs your patient is taking as well as their dosages and possible adverse effects. Stress the importance of not stopping the drugs without consulting with his physician. Urge your patient to keep all follow-up medical appointments, and explain that he will have his blood drawn periodically to check for toxic levels, liver and kidney dysfunction, and electrolyte imbalances.

Atrial tachycardia

In atrial tachycardia, one or more atrial pacemakers produce an atrial rate above 100 bpm. This condition differs from sinus tachycardia in that the pacemaker site isn't the SA node but is an ectopic focus in the atria. You may encounter three types of atrial tachycardia: atrial tachycardia with block, multifocal atrial tachycardia, and paroxysmal atrial tachycardia.

In atrial tachycardia with block (missed ventricular response), the patient has a single ectopic pacemaker. In multifocal atrial tachycardia, the rhythm results from more than three atrial foci. Consequently, the patient's ECG will show the same number of morphologically different P waves.

Paroxysmal atrial tachycardia occurs suddenly as a burst of rapid atrial rhythm during a normal sinus rhythm. And it generally ends just as abruptly as it begins. Use of the term typically relates more to the patient's history and signs and symptoms than from ECG evidence.

Pathophysiology

The usual cause of atrial ectopy is an elevation in cardiac preload as a result of an enlarged left or right atrium, electrolyte disturbances, and hypoxia. It also can result from enhanced automaticity that causes triggered activity and reentry. In triggered activity, a trigger or stimulus irritates the atria into ectopic activity. Examples of such triggers include increased circulating blood catecholamines—from fever, anxiety, exertion, or thyrotoxicosis, for instance—or increased sympathetic activation from myocardial ischemia or a toxic reaction to a digitalis glycoside.

Hyperkalemia, hypercalcemia, and use of alcohol can trigger enhanced automaticity because these conditions cause intracellular calcium to accumulate, which enables the atria to depolarize during an action potential.

Alcohol is an indirect trigger because, although it depresses the nervous system, it produces a rebound surge of catecholamines when blood levels of alcohol drop, irritating the atria as a result. Also, alcohol abuse can disrupt normal conduction through the impaired synthesis or accelerated degradation of contractile proteins in the myocardium.

Atrial tachycardia also can result if the SA node fails because occlusion of the right coronary artery interrupts blood flow to the node. Failure of the normal conductive pathway can also result from diseases that infiltrate the myocardium with abnormal connective tissue, such as amyloidosis and sarcoidosis. Multifocal atrial tachycardia occurs most commonly in patients with severe pulmonary disease such as emphysema, pulmonary hypertension, and incompetent pulmonary valves.

Signs and symptoms

Signs and symptoms of atrial tachycardia vary with the patient's ventricular response rate and cardiac health. An otherwise healthy person who develops atrial tachycardia may have no signs or symptoms or may feel palpitations, nervousness, light-headedness, or shortness of breath. A patient with CAD may experience angina, dyspnea, diaphoresis, and nausea because his decreased ventricular filling time reduces his CO.

Characteristics of atrial tachycardias

Atrial tachycardia with block

Atrial rate: 150 to 250 beats per minute (bpm)
Ventricular rate: one-half of atrial rate
Rhythm: regular; irregular if block is variable
P wave: flattened, notched, or hidden
PR interval: 0.12 to 0.2 second
QRS complex: < 0.2 second

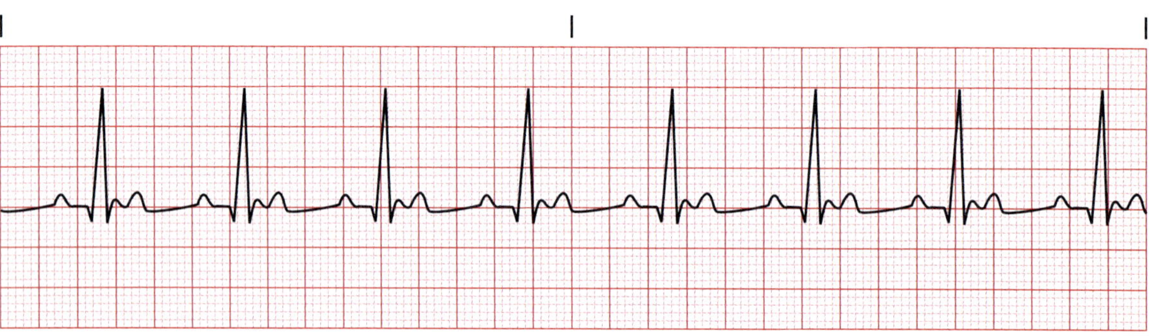

Multifocal atrial tachycardia

Rate: 150 to 250 bpm
Rhythm: irregular
P wave: flattened, notched, or hidden
PR interval: 0.12 to 0.2 second
QRS complex: < 0.12 second

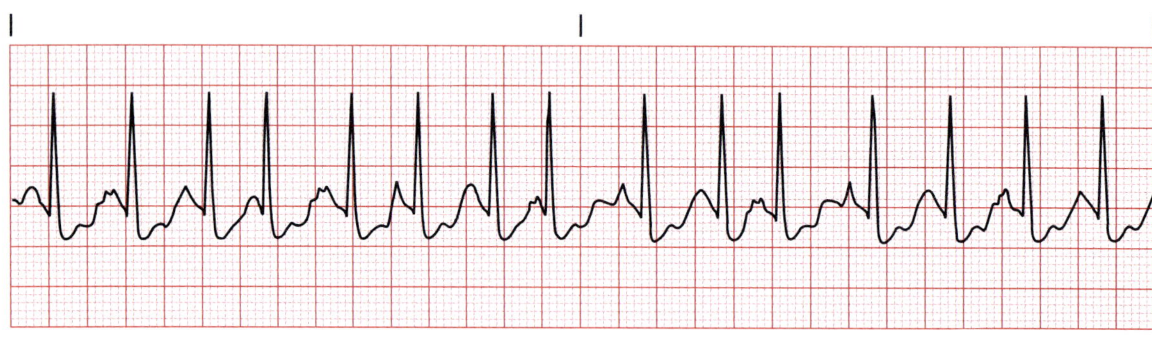

(continued)

When examining the patient, you'll find that he has a pulse rate above 100 bpm. If he has heart failure, you may hear an S_3 or crackles.

Signs of atrial tachycardia on the patient's ECG include an accelerated rate and changes involving the P waves. Usually, the rhythm is regular, although irregularities can develop if the pacemaker site moves among the SA node, the lower atria, and the AV node, as in multifocal atrial tachycardia (see *Characteristics of atrial tachycardias*).

The rate accelerates because rapid firing of an ectopic atrial focus induces overdrive suppres-

Characteristics of atrial tachycardias (continued)

Paroxysmal atrial tachycardia

Rate: 150 to 250 bpm
Rhythm: regular
P wave: flattened, notched, or hidden

PR interval: 0.12 to 0.2 second
QRS complex: usually < 0.12 second; may be aberrant

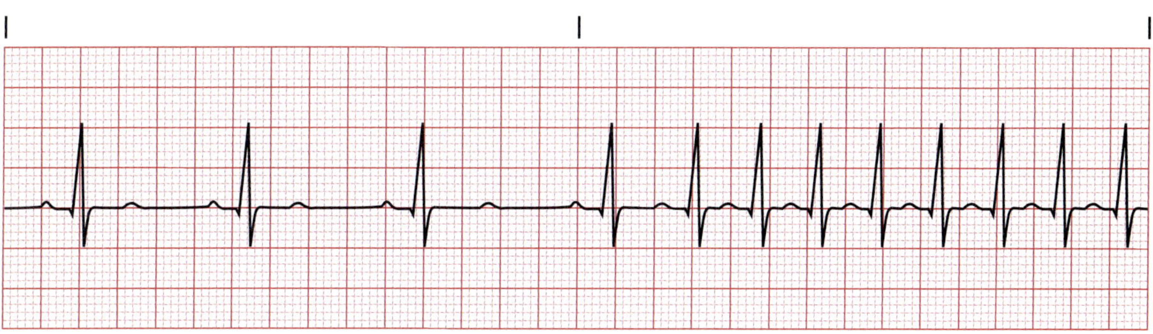

sion of the SA node. In other words, the focus with the highest inherent rate suppresses and paces other foci with slower rates. The atrial rate in atrial tachycardia is 150 to 250 bpm.

Except in multifocal atrial tachycardia, the patient's P waves will all look alike, which indicates a unifocal pacemaker. However, they'll all also look abnormal. In atrial tachycardia, P waves are generally indistinguishable because of an accelerated ventricular response rate, which is usually greater than 130 bpm. Ectopic atrial beats result in an abnormal P-wave configuration characterized as P prime (P′). On a 12-lead ECG, they're inverted in leads I, II, and aV_F, and upright in lead aV_R—the opposite of normal P waves.

In multifocal atrial tachycardia, the P waves differ from each other based on the number of foci producing them. Conduction time through the atria to the AV node differs for each one, resulting in varying PR intervals. For the same reason, P-P and R-R intervals differ and the arrhythmia produced is generally irregular.

The R-R intervals typically are regular unless the patient has a variable AV block. The QRS complex may appear normal or abnormal on the ECG. A normal duration of 0.1 second or less indicates a focus above the ventricles. However, atrial tachycardia with aberrant conduction produces a QRS complex widened to more than 0.1 second.

Treatment

Because atrial tachycardias typically result either from an underlying myocardial problem or from excessive exogenous or endogenous stimulation, treatment focuses on resolving the underlying problem. Exogenous stimulants include caffeine, beta-agonists (such as albuterol and theophylline), and recreational drugs.

Endogenous stimulants include the catecholamines epinephrine and norepinephrine. They may be secreted in normal amounts or, in a condition such as pheochromocytoma, in abnormal amounts. Pheochromocytoma can be confirmed through a urine test.

Check your patient's blood digoxin level and blood potassium and magnesium levels, and correct them, as necessary. If the patient receives digoxin, discontinue the drug, as ordered.

Also, evaluate the patient's thyroid function to determine whether it could be causing the arrhythmia. In patients with endocrine dysfunction, the ventricular rate should be controlled until the problem can be corrected.

Antiarrhythmic drugs

When underlying causes can't be corrected, the patient most likely will need drug treatment. Atrial tachycardias not caused by a toxic reaction to a digitalis glycoside can be treated with a beta-blocker or a calcium channel blocker, usually delivered by the I.V. route. A sodium channel blocker or a potassium channel blocker can be added if the atrial tachycardia persists.

Beta-blockers

Beta-blockers provide an optimal choice for treating atrial tachycardia because they prohibit the binding of blood catecholamines to beta-adrenergic receptors on the myocardial cells, thus suppressing automaticity. Suppression of automaticity also helps to abolish reentrant AV nodal tachyarrhythmias.

The therapeutic goal of beta-blockade is to hold the ventricular response rate at less than 100 bpm while maintaining blood pressure within normal ranges. In patients with ischemic heart disease, the desired goal is lower still, at 60 to 70 bpm.

Metoprolol: Give 5 mg of metoprolol I.V. every 5 minutes until you've given a total of 15 mg. With the ventricular rate in control, start giving oral metoprolol, 50 to 100 mg twice daily, preferably 8 to 12 hours apart. For maintenance therapy, instruct your patient to take 20 to 40 mg two to four times daily, as prescribed.

Atenolol: Because atenolol allows once-daily dosing, it may increase patient compliance. Instruct your patient to take 50 to 200 mg/day as ordered.

Propranolol: A nonselective beta-blocker, propranolol also is considered a class Ib antiarrhythmic because of its membrane-stabilizing properties. Give 1 mg of propranolol I.V. slowly over 1 minute. If that doesn't control the ventricular rate, repeat the dose as needed up to a total of 5 mg. Oral doses are 10 to 80 mg every 6 to 8 hours. Propranolol is contraindicated in uncompensated heart failure, chronic bronchitis, and emphysema.

Potassium channel blockers

Amiodarone is the most commonly used potassium channel blocker for atrial tachycardias. Give 600 mg orally for 1 week, followed by 400 mg/day for 2 weeks. If the atrial tachycardia converts to a sinus rhythm, switch to maintenance dosing at 200 mg/day. Keep in mind, however, that the drug may not convert or suppress the arrhythmia for 4 to 6 weeks.

Calcium channel blockers

Because the SA and AV nodes depend on slow-channel activity, calcium channel blockers are well suited for treating supraventricular tachycardias. These drugs include adenosine, diltiazem, and verapamil.

Adenosine: Available only in I.V. form, adenosine is a rapid-acting calcium channel blocker that commonly halts atrial tachycardia immediately when caused by AV node reentry and accessory pathway conduction (see *Treating atrial tachycardias with adenosine*). If the patient doesn't respond to the first dose within about 2 minutes, you may need to give a second dose.

Adenosine is contraindicated in patients with second-degree or third-degree AV block, sick sinus syndrome, an MI, or cerebral hemorrhage. Adenosine does not convert atrial flutter, atrial fibrillation, or ventricular tachycardia to a normal sinus rhythm, although slowing of the ventricular response may be noticed after administration. If adenosine is contraindicated for your patient, anticipate giving diltiazem, verapamil, or digoxin I.V. instead to treat hemodynamically stable atrial tachycardia.

Diltiazem: Give 0.25 mg/kg of diltiazem I.V. over 2 minutes. If the patient's ventricular rate stays above 100 bpm, give a second bolus of 0.35 mg/kg over 2 minutes. Then switch to a maintenance infusion, as ordered, at 5 to 15 mg/hour. To determine the appropriate oral maintenance dose, multiply the cumulative 24-hour I.V. dose by 150%. Maintenance oral dosing is available in regular-release, sustained-release, and once-daily doses.

Contraindications to diltiazem include hypotension, sick sinus syndrome, and cardiogenic shock.

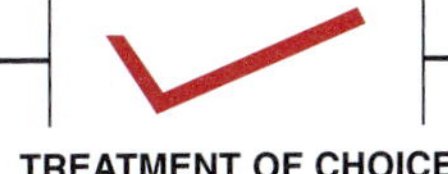

TREATMENT OF CHOICE

Treating atrial tachycardias with adenosine

Adenosine is a rapid-acting calcium channel blocker available only for I.V. administration. Because adenosine depresses conduction through the atrioventricular (AV) node, prolongs the AV node's refractory period, and inhibits sinoatrial node automaticity, it's the treatment of choice for several atrial tachycardias.

You'll most likely give a 6-mg bolus of adenosine rapidly, using a large vein, preferably the brachiocephalic vein, followed by a 10-ml to 30-ml saline flush. Usually, the patient's tachycardia stops immediately. If it doesn't, give a second bolus of 12 mg, as ordered, after 1 to 2 minutes.

Keep in mind that large doses of adenosine can induce frequent premature atrial contractions and atrial fibrillation. The drug is contraindicated in patients with a known hypersensitivity, symptomatic bradycardia, second-degree or third-degree AV block, or sick sinus syndrome without a permanent pacemaker in place. Always recheck your patient's electrocardiogram before giving the drug.

Also, be aware that sinus pauses up to 6 seconds long are common after giving adenosine. If your patient is receiving dipyridamole, the physician probably will reduce the dose by 25%. That's because dipyridamole blocks the cellular uptake of adenosine, increasing its effects. In contrast, methylxanthines—such as theophylline and caffeine—block the adenosine receptors in myocytes, rendering the drug ineffective.

It also is contraindicated in atrial flutter with an accessory bypass tract, as in WPW syndrome and short PR-interval syndrome. Giving diltiazem or verapamil in these preexcitation syndromes can result in 1:1 conduction of atrial impulses, possibly yielding ventricular rates up to 350 bpm.

Verapamil: Give 2.5 to 5 mg of verapamil I.V. over 2 minutes. Repeat the dose once after 5 minutes if the patient's ventricular rate doesn't respond quickly. Keep in mind that I.V. administration commonly leads to hypotension. Regular-release and sustained-release preparations are available for maintenance oral dosing; give 120 to 480 mg per 24 hours, as prescribed.

Verapamil is contraindicated if your patient has an ejection fraction under 30%, hypotension, sick sinus syndrome, or atrial flutter or fibrillation with WPW syndrome. Because verapamil is highly protein bound, it can increase blood digoxin levels by 50% to 75%.

Electrical cardioversion

If drug treatment fails to control your patient's signs and symptoms, he may need synchronized direct-current cardioversion. This procedure works by depolarizing or capturing all receptive parts of the myocardium, including those of the reentry circuit, which is made nonreceptive to the returning impulse from the reentry loop.

Before electrical cardioversion begins, make sure you have resuscitative equipment immediately available in case your patient needs intubation or supplemental oxygen. Also, establish reliable large-bore I.V. access.

Typically, atrial tachycardia is treated with a current of 25 to 100 joules. Cardioversion pads should be strategically placed for the most effective current delivery. For atrial tachycardia, the anterior pad should be placed firmly against the patient's skin at the left sternal border between the third and fourth intercostal spaces; the posterior pad should be placed slightly below the left scapula. Pads should be placed at least 6 cm from permanent pacers or automatic implantable cardioverter-defibrillators. Synchronous mode must be reset after each discharge.

During and after cardioversion, monitor your patient's rhythms closely. Transient atrial, nodal, and ventricular escape beats can occur. Rhythms other than atrial tachycardia can result from the release of catecholamines, acetylcholine, and potassium after delivery of the electrical current.

Assess the results of your patient's laboratory tests, as indicated, possibly including blood LD, AST, and isoenzymes of CK. Recall that CK-MB isoenzyme is specific to myocardial cells. The MB fraction usually doesn't rise until the patient has received a cumulative discharge of 425 joules.

Carotid sinus massage

The physician may use carotid sinus massage to help reduce the heart rate in a patient with hemodynamically stable atrial tachycardia. Carotid sinus massage is the most widely recommended of what are called vagal maneuvers. It involves applying gentle pressure to one carotid artery for 5 to 10 seconds. Successful carotid sinus massage slows the rate of atrial tachycardias by interrupting input from cranial nerve X to the myocardium.

Complications of carotid sinus massage are rare; however, the procedure may raise the risk of asystole or VF in some patients. The procedure is contraindicated in patients with a carotid bruit because athlerosclerotic plaque could become dislodged, resulting in cerebral ischemia or an embolism. Simultaneous pressure to both carotid arteries should never be applied because this completely obstructs cerebral blood flow.

Complications

A rapid ventricular rate prevents the ventricles from filling properly, thus leading to reduced CO. Most patients with chronically increased heart rates have activity intolerance. Patients with chronic atrial tachycardia usually complain of shortness of breath and easily develop dyspnea upon exertion. The chronic decrease in CO introduces the risk of ischemic peripheral vascular disease. Your patient may experience cyanosis of the nail beds or toes. He may also develop venous stasis ulcers from poor blood flow to high-pressure areas.

If your patient's blood pressure drops significantly and you have trouble palpating his distal pulses, he needs immediate intervention to prevent cardiovascular collapse. Should your patient start to experience cardiovascular collapse, expect to see the following signs and symptoms:

- a change in mental status
- hypotension
- cold, clammy extremities
- faint or absent peripheral pulses.

Be prepared to lower the head of the bed to increase cerebral perfusion. Notify the physician immediately of the change in your patient's condition. Assess your patient for signs of further deterioration, such as poor respiratory effort or loss of consciousness. Be prepared to begin I.V. fluid therapy with 0.9% sodium chloride solution, as prescribed. Have emergency equipment available for cardiopulmonary resuscitation, as necessary.

Nursing considerations

To effectively manage atrial tachycardia with aberrant conduction, you must be able to distinguish it from VT. The two disorders can cause similar signs and symptoms, including angina, dyspnea, and syncope. Although you can assume that a patient with a history of CAD and an MI is more likely to experience VT than atrial tachycardia, the ECG provides virtually the only objective means of distinguishing one condition from the other.

Aberrancy is the temporary abnormal intraventricular conduction of impulses originating above the ventricles. The significance of aberrant conduction is that it widens the QRS complex and simulates ventricular ectopic beats.

A preceding P′ wave and a pattern of right bundle-branch block in lead V_1 or a contour of rSR′ (a type of QRS complex with two R waves and an S wave but no Q wave) in leads V_1 and V_6 are the hallmarks of supraventricular tachycardia with aberrant conduction. The rhythm must be regarded as supraventricular tachycardia because the widened QRS complex could mean that the pacemaker site is below the atria. The duration of the QRS complex is usually less than 0.14 second in atrial tachycardia with aberrancy, and greater than 0.14 second in VT. Several findings are common in VT but not in atrial tachycardia with aberrancy, including an RS interval greater than 0.1 second and capture and fusion beats.

Fusion beats result from a combination of two different foci depolarizing the myocardium at once. The ventricle is partly depolarized from a sinus-conducted impulse and partly from a ventricular impulse. A fusion beat is a blending of a normal QRS complex with a premature ventricular-type complex. The atrial depolarization travels only to where the ventricle is simultaneously depolarizing. It's the ventricular impulse that captures the ventricle. Capture beats are produced when the atrial portion of the depolarization conducts through to the ventricle and produces a normal QRS complex. In this case, the atrial depolarization captures the ventricle.

Comparing QRS complexes of the rhythm in question with tracings of pretachycardic rates or sinus rhythm can help you differentiate between atrial tachycardia and VT. If the QRS complexes appear similar, the diagnosis of atrial tachycardia with aberrancy is almost certain. Finding P waves in the atrial lead point also confirms the arrhythmia as supraventricular in origin.

Vagal maneuvers such as carotid sinus massage may slow the ventricular rate in atrial tachycardia to reveal P waves. However, carotid sinus massage either has no effect on atrial tachycardia or immediately converts it to sinus rhythm. Upon cardiac auscultation of your patient with atrial tachycardia with aberrancy, an S_1 will not vary in intensity as it does in VT.

Patient teaching

Teach your patient about his arrhythmia and the tests, procedures, and treatments he'll undergo. Make sure he understands the doses, therapeutic effects, and adverse effects of his drugs. Show him how to check his pulse, and explain which abnormalities he should report to his physician, such as dizziness, chest pain, palpitations, and shortness of breath. If his arrhythmia is caused by an underlying condition, such as emphysema or heart failure, stress the importance of following his prescription and continuing treatment unless his physician tells him to stop.

If he takes drugs that can cause hypotension, caution him to sit and stand slowly, especially when getting out of bed in the morning. If he's receiving amiodarone, encourage him to obtain chest X-rays, pulmonary function tests, thyroid function tests, and eye examinations at prescribed times to detect signs of a toxic reaction. Warn him that his skin may turn slightly blue and that he must use sunscreen and wear protective clothing when outdoors.

Make sure your patient writes down the dates and times of his follow-up appointments. Reinforce the need to keep all follow-up visits and to have blood work done at regular intervals.

Encourage your patient to try to reduce anxiety and stress in his life. Teach him how to perform breathing exercises and instruct him to eat a low-fat, low-sodium diet. Also, urge him to stop smoking and to avoid caffeine and alcohol.

Wandering atrial pacemaker

A wandering atrial pacemaker occurs when many irritable sites compete for control of the heart rhythm. The multiple pacemaker sites originate in and shift around in the atria, SA node, and AV node. Only one site fires at a time. If the patient's ECG shows P waves with three or more different shapes from the same lead, he has a wandering atrial pacemaker.

Pathophysiology

Although a wandering atrial pacemaker may be a normal finding in young people, athletes, and even the elderly, it also is a common abnormal finding in patients with chronic heart failure. The most common cause of wandering atrial pacemaker is the inhibitory vagal effect of respiration on the SA node. Vagal stimulation prolongs SA node conduction, which causes sinus slowing, increases intranodal conduction time, and lengthens the effective and relative refractory periods of the SA node.

The large artery of the SA node has significant perfusion pressures that can affect the SA node. Distention of this artery slows the sinus rate, which may allow faster atrial foci to take over as pacemakers for the heart. Normally, the heart rate is under extrinsic control of the autonomic nervous system, predominantly the parasympathetic nervous system. Parasympathetic control keeps the heart rate stable at 60 to 100 bpm. However, cardiac decompensation and changes in vascular tone associated with chronic heart failure cause the sympathetic nervous system to dominate. Sympathetic dominance leads to faster heart rates and increased myocardial irritability.

Wandering atrial pacemaker also may be triggered by digoxin if I.V. administration is too fast. Digoxin should be administered in a 4:1 dilution of sterile water or 0.9% sodium chloride solution over a period of 5 minutes or longer. Rapid administration can cause vasoconstriction of the coro-

Characteristics of wandering atrial pacemaker

Rate: 60 to 100 beats per minute
Rhythm: slightly irregular
P wave: at least three different shapes
PR interval: < 0.2 second
QRS complex: < 0.12 second

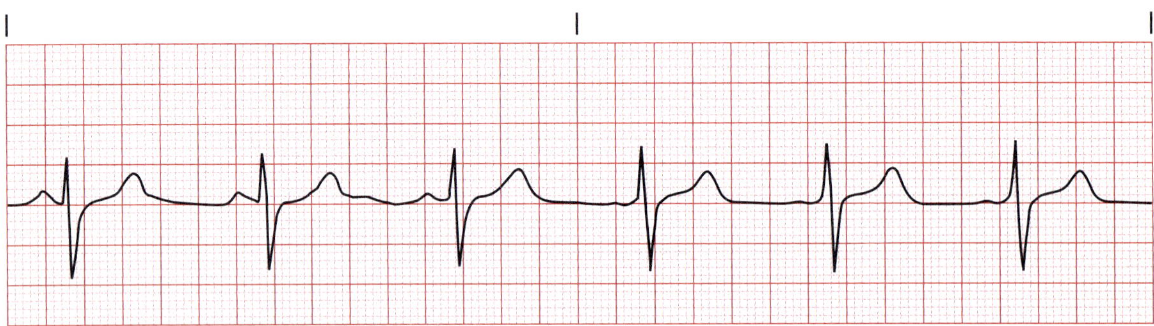

nary arteries, affecting blood flow to the SA node. When the heart rate slows excessively, both the signs and symptoms and the management are the same as those for symptomatic sinus bradycardia.

Any condition that increases parasympathetic tone, such as rheumatic heart disease, atrial hypertrophy, or an MI, can aggravate your patient's wandering atrial pacemaker rhythm, leading to symptomatic bradycardia or heart block. Other factors that can cause or aggravate wandering atrial pacemaker include the use of theophylline and other sympathetic stimulants, electrolyte imbalances, acid-base imbalances, and hypoxemia.

Signs and symptoms

A patient with a wandering atrial pacemaker typically has no signs or symptoms. Physical assessment findings include an irregular pulse and auscultatory variations in the intensity of S_1.

If your patient's heart rate deteriorates into an arrhythmia with a rate above 100 or below 60 bpm, his CO may drop. If this happens, he may experience some or all of the following signs and symptoms:

- hypotension
- shortness of breath
- chest pain
- pulmonary crackles
- decreased level of consciousness
- dizziness.

If you detect signs or symptoms of reduced CO, notify the patient's physician. Check the ECG for ST-segment and T-wave changes that may suggest ischemia. To determine whether your patient has wandering atrial pacemaker, examine the P waves carefully.

In wandering atrial pacemaker, the heart rate is 60 to 100 bpm. By definition, wandering atrial pacemaker involves at least three different pacemaker sites. Impulse generation shifts back and forth among the SA node, the AV node, and the atria. Depending exactly where those pacemaker sites are located, the heart rate can vary from faster than normal, when an impulse is discharged from the atria, to slower than normal, when the impulse originates in the AV node (see *Characteristics of wandering atrial pacemaker*).

Because the sites of impulse generation vary, wandering atrial pacemaker usually produces an irregular rhythm. However, in rare instances the rhythm may be regular.

Because at least three different pacemaker

sites are involved, the ECG shows P waves with at least three different shapes, sizes, and directions in the same lead, and an isoelectric baseline between the P waves. P waves originating in the SA node appear smooth, rounded, and rarely more than 2 mm in height. The normal P-wave duration is 0.1 second or less. P waves originating in the atria usually fire much faster than those coming from the SA node and therefore appear less rounded on the ECG. P waves originating in the AV node or the left atrium may be biphasic, peaked, or inverted. You should notice that the P waves gradually change in shape and size over the duration of several beats.

The length of the PR interval varies because of the different pacemaker sites in the atria. The length decreases from 0.2 to 0.12 second as the pacemaker site changes from the SA node to the AV node or the lower part of the atria. If conduction through and beyond the AV node is normal, the QRS complex is 0.1 second or less. If, however, your patient has a bundle-branch block or an AV conduction defect, the QRS complex is prolonged.

Treatment

If your patient with wandering atrial pacemaker is stable and doesn't have any significant signs or symptoms, he usually won't require treatment. Therefore, management should focus on correct identification of the arrhythmia and continuous assessment for changes that may indicate a deterioration in his condition.

Assess your patient's cardiovascular status to establish a baseline, including his vital signs, heart rate and rhythm, breath sounds, skin color and temperature, capillary refill, urine output, and level of consciousness. Ask your patient whether he's experiencing any chest pain. Always quantify pain by having your patient rate it on a scale of 0 to 10, with 0 being no pain and 10 being the worst pain possible. Also, assess complaints of dizziness and shortness of breath.

Preventive measures, such as correcting electrolyte abnormalities and treating heart failure, may be indicated for your patient with a wandering atrial pacemaker rhythm. Administer bronchodilators as prescribed. Be aware that theophylline and sympathomimetic bronchodilating drugs, such as isoproterenol, can switch your patient's rhythm to multifocal atrial tachycardia. If he develops an irregular pulse, obtain a 12-lead ECG and begin continuous monitoring, as prescribed.

Antiarrhythmic drugs

If multifocal atrial tachycardia develops and your patient becomes clinically unstable, he may require antiarrhythmic drugs appropriate for that disorder to control his rapid heart rate.

If your patient has a change in heart rate to greater than 100 bpm, anticipate insertion of an I.V. catheter to administer antiarrhythmic drugs such as metoprolol, verapamil, or amiodarone, as prescribed. Monitor the patient's ECG continuously while giving these I.V. drugs and monitor his cardiovascular status carefully, especially if he has heart failure.

When administering metoprolol, watch your patient for adverse effects, such as hypotension; the onset of new arrhythmias, including bradycardia and heart block; and respiratory difficulties, such as bronchospasm, dyspnea, and wheezing. Metoprolol can mask hypoglycemia, so monitor blood glucose levels closely if your patient is diabetic. Verapamil can cause hypotension, bradycardia, heart block, and heart failure. Monitor your patient receiving amiodarone for adverse effects such as hypotension, nausea, anorexia, weakness, insomnia, corneal deposits, bluish skin color, photosensitivity, toxic pulmonary reaction, and thyroid dysfunction.

Complications

Your patient with wandering atrial pacemaker won't have acute problems associated with the arrhythmia itself. However, because the condition can deteriorate and your patient can become hemodynamically unstable, monitor his cardiovascular status frequently and report signs and symptoms of decompensation to the physician.

Emphysema and heart failure are chronic disorders that tend to worsen with time. If your patient has one of these disorders, expect him to have continual or recurrent episodes of wandering atrial pacemaker. Although the arrhythmia causes no chronic debilitating effects, it does create a chronic increased risk of cardiac conduction defects.

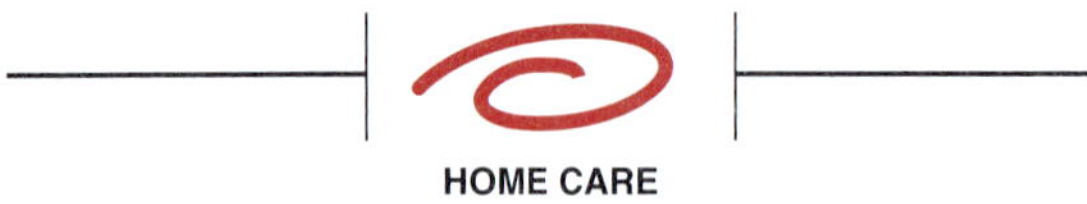

HOME CARE

Teaching your patient to take his pulse

To help your patient quickly detect changes in his heart rate or rhythm, teach him to check his own pulse. Start by explaining what a pulse is and why he should monitor it at home.

Show him how to find his radial pulse. Tell him to place his index and middle fingers on the bony prominence of the thumb side of his wrist. Then have him slide his fingers inward toward the middle of his wrist until he can feel the beating, as shown.

Demonstrate how to use the pads of the first and second fingers to feel the beats and tell the patient to avoid using his thumb. Explain that he should press just hard enough to feel the pulse; pressing too hard can stop the pulse and pressing too lightly can prevent him from feeling it.

When you know he can feel his pulse, explain what he's feeling and tell him that the beats should form a regular pattern. As appropriate for the patient's arrhythmia, explain what he should do if he feels an irregular pattern. Tell him to count his pulse for 1 full minute and to report to his physician a change of 10 beats per minute or more.

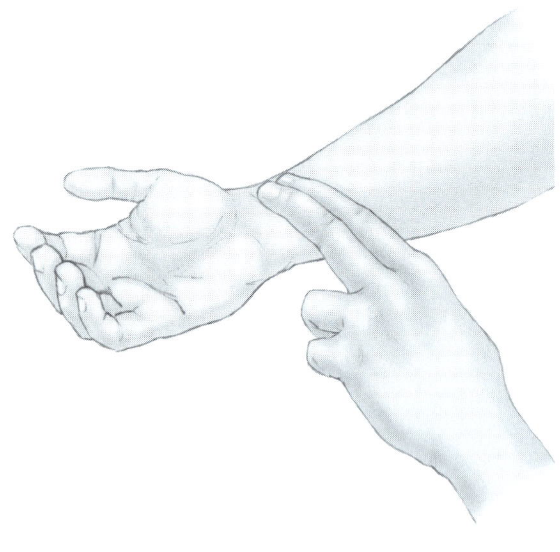

Nursing considerations

Assist in treating the underlying condition that may be causing your patient's arrhythmia. If your patient's arrhythmia results from heart failure, anticipate administering oxygen, an inotropic drug, a vasodilator, and a diuretic. Follow fluid restrictions and place your patient on a low-sodium diet, if indicated. Monitor him for signs and symptoms of a toxic reaction to a digitalis glycoside, such as anorexia, nausea, vomiting, diarrhea, and blurred or yellow vision. If you suspect that your patient has wandering atrial pacemaker as a result of digoxin administration, withhold the drug while you notify the physician. Obtain orders for an immediate determination of the blood digoxin level to confirm your assessment findings.

A toxic reaction to digoxin is more likely in a patient who's also hypokalemic. Obtain blood potassium levels and report abnormal values immediately. Anticipate orders for electrolyte replacement because electrolyte imbalances can cause wandering atrial pacemaker. Measure blood drug levels to make sure antiarrhythmic drugs are within their therapeutic ranges and haven't reached toxic levels. Prepare to increase or decrease antiarrhythmic drug doses based on these results.

Patient teaching

Explain to your patient and his family the purpose of all monitoring equipment, procedures, and treatment. Teach your patient about his arrhythmia. Make sure he understands that he needs no treatment unless he has bothersome signs or symptoms or his heart rate goes above 100 bpm or below 60 bpm.

Show your patient how to check his radial pulse. Explain that he should report any change in rhythm or significant change in rate to his physician (see *Teaching your patient to take his pulse*). Tell your patient to report dizziness, chest pain, and shortness of breath as well.

Educate your patient about the drugs he'll be taking at home, including their names, dosages, and adverse effects. If the arrhythmia stems from an underlying condition, such as heart failure, make sure your patient understands the importance of taking his drugs and following treatment guidelines faithfully. Make sure he knows the danger of stopping any of his drugs without consulting his physician.

If your patient takes drugs known to cause hypotension, caution him to sit up and stand up slowly, especially when first getting out of bed in the morning. If he's receiving amiodarone, advise him that he requires follow-up chest X-rays, pulmonary function tests, thyroid function tests, and eye examinations to detect signs and symptoms of a toxic reaction. Warn him that his skin may take on a bluish color and that he needs to use sunscreen and protective clothing when outdoors.

Make sure your patient knows the date and time of his follow-up appointments. Reinforce the importance of keeping all follow-up visits and having blood work done at regular intervals.

Assess your patient's level of anxiety and his fears about having an arrhythmia. Administer sedatives, as prescribed, to help reduce his anxiety. Encourage your patient with a history of cardiopulmonary disease to perform breathing exercises and to eat a low-fat, low-sodium diet. Also, urge him to stop smoking and to avoid the use of caffeine and alcohol.

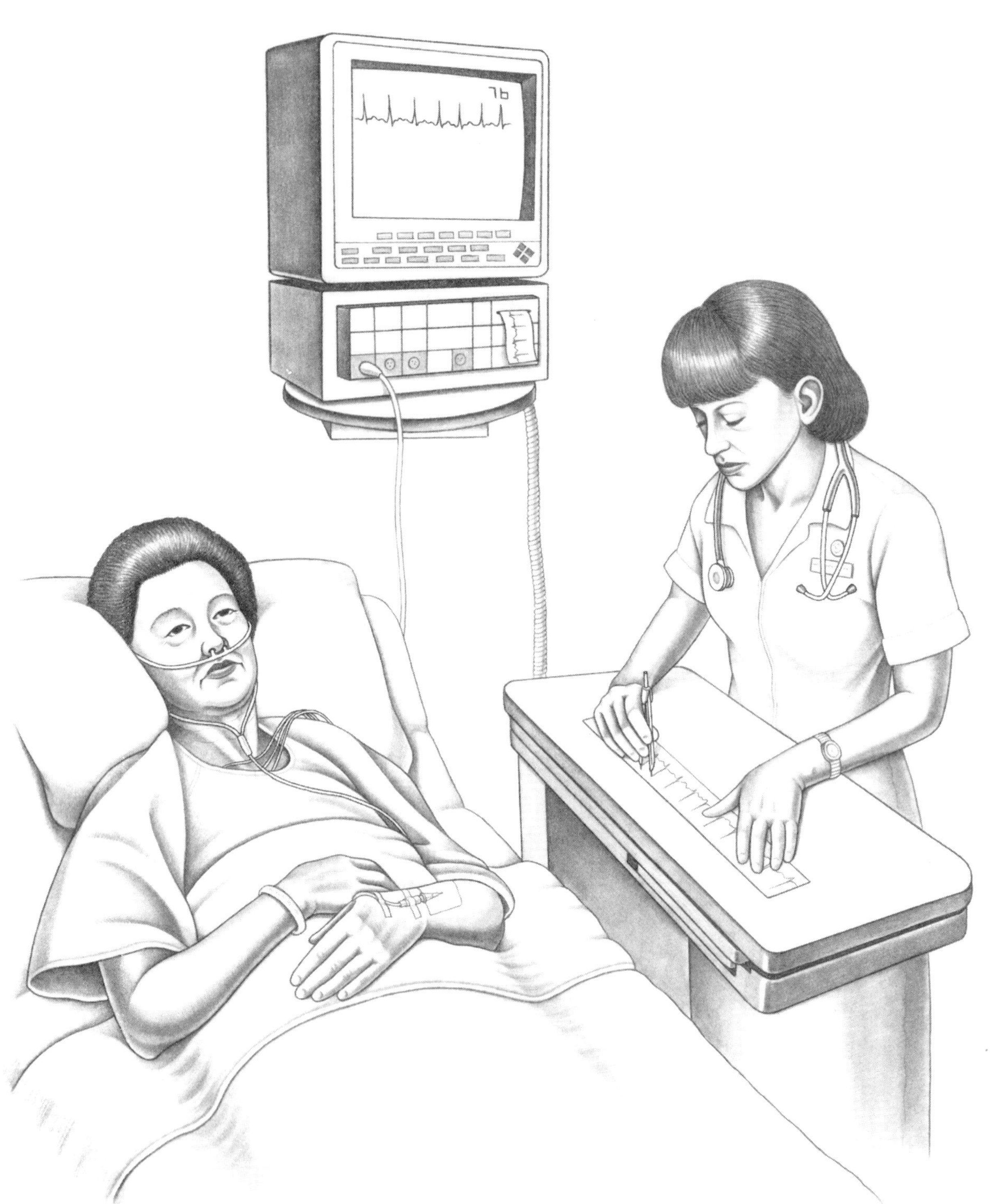
76

5

Junctional Arrhythmias

Normally, electrical impulses generated in the sinoatrial (SA) node travel through the internodal pathways, stimulating atrial contractions. Then, the impulses stimulate the junctional area, which contains the atrioventricular (AV) node and the bundle of His, triggering ventricular contractions.

But if the junctional area spontaneously generates its own electrical impulses without stimulation from the SA node, the result can be one of several junctional arrhythmias—arrhythmias that can cause life-threatening complications for your patient.

In this chapter, you'll find a review of the four most common junctional arrhythmias: premature junctional contractions, junctional escape rhythm, accelerated junctional rhythm, and paroxysmal junctional tachycardia.

Premature junctional contractions

A premature junctional contraction is an ectopic beat generated by the junctional area of the heart. This beat occurs earlier in the cardiac cycle than a normal sinus beat.

In this arrhythmia, the AV junction generates a spontaneous impulse from one of several sites: specialized tissue of the lower atrium, tissue surrounding the AV node, the AV node itself, or the bundle of His (see *Where junctional arrhythmias originate,* page 80). The impulse then travels into the atria and ventricles, causing atrial and ventricular contractions. These contractions create an extra beat before the SA node generates the normal beat.

Pathophysiology

Although premature junctional contractions are rare in healthy people, they may occur as a normal reaction to stress. Other conditions that contribute to the formation of premature junctional contractions include a toxic reaction to a drug, diet habits, vagal stimulation, and certain diseases.

In many cases, premature junctional contractions are an early sign of a toxic reaction to a digitalis glycoside, usually digoxin. Digoxin delays AV conduction and enhances AV junction automaticity, resulting in irritability of the junctional tissue. Other drugs—such as beta-blockers, calcium channel blockers, procainamide, and quinidine—also affect AV conduction and AV automaticity.

Caffeine, alcohol, nicotine, and amphetamines can cause premature junctional contractions. And vagal maneuvers—such as straining during a bowel movement, vomiting, or coughing—may slow

Where junctional arrhythmias originate

If the atrioventricular junctional area of the heart generates spontaneous impulses, a junctional arrhythmia may result. Typically, the arrhythmia originates in an irritable focus at one of the four junctional sites shown.

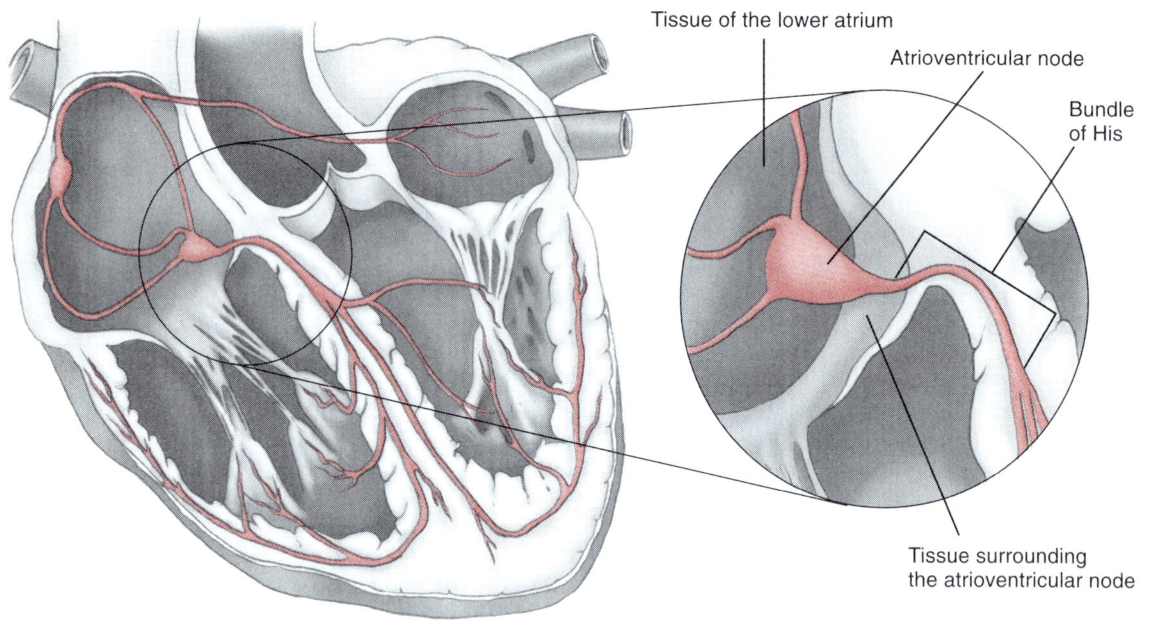

the heart rate, thus stimulating the AV junction to generate spontaneous impulses.

Cardiovascular disorders such as coronary artery disease, heart failure, pericarditis, and valvular heart disease can cause premature junctional contractions. Also, myocardial ischemia and myocardial infarction (MI) may damage tissue in the SA node or conduction pathways, causing the AV node to generate extra impulses.

Premature junctional contractions can result from asthma, emphysema, and chronic respiratory difficulty. In these respiratory disorders, poor gas exchange can lead to irritation of AV junctional tissue.

Disorders such as hyperthyroidism and electrolyte imbalances also can cause premature junctional contractions by irritating junctional tissues.

Signs and symptoms

Usually, a patient with intermittent premature junctional contractions won't have any signs or symptoms. This arrhythmia is generally benign and causes signs and symptoms only when it occurs often enough to affect cardiac output (CO).

Frequent premature junctional contractions can reduce your patient's CO. The arrhythmia causes the atria to relax at abnormal times during the cardiac cycle, causing asynchrony with the ventricles. Thus, the atria pump less blood into the ventricles, and the ventricles, in turn, pump less blood to the coronary arteries and major organs. This decreased CO may cause your patient to experience chest pain, hypotension, weakness, dizziness, syncope, decreased urine output, and cool, clammy skin.

Characteristics of premature junctional contractions

Rate: depends on underlying rhythm
Rhythm: usually regular
P wave: peaked or inverted; before, after, or buried in QRS complex
PR interval: < 0.12 second
QRS complex: < 0.12 second

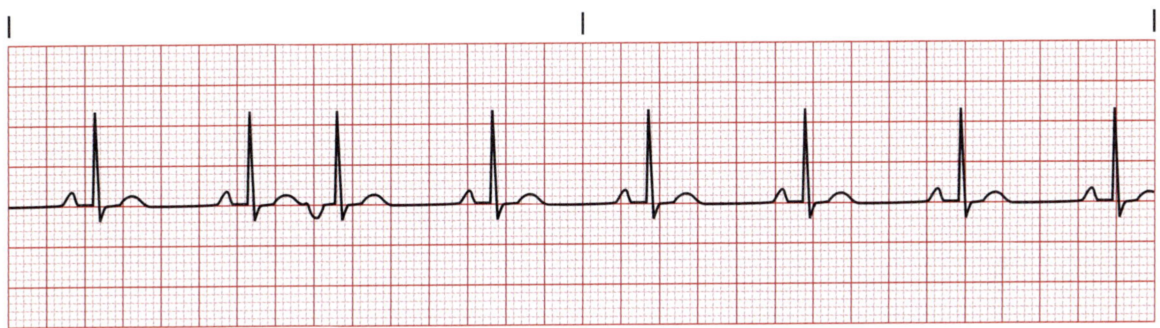

On the electrocardiogram (ECG) of your patient with premature junctional contractions, the rate will depend on the underlying rhythm. If the arrhythmia occurs intermittently, her rhythm may be normal or nearly normal. Thus, her rate will also be normal, from 60 to 100 beats per minute (bpm). If the arrhythmia occurs frequently, her rhythm will be irregular. And her rate will change (see *Characteristics of premature junctional contractions*).

If your patient's rhythm is irregular, her ECG will show premature junctional beats with noncompensatory pauses. These premature beats may appear in the following patterns:

- bigeminal (every other cardiac cycle)
- trigeminal (every third cardiac cycle)
- quadrigeminal (every fourth cardiac cycle)
- coupled (in pairs).

You may observe P waves on your patient's ECG. If P waves are present, their shape will be abnormal, and their deflection may be peaked or inverted. On a 12-lead ECG, you'll see inverted P waves in leads II, III, and aV_F as a result of retrograde conduction from the AV junctional site up through the atria.

Of course, premature junctional contractions also cause antegrade conduction from the AV junctional site down through the ventricles. Because the arrhythmia causes both retrograde and antegrade conduction, the atria may contract before the ventricles, simultaneously with the ventricles, or after the ventricles.

If the atria contract before the ventricles, the P wave will appear before the QRS complex. If the atria and ventricles contract simultaneously, the P wave will be buried within the QRS complex. If the atria contract after the ventricles, the P wave will follow the QRS complex and may distort the ST segment or the T wave.

With premature junctional contractions, the time during the cardiac cycle when the AV junctional site generates an impulse determines the sequence of atrial and ventricular contractions. This timing may be further influenced by the speed at which the impulse travels along the conduction pathways. Structural defects within the conduction system may slow an impulse before it reaches the atria or ventricles. Electrolyte imbalances may also affect the speed at which the impulse travels.

When measurable P waves accompany premature junctional contractions, the PR interval is less than 0.12 second. This shortened PR interval is caused by the reduction in time required for a normal impulse to travel from the SA node to the AV node.

Because premature junctional contractions cause extra beats in the cardiac cycle, your patient's ECG may have short and long R-R intervals. The R-R interval between a normal sinus beat and a premature junctional contraction will be shorter than the R-R interval between the premature junctional contraction and the next sinus beat. This longer interval between the premature junctional contraction and the sinus beat results from a noncompensatory pause—the time required for the SA node to reset before the next atrial contraction—that occurs after the premature beat.

If the ventricular conduction pathway is intact, the QRS complex of a premature junctional contraction looks the same as the normal sinus beat because the junctional impulse follows the normal pathway for ventricular depolarization. The QRS complex of the arrhythmia will appear before the normal sinus beat on your patient's ECG.

If the impulse is slowed along the ventricular pathway, you may see an abnormal QRS complex where atrial and ventricular depolarization occur almost simultaneously. In such cases, the P wave will be buried in the QRS complex, producing a distorted Q wave.

Treatment

Usually, a patient with intermittent premature junctional contractions will be asymptomatic, and she won't require treatment for the arrhythmia. However, if her arrhythmia occurs frequently, she may begin to show the signs and symptoms of reduced CO. The physician may prescribe atropine to increase her heart rate and CO. He may also insert a temporary pacemaker.

Atropine

Usually, a physician prescribes atropine to increase CO in a patient with symptomatic premature junctional contractions. By blocking the action of acetylcholine in the SA node, atropine allows the patient's normal sinus rhythm to override the junctional pacemaker that's causing the arrhythmia.

Typically, if your patient's heart rate is less than 60 bpm and she becomes symptomatic, you'll give I.V. atropine. The usual dose is a 0.5-mg to 1-mg I.V. push, repeated every 5 minutes to a total of 2 mg or until symptoms are relieved.

When giving atropine, monitor your patient for tachycardia. Other adverse effects of the drug include urine retention, dry mucous membranes and skin, and decreased bronchial secretions. And remember that doses of less than 0.5 mg can cause a paradoxical bradycardia.

Because atropine increases the heart rate, it also may intensify myocardial oxygen demand. During treatment, monitor your patient's heart rate, rhythm, vital signs, and urine output.

Atropine is contraindicated in patients with glaucoma because the drug dilates the pupils of the eye and can cause blurred vision and severe ocular pain. Use atropine with caution in very young and elderly patients because they're highly sensitive to the drug's adverse effects.

Pacemaker

If drug therapy doesn't help your patient maintain an adequate heart rate, a physician may insert a temporary cardiac pacemaker. The pacemaker will increase your patient's heart rate and allow the SA node to reestablish control of her heart's rhythm.

Complications

Although complications from premature junctional contractions are rare, frequent premature contractions may precede more dangerous arrhythmias such as junctional escape rhythm, paroxysmal junctional tachycardia, and AV block. If acute complications occur, they usually result from decreased CO, which is treated with atropine or a temporary pacemaker.

Atropine may also be used to treat the most common chronic problem of premature junctional contractions—a patient's anxiety from having a cardiac arrhythmia. Anxiety can cause the release of acetylcholine, which increases the frequency of premature contractions. But atropine helps the SA node regain control of the cardiac rhythm.

Nursing considerations

Evaluate your patient's drug regimen to determine whether a drug is causing her arrhythmia. A beta-blocker, a calcium channel blocker, quinidine, procainamide, or digoxin may cause premature junctional contractions. If your patient is taking one of these drugs, her physician may decide to withhold it or adjust the dosage to correct the arrhythmia.

If your patient is experiencing frequent ectopic beats, assess her for the signs and symptoms of decreased CO. Check her level of consciousness, skin color, skin temperature, heart rate, blood pressure, and urine output. Also, ask if she's experiencing chest pain or shortness of breath.

Auscultate her lungs for abnormal sounds, such as crackles, which may indicate cardiac compromise. And monitor her laboratory test results, including her electrolyte, drug, and arterial blood gas levels.

Patient teaching

Teach your patient about the possible causes of her arrhythmia. If appropriate, explain that alcohol, caffeine, nicotine, and amphetamines affect cardiac rhythm and may contribute to her condition. Tell her that she may need to make lifestyle changes such as reducing her alcohol intake, improving her diet, and quitting smoking. To encourage her compliance with these lifestyle changes, include her family or caregivers in your teaching.

Provide your patient with information about relaxation techniques. Explain that anxiety about her condition may contribute to it. Also, encourage her to ask questions and allow time for her to express her fears.

Teach your patient how to check her pulse at home. Teach her the signs and symptoms of decreased CO and tell her to contact her physician if she experiences them.

Junctional escape rhythm

Junctional escape rhythm, a normal protective mechanism of the cardiac conduction system, occurs when an ectopic focus in the AV junctional tissue paces the heart. Normally, the firing of the SA node overrides AV junctional impulses. But, if the SA node doesn't produce a heart rate of at least 60 bpm, the junctional area of the heart provides a backup pacemaker, which can maintain a heart rate of 40 to 60 bpm.

Junctional escape rhythm also may develop if impulses generated in the SA node don't reach the AV node. The AV junctional tissue, acting as if the SA node has failed, may begin to automatically generate its own impulses to pace the heart.

Pathophysiology

As described, junctional escape rhythm occurs when impulses from the SA node fail to reach the AV node within a normal time frame. This failure may occur because of damage to the SA node, which prevents it from pacing the heart, or because of damage or alterations to the cardiac conduction system, which may slow or block impulses from the SA node.

Ischemia and tissue trauma can damage the SA node directly, preventing it from generating impulses. And an MI can damage the SA node indirectly by reducing blood flow through the right coronary artery, which supplies blood to the SA node.

Tricuspid and mitral valve diseases can damage the SA node. Also, if your patient has undergone cardiac surgery, she's at risk for developing junctional escape rhythm because of postoperative edema around the SA node. However, as the edema subsides, normal sinus rhythm usually returns.

Junctional escape rhythm may occur with arrhythmias such as sinus bradycardia, sick sinus syndrome, premature atrial contractions, and second-degree AV block. In sinus bradycardia, the long pauses between sinus beats allow time for a junctional escape beat to fire. The compensatory pause following a premature atrial contraction enhances junctional automaticity. And the dropped beat of second-degree AV block may leave time for a junctional impulse to fire.

Vagal stimulation may cause junctional escape rhythm if the heart slows enough to allow a junctional ectopic focus to take over as pacemaker. You should caution your patient about vagal maneuvers that may reduce her heart rate, such as coughing, vomiting, or straining during a bowel movement.

A toxic reaction to a drug, particularly digoxin, also is a common cause of junctional escape rhythm. Digoxin promotes irritability of the AV junctional pacemaker tissue and reduces impulse conduction from the SA node.

Other drugs that reduce impulse conduction and alter cardiac action potentials may cause the arrhythmia. These drugs include beta-blockers, calcium channel blockers, procainamide, and quinidine.

Junctional escape rhythm also may be intentionally induced as an alternative to more dangerous arrhythmias such as rapid atrial fibrillation. In a procedure called nodal ablation, a physician uses a radiofrequency catheter to block SA

Characteristics of junctional escape rhythm

Rate: 40 to 60 beats per minute
Rhythm: regular
P wave: if visible, is usually inverted; before, after, or buried in QRS complex
PR interval: < 0.12 second
QRS complex: < 0.12 second

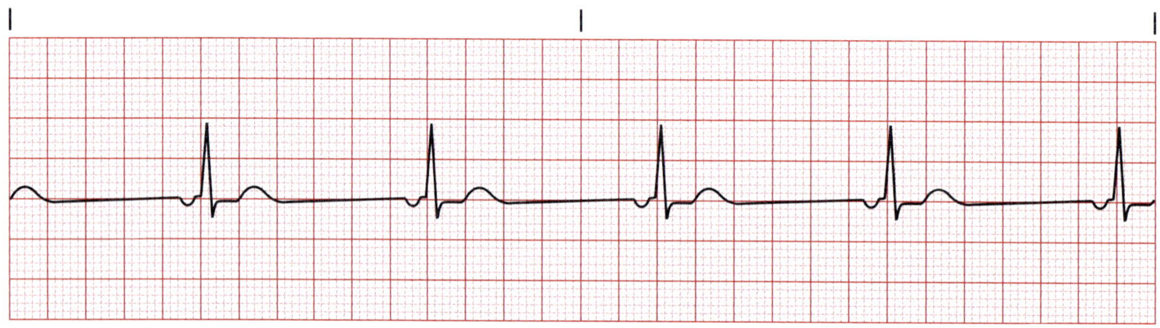

node impulses before they reach the AV node, causing the patient's AV junctional tissue to take over as the heart's pacemaker.

Signs and symptoms

Despite the slow heart rate produced by junctional escape rhythm, most patients tolerate the arrhythmia well. However, if your patient has other health problems, the arrhythmia may cause her to experience the signs and symptoms of reduced CO, such as hypotension, chest pain, dyspnea, syncope, confusion, weakness, decreased urine output, and cool, clammy skin.

On a patient's ECG, the rate of a junctional escape rhythm inherently is 40 to 60 bpm. Normally, this rate prevents the AV junctional pacemaker from overcoming the SA node when the SA node impulses are merely delayed from reaching the AV node. However, if a damaged SA node isn't generating impulses, the AV junctional pacemaker may take over completely, and the heart rate may be as slow as 40 bpm (see *Characteristics of junctional escape rhythm*).

With junctional escape rhythm, the patient's rhythm usually is regular. The arrhythmia becomes recognizable on the ECG when six or more escape beats occur in succession.

P waves may or may not be visible, depending on when the ectopic impulse stimulates atrial contraction. Because the AV impulses travel both forward and backward, atrial contractions may occur before, during, or after ventricular contractions.

The retrograde conduction that causes atrial contractions changes the appearance of the P wave on the ECG, giving it an abnormal shape and an inverted deflection. On a 12-lead ECG, inverted P waves appear in leads II, III, and aV_F. You'll see one P wave for each QRS complex, although a P wave hidden in a QRS complex may be difficult to identify.

If the atrial contractions occur before the ventricular contractions, the P wave will appear before the QRS complex. If the atria and ventricles contract simultaneously, the P wave will fall within the QRS complex. If the ventricles contract before the atria, the P wave will follow the QRS complex and may distort the ST segment or the T wave.

With junctional escape rhythm, the PR interval is short (less than 0.12 second) or absent. Usually, the R-R interval is regular.

If your patient's ventricular conduction pathway is intact, her QRS complex will be normal. But if the ventricular conduction pathway is interrupted or if simultaneous atrial and ventricular contractions bury the P waves in the QRS complex, the QRS complex will appear abnormal on your patient's ECG.

Treatment

Many patients tolerate junctional escape rhythm without experiencing any of the signs or symptoms of the arrhythmia, and such patients don't require treatment for the condition. However, if the arrhythmia reduces your patient's CO, she'll require treatment.

Usually, if junctional escape rhythm reduces a patient's CO, a physician will prescribe drug therapy with atropine or isoproterenol. If drug therapy doesn't increase the patient's CO, the physician may insert a pacemaker.

Drug therapy and pacemaker insertion will help increase your patient's CO by increasing or regulating her heart rate. However, treatment for junctional escape rhythm should never suppress the AV junctional rhythm, particularly if the AV junction is pacing the heart without the aid of the SA node. Suppressing the AV junctional rhythm could cause ventricular asystole, a potentially fatal condition.

Atropine

A physician may prescribe atropine to stimulate SA node activity, increase AV conduction, and suppress vagal activity, thus increasing your patient's heart rate and CO.

Administer atropine as prescribed. The usual dose is 0.5 mg to 1 mg by I.V. push. This dose can be repeated every 5 minutes up to a total of 2 mg to achieve a heart rate of 60 to 100 bpm or to relieve your patient's signs and symptoms.

When giving atropine, monitor your patient for tachycardia. Other adverse effects of the drug include urine retention, dry mucous membranes and skin, and decreased bronchial secretions.

Because atropine increases the heart rate, the drug may also increase myocardial oxygen demand. Throughout treatment, monitor your patient's heart rate, rhythm, vital signs, and urine output.

Isoproterenol

If atropine doesn't increase your patient's heart rate and she continues to show the signs and symptoms of reduced CO, the physician may prescribe isoproterenol. By stimulating $beta_1$ and $beta_2$ receptors, isoproterenol increases the heart's rate and contractility. The drug also enhances the pacemaker function of the SA node and improves AV conduction.

When giving I.V. isoproterenol, monitor your patient closely for adverse effects. Your patient's heart rate may increase significantly in response to the decreased peripheral vascular resistance caused by isoproterenol. Be alert for the signs and symptoms of myocardial ischemia. Premature ectopic beats commonly occur in patients receiving isoproterenol. An increased heart rate increases oxygen demand, but because isoproterenol reduces diastolic blood pressure and coronary artery perfusion, oxygen supply decreases.

Other adverse effects include headache, nausea, flushed skin, diaphoresis, angina, dizziness, and weakness.

Pacemaker

If drug therapy fails to increase your patient's CO, the physician may insert a pacemaker, which will increase the heart rate by overriding the junctional arrhythmia. Usually, the pacemaker insertion is temporary. However, if the patient's junctional escape rhythm causes hemodynamic instability and isn't expected to improve, she may need a surgically implanted permanent pacemaker.

Depending on your patient's condition, the physician may use either a fixed-rate pacemaker or a demand pacemaker. A fixed-rate pacemaker delivers an electrical impulse at a preset rate that's independent of the patient's cardiac activity. A demand pacemaker delivers an electrical impulse only when the patient needs it, so the device doesn't compete with the patient's natural cardiac rhythm.

Complications

As you know, most patients tolerate junctional escape rhythm well and don't suffer complications of the arrhythmia. However, if complications do occur, they're usually related to decreased CO, which may aggravate other underlying health problems such as myocardial ischemia and peripheral vascular disease. A decrease in CO may result from frequent interruptions in the regular heart rhythm caused by the premature junctional contractions (see *At risk for myocardial ischemia,* page 86).

If junctional escape rhythm causes asynchrony between your patient's atrial and ventricular contractions, she also may develop thromboembo-

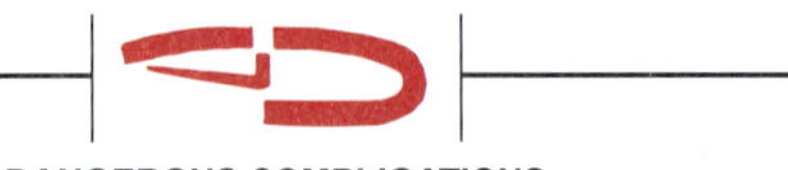

DANGEROUS COMPLICATIONS

At risk for myocardial ischemia

Junctional escape rhythms are inherently less efficient than rhythms originating in the sinoatrial node. And the slower heart rate and reduced cardiac output (CO) that the arrhythmia causes can put your patient at risk for myocardial ischemia.

If your patient has reduced CO, her myocardium receives less blood and, of course, less oxygen and nutrients. As myocardial metabolism becomes anaerobic, the boundaries between myocardial cells begin to deteriorate. Eventually, ischemia may lead to an infarction, in which some myocardial cells become functionally and electrically silent.

Spotting trouble

If your patient's junctional escape rhythm causes myocardial ischemia, she may experience chest pain, palpitations, shortness of breath, diaphoresis, nausea, and weakness. If she complains of chest pain, obtain an electrocardiogram (ECG). If she has myocardial ischemia, the ECG will show changes to the ST segment, such as an elevation or a slight depression from the baseline.

lism. Asynchrony may cause blood to pool within the atria, providing a setting for thrombus formation. Atrial and ventricular contractions then may move the clot into her peripheral circulation, causing a cerebrovascular accident (CVA), pulmonary embolism, and other embolic disorders.

Nursing considerations

Evaluate your patient's drug regimen to assess whether it's causing her arrhythmia. Antiarrhythmic drugs may induce junctional escape rhythm. If your patient develops this arrhythmia while taking a beta-blocker, a calcium channel blocker, quinidine, procainamide, or digoxin, report this to her physician. The physician may withhold the drug or adjust its dosage to control the arrhythmia.

Monitor your patient for the signs and symptoms of reduced CO. Also, monitor her for the signs and symptoms of myocardial ischemia. In particular, watch for ST-segment changes on her ECG, which may indicate myocardial ischemia.

If your patient's junctional escape rhythm results from vagal stimulation, teach her how to avoid stimulating the vagal response. Provide information on relaxation techniques, including music therapy and guided imagery, and lifestyle changes, such as diet modifications and exercise, that may help control her cardiac status.

Accelerated junctional rhythm

In accelerated junctional rhythm, also called accelerated junctional tachycardia, an irritable focus in the AV junction speeds up to override the SA node for control of the heart. Ectopic beats may be generated by junctional tissues within the lower part of the right atrium, surrounding the AV junction, in the AV node, and within the bundle of His.

Normally, the inherent rate of the AV node is 40 to 60 bpm. But with accelerated junctional rhythm, the AV junctional pacemaker can produce a heart rate of 60 to 100 bpm, matching the SA node's pace. And when excited, the AV pacemaker may even conduct impulses as rapidly as 150 bpm. However, even at this pace, the rate of atrial and ventricular contractions remains equal.

Pathophysiology

Like other junctional arrhythmias, accelerated junctional rhythm usually occurs because the AV node isn't receiving impulses from the SA node. However, accelerated junctional rhythm also involves an irritable focus in the AV junctional tissue, which results in a faster heart rate than the SA node normally produces.

Digoxin, a digitalis glycoside, commonly causes accelerated junctional rhythm. Used to treat certain atrial arrhythmias and heart failure, digoxin slows the atrial conduction of SA node impulses by inhibiting the action of the sodium-potassium pump. Digoxin also prolongs the refractory period in the AV node and surrounding tissue, leading to increased automaticity.

Characteristics of accelerated junctional rhythm

Rate: 60 to 100 beats per minute
Rhythm: regular
P wave: if visible, is usually inverted; before, after, or buried in QRS complex
PR interval: < 0.12 second
QRS complex: < 0.12 second

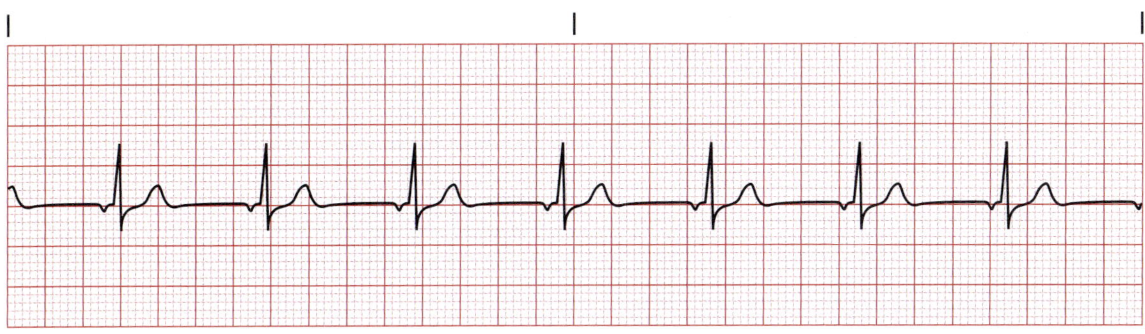

Accelerated junctional rhythm also may result from the toxic effects of other antiarrhythmic drugs, such as beta-blockers, calcium channel blockers, quinidine, and procainamide. That's because these drugs slow conduction through the atria, giving junctional ectopic foci time to take over pacemaker control of the heart.

Accelerated junctional rhythm may result from any form of heart disease or cardiac trauma that decreases blood flow to the SA node and AV junction. Decreased blood flow can be caused by the trauma of open-heart surgery. It also commonly results from the following conditions:

- an inferior-wall MI
- myocarditis
- heart failure
- valvular heart disease
- rheumatic fever.

Signs and symptoms

Your patient with accelerated junctional rhythm may experience no signs or symptoms, mild discomfort, or severe signs and symptoms, depending on the cause of her arrhythmia and her overall health.

Increased physical activity and stress may affect your patient's ability to tolerate the arrhythmia. As with other junctional arrhythmias, accelerated junctional rhythm may cause your patient to experience the signs and symptoms of myocardial ischemia and decreased CO, such as hypotension, syncope, dizziness, confusion, weakness, decreased urine output, and cool, clammy skin.

With accelerated junctional rhythm, your patient's ECG usually shows a normal rhythm and a heart rate of 60 to 100 bpm (see *Characteristics of accelerated junctional rhythm*).

Your patient's P waves may not be visible. But if they are, they may be upright or inverted. They may appear before the QRS complex, be buried within it, or come after it.

Typically, one P wave appears for each QRS complex. If the P wave precedes the QRS complex, the PR interval usually is shorter than normal—that is, less than 0.12 second.

Your patient with accelerated junctional rhythm usually will have normal R-R intervals and QRS complexes because the electrical impulses for ventricular contractions follow the regular route along the ventricular conduction pathways. However, if her ventricular conduction pathways

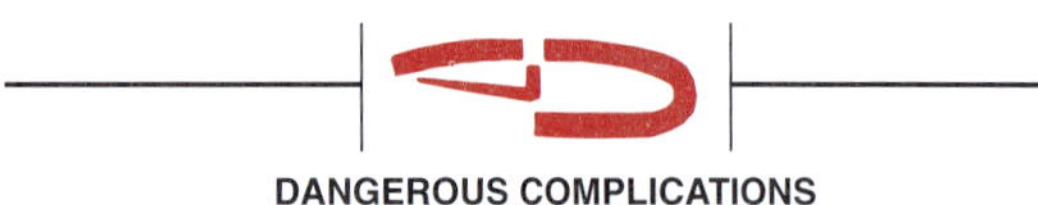

DANGEROUS COMPLICATIONS

Hypokalemia: Causes and effects

Potassium, an intracellular cation appearing mainly in muscle tissue, is essential for the impulse conduction that causes myocardial contractions. Normally, your patient's blood potassium level should be 3.5 to 5 mEq/L.

Common causes of hypokalemia include vomiting and diarrhea. Hypokalemia also may result from the following:

- digoxin immune FAB
- potassium-wasting diuretics
- potassium-free fluid infusions
- corticosteroids
- increased aldosterone secretion
- decreased potassium intake.

Mild hypokalemia may cause your patient to experience slow and irregular heart rhythms, muscle cramps, paresthesia, weakness, nausea, and confusion. Severe hypokalemia can induce cardiac arrest.

Because hypokalemia can also cause ventricular arrhythmias, be sure to monitor your patient's electrocardiogram for a depressed, prolonged ST segment, a depressed or inverted T wave, and a U wave.

are damaged, her QRS complex may appear abnormal. A P wave buried within the QRS complex also may cause the QRS complex to appear abnormal.

Treatment

Typically, a physician treats accelerated junctional rhythm by treating the arrhythmia's underlying cause. For example, if your patient's arrhythmia results from a toxic reaction to digoxin, the physician may withhold the drug until the patient achieves a normal sinus rhythm. Then, the physician may reinstitute the drug at a lower dose or longer dosage interval to maintain your patient's normal sinus rhythm.

If digoxin causes life-threatening signs and symptoms, the physician may prescribe digoxin immune FAB to quickly decrease your patient's blood digoxin level. Typically, you'll administer digoxin immune FAB as an 800-mg I.V. push.

If your patient was receiving digoxin for heart failure or atrial fibrillation, monitor her closely for a recurrence of these conditions when administering digoxin immune FAB. The drug may also reduce your patient's blood potassium level. So when giving digoxin immune FAB, also monitor your patient for the signs and symptoms of hypokalemia, which could lead to more serious arrhythmias and cardiac arrest (see *Hypokalemia: Causes and effects*). Be prepared to administer potassium supplements, as prescribed.

If your patient is taking a beta-blocker, a calcium channel blocker, quinidine, or procainamide, notify her physician. These drugs can accelerate a junctional escape rhythm. The physician may decide to withhold the drug until your patient achieves a normal sinus rhythm.

Complications

Most patients with accelerated junctional rhythm tolerate the arrhythmia well. However, some patients may experience the signs and symptoms of decreased CO. With this arrhythmia, decreased CO results from absence of the atrial kick.

Normally, atrial kick occurs when the atria contract, pumping blood into the ventricles. Atrial kick accounts for about 25% of the total stroke volume—the blood that's ejected from the heart with each beat.

However, when atrial contractions are late, the ventricles may not simultaneously relax, and atrial kick doesn't occur. Thus, stroke volume and CO may be reduced, resulting in severely decreased blood flow to the coronary arteries and organs.

Nursing considerations

Monitor your patient with accelerated junctional rhythm for the toxic effects of digoxin, including abdominal pain, nausea, vomiting, anorexia, weakness, headache, drowsiness, confusion, and visual disturbances. If your patient experiences these signs or symptoms, report them to her physician.

Administer digoxin immune FAB, as prescribed. And monitor your patient for the recurrence of heart failure and atrial fibrillation, for which she may have been receiving digoxin. Also, monitor her blood potassium level and be alert for the signs and symptoms of hypokalemia.

After your patient achieves a normal sinus rhythm, discuss the causes of the arrhythmia with her. As appropriate, teach her the signs and symptoms of a toxic reaction to digoxin and of decreased CO. Also, instruct her to take her pulse daily to monitor herself for changes in rate or rhythm. If she experiences any of these signs or symptoms, tell her to report them to her physician immediately.

Paroxysmal junctional tachycardia

Paroxysmal junctional tachycardia, like accelerated junctional rhythm, originates in an irritable AV junctional focus that overtakes the SA node for pacing the heart. However, with paroxysmal tachycardia, the AV focus is repeatedly reexcited, resulting in a more rapid heart rate than that produced by accelerated junctional rhythm.

Paroxysmal junctional tachycardia also has a rapid onset. When it begins, the arrhythmia may last for only a few seconds or much longer. And it usually ends as quickly as it begins.

The rapid rate produced by this arrhythmia can significantly decrease your patient's CO. Eventually, it can also damage cardiac cells, decreasing their conductivity and causing an increased risk of cardiac arrest.

Pathophysiology

As with other junctional arrhythmias, the digitalis glycoside digoxin may cause paroxysmal junctional tachycardia. Digoxin inhibits sinus impulse conduction, thus irritating junctional pacemaker tissue.

Paroxysmal junctional tachycardia may also result from the reentry phenomenon and from enhanced automaticity, which can cause the heart to accelerate to a rate of more than 150 bpm.

Reentry phenomenon

The reentry phenomenon, which can trigger junctional tachycardia, results from a unidirectional block that allows electrical impulses to reenter and stimulate cardiac cells that have recovered from depolarization. This restimulation creates a circular pattern of electrical activity called the reentry loop.

If an impulse travels the reentry loop only once, it causes a single premature beat. However, if the restimulated cardiac cells have a slow conduction velocity and a short refractory period, an impulse can travel the reentry loop numerous times, causing a run of premature beats or sustained tachycardia.

Usually, reentry rhythms occur in the AV junction and in the Purkinje fibers. But, if the reentry phenomenon affects a sufficiently large group of cells, an uncontrolled rhythm may take over the heart's entire conduction system, worsening the tachycardia. Because tachycardia caused by the reentry phenomenon doesn't allow cardiac cells to rest and fully repolarize, the cells may weaken and be unable to generate and conduct impulses. Eventually, this condition may result in cardiac arrest.

Enhanced automaticity

Enhanced automaticity can cause paroxysmal junctional tachycardia by increasing the rate at which AV pacemaker cells generate impulses. Normally, these cells generate impulses only if the SA node, which is the dominant pacemaker, fails to generate impulses and pace the heart. But certain conditions such as ischemia, hypoxia, hyperkalemia, and a toxic reaction to digoxin can decrease the resting potential of AV pacemaker cells. These conditions also can increase the rate of diastolic depolarization. Decreased resting potential and increased depolarization cause the AV pacemaker cells to generate impulses more rapidly than the SA node, resulting in tachycardia.

Signs and symptoms

Initially, your patient with paroxysmal junctional tachycardia may experience an increased CO. However, as the arrhythmia progressively weakens the cardiac cells, she may experience the signs and symptoms of decreased CO and myocardial ischemia, including dyspnea, hypotension, weakness, dizziness, syncope, chest pain, and cool, clammy skin. As with accelerated junctional rhythm, paroxysmal junctional tachycardia decreases CO because the arrhythmia's rapid, unstable heart rate results in a loss of atrial kick.

Characteristics of paroxysmal junctional tachycardia

Rate: 100 to 180 beats per minute
Rhythm: regular or irregular
P wave: if visible, is usually inverted; before, after, or buried in QRS complex
PR interval: < 0.12 second or can't be determined
QRS complex: < 0.12 second

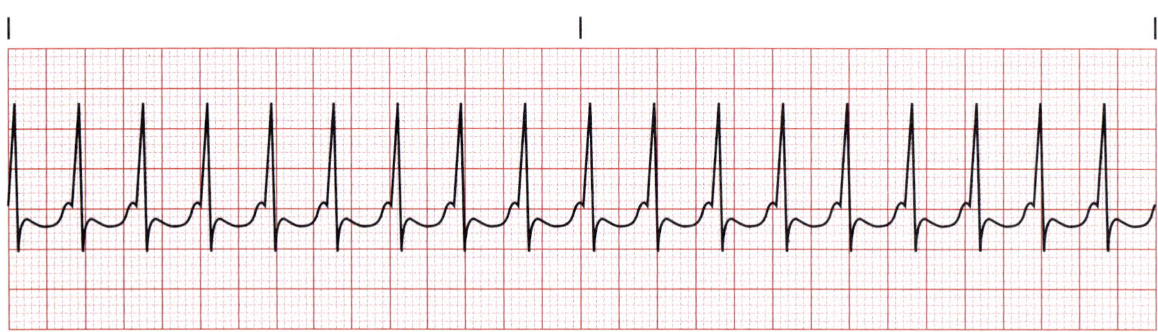

The ECG of a patient with paroxysmal junctional tachycardia will usually show a heart rate between 100 and 180 bpm. Even at the most accelerated rates produced by the arrhythmia, a patient's rhythm usually is regular (see *Characteristics of paroxysmal junctional tachycardia*).

P waves may be absent, inverted, or buried within the QRS complex. They also may follow the QRS complex. But because of the rapid heart rate produced by this arrhythmia, the P waves are less evident than in the ECGs of slower junctional arrhythmias. If P waves are evident, one will appear for each QRS complex.

Usually, if the P wave precedes the QRS complex, the PR interval is shorter than normal, less than 0.12 second. If the P wave follows the QRS complex, the PR interval may be less than 0.2 second.

Unless your patient has an idioventricular conduction defect, her R-R intervals and QRS complexes should be normal, with the QRS complexes occurring about every 0.12 second or less.

Treatment

Typically, a physician begins treatment for paroxysmal junctional tachycardia by treating the underlying cause of the arrhythmia. For example, if a toxic reaction to digoxin is causing your patient's arrhythmia, the physician may withhold the drug until the patient regains a normal sinus rhythm. The physician also may prescribe digoxin immune FAB to reduce your patient's blood digoxin level.

However, in some patients, paroxysmal junctional tachycardia produces a heart rate so rapid that the physician must treat the arrhythmia itself. Usually, a physician uses electrical cardioversion to reduce the patient's heart rate. And for a patient with chronic junctional paroxysmal tachycardia, a physician may use ablation therapy and rapid atrial pacing to suppress the arrhythmia.

Electrical cardioversion

If your patient has an extremely high heart rate and an unstable rhythm, the physician may use electrical cardioversion to produce a slower rate and a more stable sinus rhythm. In synchronized cardioversion, a defibrillator is synchronized with a cardiac monitor to fire an electrical impulse during the patient's QRS complex. This impulse causes all of the cardiac cells to depolarize simultaneously, thus enabling the SA node to regain control of the heart's pacing (see *How synchronized cardioversion works*).

After this procedure, the patient's rhythm usually improves. And she has improved peripheral pulses and a stable blood pressure.

Ablation therapy

If your patient's chronic paroxysmal junctional tachycardia results from the reentry phenomenon, the physician may use radiofrequency catheter-induced ablation to treat the arrhythmia. During this procedure, which is performed in an electrophysiology laboratory, the physician is able to determine the site of the arrhythmia's focus and the extra conduction pathways that allow impulse reentry.

To locate the site of the irritable junctional focus, the physician inserts a catheter, usually into the femoral artery, and moves it through the superior vena cava and into the right atrium. When the catheter reaches the site that's causing the arrhythmia, the physician uses high-frequency impulses to cauterize the site. This cauterization eliminates the irritable junctional focus and allows the SA node to begin pacing the heart in a normal sinus rhythm (see *Treating tachycardia with radiofrequency catheter-induced ablation,* page 92).

After the procedure, the patient will have some restrictions for about 72 hours. In particular, she should avoid lifting, sitting for extended periods, and engaging in other activities that require leg bending.

Radiofrequency catheter-induced ablation is a fairly low-risk procedure. Fewer than 1% of patients who undergo the procedure experience complications. But when complications occur, they tend to be serious and may include an MI, a cardiovascular accident, bleeding at the catheter insertion site, thromboembolism, and myocardial perforation.

Rapid atrial pacing

A physician may use rapid atrial pacing to suppress paroxysmal junctional tachycardia in a patient who has undergone cardiac surgery. With this procedure, an electronic cardiac pacemaker is inserted to artificially stimulate the heart muscle.

The pacemaker is made up of a pulse generator and a catheter with electrodes. A lead wire in the catheter senses the patient's heart rhythm and transmits this information to the pulse generator, which generates an impulse. Then, the impulse travels to the heart via the lead wire and electrodes.

Usually, with paroxysmal junctional tachycardia, the pacemaker paces the atria more quickly than the AV junctional focus that's causing the arrhythmia. Normally, the pacemaker is set at a rate 10 beats faster than the junctional rate.

As indicated by the physician, you may need to slowly increase the pacemaker's output, either until pacing spikes can be seen on the ECG or until the patient achieves a sinus rhythm. Then, the physician will order a decrease to the minimum output needed to achieve a normal heart rate.

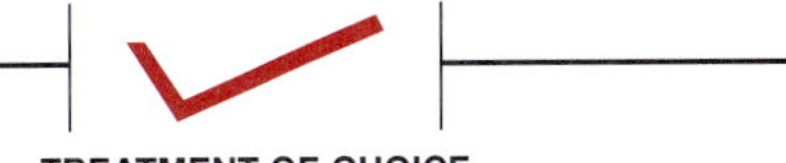

TREATMENT OF CHOICE

How synchronized cardioversion works

Synchronized cardioversion can convert a hemodynamically unstable rhythm, such as paroxysmal junctional tachycardia, into a normal sinus rhythm.

To perform the procedure, the physician places electrodes or paddles on the patient's chest and uses a defibrillator to deliver a low-energy current to her heart. Because the defibrillator delivers this current only when it senses the patient's own ventricular depolarization, it ensures simultaneous depolarization of all cardiac cells. Thus, the current stops the arrhythmia and allows the sinoatrial node to regain control of the heart and establish a normal rhythm.

The defibrillator detects the patient's ventricular depolarization by sensing the peak of her R wave on the electrocardiogram. At that precise moment, the defibrillator delivers its current. This synchronization ensures that the current doesn't reach the heart during ventricular repolarization—a period in which forced depolarization could trigger life-threatening ventricular tachycardia and ventricular fibrillation.

Complications

As with other junctional arrhythmias, paroxysmal junctional tachycardia can cause reduced CO. But with this arrhythmia, the onset may be sudden and the effects much more severe than with other slower junctional arrhythmias.

Typically, paroxysmal junctional tachycardia

Treating tachycardia with radiofrequency catheter-induced ablation

A nonsurgical procedure, radiofrequency catheter-induced ablation is used to treat atrial and junctional tachycardias that result from the reentry phenomenon.

Performed in an electrophysiology laboratory, the treatment takes 3 to 6 hours. First, the physician performs an electrophysiology study to pinpoint the area of irritable focus that's producing the patient's arrhythmia. During the study, the physician induces the arrhythmia and maps the internal cardiac structures to locate the site of the extra conduction pathway.

During radiofrequency catheter-induced ablation, the physician inserts a catheter into a selected vein and guides it into the heart. He then positions the catheter near the irritable focus and uses high-frequency energy impulses to cauterize it, as shown.

Depending on the size of the irritable focus, a single application of heat may be sufficient, or several may be needed. If the first procedure doesn't eliminate the arrhythmia, the physician usually makes a second attempt.

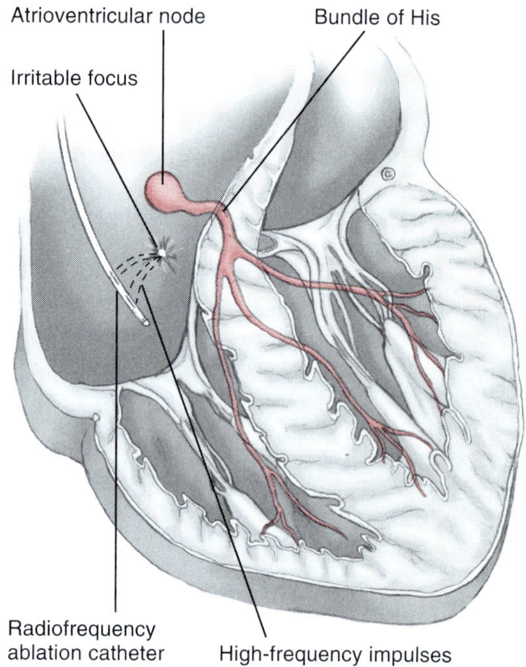

reduces atrial kick and causes asynchrony between the atria and ventricles. This condition reduces blood flow to the lungs, organs, and heart muscle, which can quickly result in myocardial hypoxia and acidosis. Hypoxia and acidosis put your patient at risk for an MI and acute respiratory distress.

Hypoxia can be particularly dangerous because it causes your patient's heart to strengthen its contractions in an attempt to increase CO. The heart's chamber walls, especially the walls of the left ventricle, become hypertrophied. And as your patient's heart weakens from the constant exertion, she may experience heart failure.

Nursing considerations

If your patient's paroxysmal junctional tachycardia results from a toxic reaction to digoxin, monitor her for signs and symptoms such as nausea, abdominal pain, and visual disturbances. Monitor your patient for the adverse effects of digoxin, including hypokalemia and a recurrence of heart failure. If the physician orders digoxin immune FAB, administer the drug, as prescribed.

If your patient with paroxysmal junctional tachycardia is scheduled to be treated with electrical cardioversion or with ablation therapy, she may be admitted to the hospital the evening before or the morning of the procedure. Perform a baseline physical assessment, including her vital signs, level of consciousness, and pulse. Be prepared to obtain a 12-lead ECG. For electrical cardioversion, withhold all solid and liquid foods for 6 to 8 hours before the procedure.

Explain the procedure to your patient and be sure informed consent has been obtained. Encourage her to ask questions. And offer emotional support to calm her fears about the procedure and her condition.

If your patient is scheduled for ablation therapy, explain that the site for catheter insertion will be shaved before the procedure. Tell your patient that the catheter may be inserted through a vein in the groin area and that the groin area will need to be shaved. Also, explain that the insertion site will be numbed with a local anesthetic before the catheter is inserted.

If your patient is scheduled for electrical cardioversion, ensure that emergency drugs and equipment necessary for pacing, intubation, and suction are readily available. Apply electrode paste to the defibrillator paddles or place gel pads on the patient's chest. If you use electrode paste, avoid using too much. Electrical current may follow the excess paste and cause burns on your patient's skin.

After ablation therapy and electrical cardioversion, record your patient's cardiac rhythm to determine whether the procedure was successful. Monitor her cardiovascular status and rhythm every 15 to 30 minutes for 2 to 3 hours after the procedure. Observe the ECG monitor closely and document any rhythm changes.

After synchronized cardioversion, also monitor your patient for the signs and symptoms of embolus formation, which occurs in about 3% of patients after the procedure has converted their arrhythmia to a normal sinus rhythm.

After ablation therapy, monitor your patient's insertion site for bleeding. Immobilize the affected limb. If a site in the groin was used, explain that she must refrain from any activities that require leg bending for 72 hours after the procedure. Although rare, severe complications from this procedure do occur in some patients. So monitor your patient for the signs and symptoms of an MI, a CVA, thromboembolism, and myocardial perforation. In general, ominous signs and symptoms may include chest pain, shortness of breath, rapid heart rate, hypotension, slurred speech, a decreased level of consciousness, hemiplegia, cyanosis, and shock.

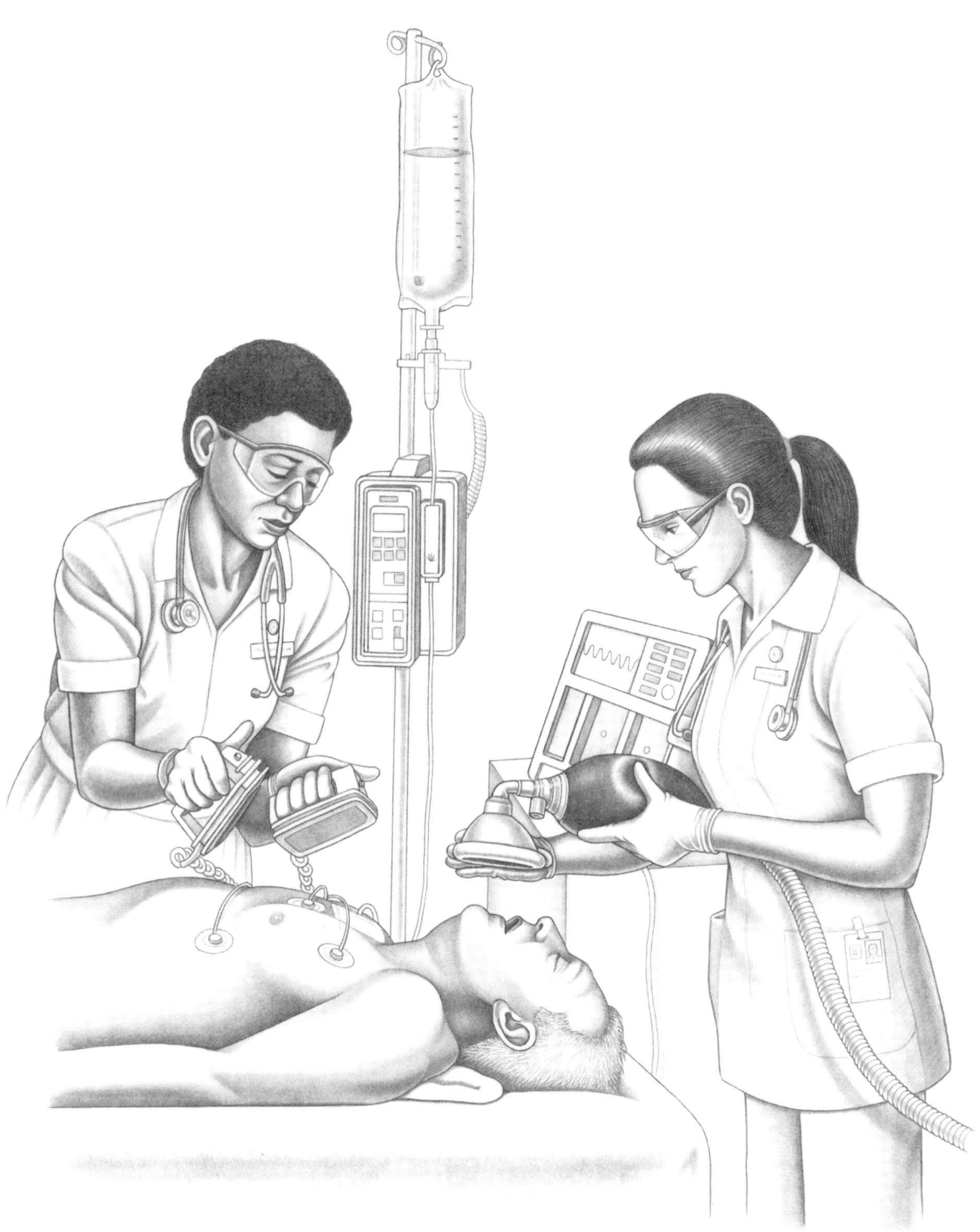

6

Ventricular Arrhythmias

Each year, over 400,000 people in the United States die of cardiac complications. And ventricular arrhythmias may be a contributing factor in most cases.

Not all ventricular arrhythmias are fatal, of course. In fact, a patient may experience a ventricular arrhythmia without having any signs or symptoms. However, all ventricular arrhythmias have the potential to lead to life-threatening complications.

In this chapter, you'll find complete descriptions of the most common ventricular arrhythmias, their causes, and their treatments. Also, the signs and symptoms and electrocardiogram (ECG) characteristics of each arrhythmia are described in detail to help you quickly identify these dangerous arrhythmias in your patients.

Premature ventricular contractions

Premature ventricular contractions (PVCs), the most common ventricular arrhythmia, result from conduction defects that produce ventricular ectopic impulses. These impulses, in turn, produce ventricular contractions earlier than normal sinus contractions.

In a healthy patient, PVCs may occur without causing any signs or symptoms. But if the arrhythmia occurs frequently, it can reduce a patient's cardiac output (CO), resulting in serious complications and even death. It also may trigger other potentially fatal arrhythmias, such as ventricular tachycardia and ventricular fibrillation.

Typically, PVCs are classified by the number of foci that produce them, their timing in the cardiac cycle, and their frequency.

If only one focus causes your patient's PVCs, the arrhythmia is called unifocal. If two or more foci cause the PVCs, the arrhythmia is called multiform or polymorphic.

A PVC may occur with or without a compensatory pause. Also, it may occur between two normal sinus rhythms or in the middle of a sinus rhythm. If a PVC occurs without a compensatory pause between two sinus rhythms, it's called an interpolated PVC. If the arrhythmia occurs simultaneously with a sinus beat, it's called a fusion beat.

As with other premature beats, PVCs are classified in the following terms according to the arrhythmia's frequency:

- salvo (a run of more than three consecutive PVCs)
- triplet (three consecutive PVCs)
- couplet (two consecutive PVCs)
- bigeminy (a PVC every other cardiac cycle)
- trigeminy (a PVC every third cardiac cycle)
- quadrigeminy (a PVC every fourth cardiac cycle).

How potassium imbalances affect the electrocardiogram

When a patient's blood potassium level rises above 5.5 mEq/L, his QRS complexes begin to widen and become markedly slurred. The QRS complexes may even widen to the point that they appear to merge with the T wave, creating a sine wave.

When a patient's blood potassium level drops below 3 mEq/L, his T wave flattens, and the smaller, usually unseen U wave becomes visible.

Hyperkalemia

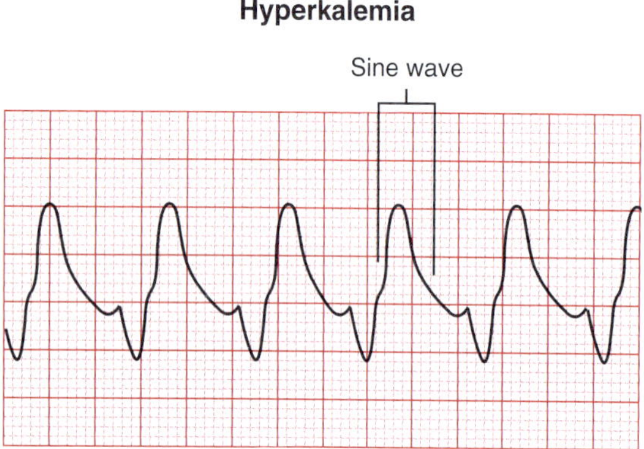

Hypokalemia

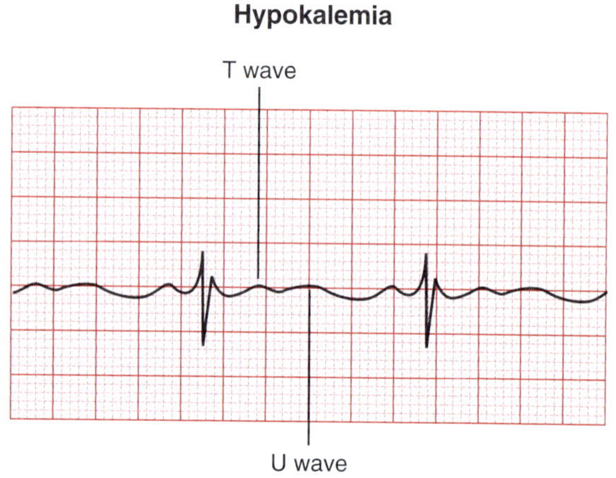

Pathophysiology

In healthy patients, PVCs may occur with no apparent cause. They may result from a sudden release of catecholamines or from increased sympathetic tone and vagal tone. A patient under severe physical and emotional stress may develop PVCs. And stimulants such as decongestants, antihistamines, coffee, tea, tobacco, and alcohol may cause PVCs even while a patient is at rest.

Typically, PVCs result from enhanced automaticity in the ventricles and abnormal impulse conduction through the ventricles. Normally, ventricular pacemaker cells in the bundle of His, bundle branches, and Purkinje fibers don't spontaneously produce their own impulses. Instead, these cells are stimulated by impulses moving down through the conduction system. However, conditions such as myocardial ischemia and beta-receptor stimulation may enhance the automaticity of these pacemaker cells, resulting in premature ventricular beats. Other conditions such as bradycardia, anemia, acidosis, and hypoxia also may stimulate or trigger enhanced automaticity and cause PVCs.

Certain procedures and devices may cause PVCs. The arrhythmia commonly occurs in patients who have a temporary pacemaker electrode in place and in those who have a displaced central venous catheter. Also, it may occur in patients during cardiac catheterization and during the postanesthesia period.

Toxic reactions to drugs and electrolye imbalances may cause PVCs. In particular, toxic reactions to drugs commonly cause bigeminal PVCs. Also, PVCs may result from potassium and calcium imbalances. Potassium and calcium are vital for the depolarization and repolarization of myocardial cells. Decreased levels of potassium and calcium affect the action potential of these cells, causing delays in impulse conduction. If impulse conduction from the sinoatrial (SA) node is delayed from reaching the ventricles, the automaticity of a ventricular focus may become enhanced enough to pace the ventricle, resulting in PVCs.

Hyperkalemia, a potassium level greater than 5.5 mEq/L, also may cause specific ECG changes that can be mistaken for PVCs. These ECG changes include a widened QRS complex, ST-segment de-

Characteristics of premature ventricular contractions

Rate: depends on underlying rhythm
Rhythm: regular or irregular
P wave: none
PR interval: none
QRS complex: ≥ 0.12 second; wide and bizarre and followed by a compensatory pause

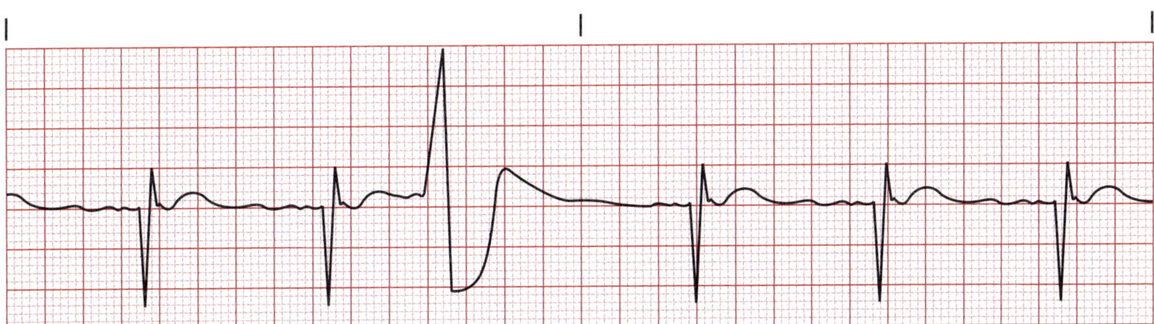

pression, and tall tent-shaped T waves (see *How potassium imbalances affect the electrocardiogram*).

Signs and symptoms

If a patient's PVCs occur infrequently, he may not experience any of the signs or symptoms of the arrhythmia. Or he may report mild signs and symptoms, such as occasionally feeling that his heart has skipped a beat. He also may experience palpitations, typically described as fluttering in the chest.

However, if PVCs occur more frequently, a patient typically will begin to experience signs and symptoms such as light-headedness, dizziness, and nausea, which result from reduced CO. His peripheral and apical pulses may be diminished or absent with each PVC. And he may experience decreased blood pressure and decreased urine output.

If your patient has heart disease, frequent PVCs may lead to chest discomfort and shortness of breath. And if his PVCs become a sustained rhythm, the arrhythmia may result in death.

On your patient's ECG, his atrial and ventricular rates may be normal for his underlying rhythm. But because PVCs interrupt the normal cardiac conduction pattern, his underlying rhythm may eventually become irregular (see *Characteristics of premature ventricular contractions*).

Usually, your patient's P waves won't be visible. But if he has retrograde conduction to the atria, his QRS complexes may be followed by retrograde or inverted P waves. With PVCs, the QRS complexes are wide, with a duration of 0.12 second or more. And they may deflect in the opposite direction of a normal QRS complex. Also, the T wave usually is large and discordant, deflecting in the opposite direction of the arrhythmia's QRS complex.

Because the P wave usually is absent with PVCs, your patient's PR interval won't be measurable. And his R-R intervals will be irregular.

Treatment

Commonly, PVCs occur in healthy people. In fact, many people experience PVCs regardless of their health. For most patients without heart disease, PVCs aren't dangerous. Basic lifestyle modifications may be sufficient for alleviating the signs and symptoms of the arrhythmia. Typically, these lifestyle modifications include reducing caffeine and alcohol intake, quitting smoking, and avoiding stress.

If your patient's PVCs occur frequently and he

begins to experience the signs and symptoms of the arrhythmia, the physician may order diagnostic testing to discover the cause of the arrhythmia and determine the correct treatment. Commonly, the arrhythmia can be alleviated by treating coexisting heart disease and electrolyte imbalances. The physician may also prescribe an antiarrhythmic drug to treat the arrhythmia directly.

If your patient's PVCs result from myocardial ischemia, he may receive supplemental oxygen and I.V. nitrates to enhance the myocardial oxygen supply. The physician may also prescribe nitroglycerin, a coronary artery vasodilator, and a peripheral vasodilator, to decrease the heart's workload.

If your patient's PVCs cause chest discomfort, the physician may prescribe morphine. Morphine, a narcotic analgesic, increases venous capacitance and decreases myocardial oxygen demand.

Your patient's PVCs also may result from treatment for coexisting heart disease. For example, PVCs commonly occur during the insertion and manipulation of invasive cardiac catheters and central venous catheters. If your patient's PVCs result from improper catheter placement, the physician will need to reposition the catheter tip to avoid irritating the myocardium.

If your patient's PVCs result from an electrolyte imbalance, the physician may alleviate the arrhythmia by treating this underlying condition. For example, if your patient is receiving diuretic therapy that decreases his blood levels of calcium and potassium, the physician may prescribe calcium and potassium supplements.

If your patient has severe hyperkalemia (a level greater than 5.5 mEq/L), the physician may prescribe an I.V. hypertonic glucose solution (50% dextrose), insulin, and sodium bicarbonate. This combination therapy drives potassium into the cells, temporarily decreasing blood potassium levels. He also may prescribe an oral cation exchange resin such as sodium polystyrene sulfonate. However, these oral drugs usually take longer to lower blood potassium levels.

Renal failure also may cause life-threatening elevations of potassium that, in turn, cause PVCs. In severe cases of hyperkalemia, dialysis may be necessary to lower blood potassium levels and alleviate the arrhythmia.

Antiarrhythmic drugs

If your patient's PVCs are life threatening, the physician may prescribe an antiarrhythmic drug. Typically, the patient receives an I.V. drug during the acute phase of the arrhythmia and then an oral drug, such as procainamide or amiodarone, for long-term control. Oral antiarrhythmics may be effective in suppressing long-term ventricular etopic beats. Many of these drugs have a narrow therapeutic range, making it difficult to avoid toxic adverse effects. Also, some of these drugs can worsen existing arrhythmias or precipitate new problems.

Complications

Commonly, PVCs trigger ventricular tachycardia or ventricular fibrillation, leading to sudden death. In some patients, a single PVC can cause a lethal arrhythmia. Left untreated, frequent PVCs can decrease your patient's CO. In elderly and medically compromised patients, decreased CO can lead to peripheral ischemia and organ damage. If your patient develops more frequent PVCs, chest pain, shortness of breath, and decreased tolerance for activity, his risk of acute complications increases.

Nursing considerations

If your patient is having PVCs, observe his ECG at least every 4 hours to document his response to therapy. Check the ECG for signs of excessive cardiac depression such as widening of QRS complexes and lengthening of the PR interval.

If the physician has prescribed an antiarrhythmic, observe your patient for adverse effects. Report any adverse effects and your patient's response to the therapy. Be prepared to alter the dose or discontinue the drug, as ordered.

Patient teaching

Teach your patient about the action and adverse effects of his antiarrhythmic drug. Tell him about possible drug interactions if he is taking more than one drug. Be sure he knows the signs and symptoms of frequent PVCs, including dizziness, chest pain, weakness, and palpitations. Also, make sure he knows the following:

- how to check his pulse
- how to check his blood pressure, if equipment is available
- when to contact his physician
- when to call an ambulance.

Ventricular tachycardia

Ventricular tachycardia, commonly referred to as V-tach, occurs when the ventricles produce several PVCs in succession. Typically, ventricular tachycardia results from a breakdown of the heart's conduction system and an increase in myocardial irritability. Your patient with ventricular tachycardia may have no pulse, and this arrhythmia can quickly deteriorate into ventricular fibrillation. Thus, ventricular tachycardia is a life-threatening condition that requires emergency intervention.

Pathophysiology

Ventricular tachycardia shortens the diastolic period, when the ventricles normally fill with blood from the atria. Also, atrial and ventricular contractions may become unsynchronized. Thus, the ventricles pump less blood, resulting in decreased perfusion to the coronary arteries, vital organs, and peripheral circulation.

A short burst of ventricular tachycardia (less than 30 seconds) is called unsustained ventricular tachycardia. Sometimes ventricular tachycardia is characterized by repetitive bursts of PVCs separated by a series of sinus beats. These short runs of ventricular tachycardia are seldom life threatening; however, they may indicate ventricular irritability and ischemia, and they may warn of sustained ventricular tachycardia.

Ventricular tachycardia that lasts more than 30 seconds is called sustained ventricular tachycardia and is considered an ominous sign. The marked reduction in CO with ventricular tachycardia produces serious hemodynamic effects for the patient. If this form of the arrhythmia is left untreated, it may degenerate into ventricular fibrillation.

Ventricular tachycardia may result from the reentry phenomenon, enhanced automaticity at a focal ectopic site, and several other causes.

The reentry phenomenon, one of the most common causes of ventricular tachycardia, occurs when an impulse travels through an area of myocardium, depolarizes it, and then reenters the same area to depolarize it again. Reentrant circuits in the ventricles may be large and involve both bundle branches, or more typically, they may be localized to a small area in the ventricles.

Patients with cardiac disease or damage to the heart's conduction system may have a prolonged QT interval, placing them at risk for R-on-T phenomenon and ventricular tachycardia. The R-on-T pattern occurs when a PVC, firing early in the cardiac cycle, is superimposed on the T wave of the preceding complex. The period when the ventricular fibers repolarize, shown on the ECG as a T wave, is the heart's most vulnerable conduction period. During this interval, some myocardial cells are only partially repolarized. If an electrical impulse enters the ventricles, it may be conducted normally in fibers that are fully repolarized and not at all in fibers that are still in their refractory period.

Ventricular tissue can develop enhanced automaticity as a result of ischemia, hypokalemia, a toxic reaction to digoxin, and beta-receptor stimulation. If automaticity increases, the ventricular fibers, which are normally slow to conduct, begin to fire impulses at an extremely rapid rate, resulting in ventricular tachycardia and other ventricular arrhythmias. Enhanced automaticity develops when a critically timed premature stimulus, such as a PVC, activates a focus in the ventricles.

Ventricular tachycardia sometimes occurs as a reperfusion arrhythmia when blood flow is suddenly restored to a previously occluded coronary artery, such as during the postthrombolytic treatment period after a myocardial infarction (MI). Reperfusion arrhythmias occur in up to 80% of MI patients who are being treated with thrombolytic drugs. The arrhythmia may also occur during coronary spasm relaxation, coronary angioplasty, or coronary artery bypass surgery.

Other conditions that can lead to ventricular tachycardia include rheumatic heart disease, coronary artery disease (CAD), mitral valve disease, heart failure, and cardiomyopathy. Ventricular tachycardia can also occur as an adverse effect of anesthesia or from hypoxia resulting from chronic pulmonary disease.

Reversible causes of ventricular tachycardia include the following:

- electrolyte imbalances
- mechanical irritants (cardiac catheters or pacemakers)
- myocarditis
- excessive adrenergic stimulation, usually caused by catecholamines
- exercise
- cocaine use
- toxic reactions to drugs such as digoxin, procainamide, isoproterenol, and quinidine.

Torsades de pointes, a type of ventricular tachy-

Identifying torsades de pointes

The French term *torsades de pointes* ("twisting of the points") refers to a type of ventricular tachycardia that's characterized by QRS complexes of changing sizes and shapes that appear to twist around the isoelectric line. The arrhythmia occurs at rates of 200 to 250 beats per minute.

Torsades de pointes results when impulses are generated by more than one ectopic ventricular focus or when impulses from the same focus follow different paths to depolarize the patient's ventricles.

This arrhythmia often appears after a prolonged QT interval during normal sinus rhythm and may occur when a premature ventricular contraction is generated during the T wave. You may see prominent U waves before the onset of torsades de pointes. Although the arrhythmia is commonly unsustained, it can degenerate into ventricular fibrillation.

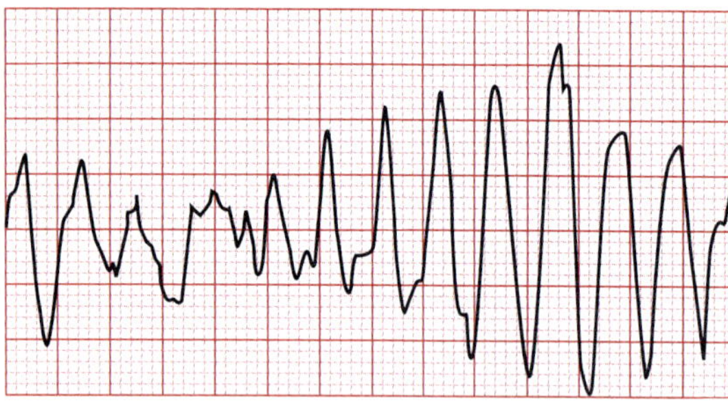

cardia, can result from any factor that prolongs the QT interval, including genetic predisposition. However, electrolyte imbalances and toxic reactions to drugs are the most common causes of torsades de pointes (see *Identifying torsades de pointes*).

Signs and symptoms

If runs of ventricular tachycardia last only a few seconds and terminate spontaneously, your patient may tolerate the arrhythmia without experiencing any related signs or symptoms. Most patients, however, are immediately aware of the sudden increase in heart rate. The patient's vital signs tend to deteriorate quickly. And he may begin to experience the signs and symptoms of reduced CO, including the following:

- syncope or dizziness
- palpitations
- confusion
- weakness
- hypotension
- cool, clammy skin
- chest pain
- dyspnea
- anxiety.

If ventricular tachycardia is sustained, your patient may lose consciousness and experience seizures, apnea, and cardiac arrest.

Check your patient's apical and peripheral pulses. The heart rate can be heard apically with a stethoscope and viewed on the ECG monitor. In many patients these beats aren't palpable. Ventricular beats generally don't perfuse to the peripheral circulation. The difference between the apical heart rate and the radial pulse rate is called the apical-radial pulse deficit. Patients who have some perfusing beats during ventricular tachycardia may experience less dramatic signs and symptoms than patients who have no distal pulses. Your patient may be alert and oriented during periods of ventricular tachycardia, or he may lose consciousness after only a few seconds of the arrhythmia.

In ventricular tachycardia, ventricular contractions usually aren't associated with atrial activity. On the ECG, the patient's QRS complexes appear wide and bizarre. Usually, the atrial rate can't be determined. The ventricular rate varies from 150 to 250 beats per minute (bpm), but it's usually greater than 140 bpm (see *Characteristics of ventricular tachycardia*).

The rhythm is usually regular. But if the ventricular tachycardia is polymorphic in origin, the rhythm may be irregular.

P waves may be absent, retrograde, or buried in the QRS complex. The PR interval can't be determined.

Typically, the R-R intervals are equal in distance because the rhythm is usually regular. In the polymorphic ventricular tachycardia of torsades de pointes, the R-R interval may be highly irregular.

The patient's QRS complex is wide and bizarre, with a duration of 0.12 second or more. The T wave is opposite the QRS deflection.

Characteristics of ventricular tachycardia

Rate: 150 to 250 beats per minute
Rhythm: usually regular
P wave: none
PR interval: none
QRS complex: ≥ 0.12 second; wide and bizarre

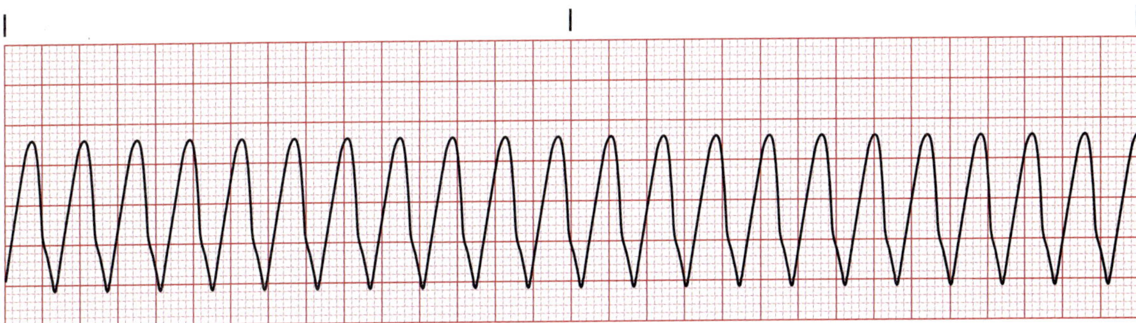

Treatment

Even in patients who don't experience the signs and symptoms of ventricular tachycardia, episodes of the arrhythmia can degenerate into ventricular fibrillation and become life threatening. Typically, the treatment for ventricular tachycardia depends on the circumstances under which it occurs, your patient's response to the arrhythmia, and the severity of the situation. Find out whether the initial episode of ventricular tachycardia was monitored or unwitnessed. For your patient who is otherwise healthy, short runs of ventricular tachycardia may require observation and investigation but no immediate treatment.

If ventricular tachycardia is witnessed on a cardiac monitor and your patient has no pulse, prompt delivery of a precordial thump may terminate the arrhythmia. If successful, the mechanical force of a blow to the chest may induce an ectopic beat that interrupts the reentrant pathway.

During the treatment for ventricular tachycardia, help isolate and correct any reversible causes of the arrhythmia. To treat ventricular tachycardia resulting from myocardial ischemia or hypokalemia, a physician may prescribe a nitrate or potassium. Ventricular tachycardia that converts to sinus bradycardia or an atrioventricular (AV) block can be corrected with 0.5 to 1 mg of I.V. atropine, a 1-μg/minute to 2-μg/minute I.V. drip of isoproterenol, or a temporary pacemaker. Monitor your patient's blood levels of drugs that cause ventricular arrhythmias, such as digoxin and quinidine.

Depending on the severity of your patient's ventricular tachycardia and whether drug therapy causes other complications, the physician may use nonpharmacologic measures to treat the arrhythmia. This treatment may include electrical cardioversion, antiarrhythmic drugs, pacing catheter insertion, ablation therapy, surgery, and implantable cardioverter-defibrillator insertion.

Electrical cardioversion

If ventricular tachycardia causes hypotension, shock, angina, or heart failure, electrical direct-current cardioversion may be used to convert the unstable rhythm into normal sinus rhythm or a more stable pattern. Electrodes or paddles are placed on the patient's chest, and a defibrillator delivers an electrical impulse to the heart. The goal is to depolarize all cardiac fibers completely and simultaneously, allowing the SA node to take control of the heart and establish a normal rhythm.

To prevent depolarization during the heart's

vulnerable period, the defibrillator's electrical impulse is synchronized with cardiac depolarization using a cardiac monitor. The monitor senses the R wave of the patient's QRS complex, and the defibrillator fires only during the safe period. Synchronized cardioversion is possible only if the patient has discernible QRS complexes to trigger the discharge. Unsynchronized cardioversion, or defibrillation, should be used only when your patient has ventricular fibrillation.

Cardioversion usually begins with 50 joules of electricity. If this is unsuccessful, the shock may be increased progressively to 100, 200, and 360 joules. Keep in mind that patients who have had a toxic reaction to digoxin don't respond well to cardioversion and should be treated with drug therapy. Make sure emergency drugs and the equipment needed for pacing, endotracheal intubation, and suction are available in case complications occur during electrical cardioversion.

Antiarrhythmic drugs

Some patients with ventricular tachycardia are hemodynamically stable with palpable pulses, fairly normal blood pressure readings, an alert level of consciousness, and no evidence of chest pain or heart failure. These patients may not require immediate cardioversion and are commonly treated with antiarrhythmic drugs.

Antiarrhythmic drugs are categorized as class I through class IV based on how they work on action potentials. Be aware that drugs within each class may differ significantly and can't be substituted for one another. Some generalizations can be made about each class of drugs. Class I drugs are subdivided into three categories based on how they work. Generally, class I drugs block sodium channels. Most antiarrhythmic drugs other than those in class Ia reduce SA node automaticity. Class II drugs antagonize adrenergic receptors, whereas class III drugs prolong repolarization. Class IV drugs generally decrease conduction by slowing the influx of calcium. All antiarrhythmic drugs, with the exception of bretylium, are capable of suppressing automaticity in ectopic foci (see *Antiarrhythmics and their effects*).

In the acute setting, lidocaine is administered I.V. as an initial bolus of 1.5 mg/kg of body weight. Boluses of 0.5 mg/kg may be given about every 5 minutes until ventricular tachycardia resolves, but the total dose shouldn't exceed 8 mg/kg. If lidocaine corrects the patient's ventricular tachycardia, expect to administer a continuous infusion of 1 to 4 mg/minute, as prescribed.

If lidocaine treatment is unsuccessful or your patient is allergic to the drug, the physician may prescribe procainamide. Procainamide is administered I.V. at 20 mg/kg/minute until either the arrhythmia is terminated; toxic effects develop, such as a widened QRS complex, hypotension, or central nervous system (CNS) effects; or 1,000 mg of the drug has been administered.

Procainamide may be administered as a continuous I.V. infusion of 1 to 4 mg/minute, titrated to the patient's response. If delivered too rapidly, procainamide can cause intraventricular conduction delays and AV block.

Bretylium may be given I.V. at 5 mg/kg over several minutes and increased to 10 mg/kg after 15 to 30 minutes. A continuous infusion of bretylium may be initiated at 1 to 2 mg/minute.

Finding the most effective long-term suppressive therapy to treat ventricular tachycardia usually involves trial and error. The goal is to find a drug that controls the arrhythmia without causing significant adverse effects. Because of their narrow therapeutic ranges and serious adverse effects, antiarrhythmic drugs are difficult to manage. The physician may order a combination of drugs with different mechanisms of action, thus allowing the patient to take low doses of two drugs rather than a high dose of one drug.

Electrophysiology studies

Because the effectiveness of drug therapy may be difficult to evaluate in patients with intermittent ventricular tachycardia, a physician may order a controlled electrophysiology study, which is performed in a cardiac catheterization laboratory. Before the procedure, your patient will probably receive conscious sedation. Multielectrode catheters are then inserted into a large vein and guided to various locations in the heart, where they're used to record the electrical activity of the myocardium. The physician also places electrodes on the patient's body for simultaneous recordings. Then, the physician uses pacing electrodes on the catheters to attempt to induce a ventricular arrhythmia. If the arrhythmia can't be reintroduced by this electrical stimulation, the drug therapy is probably effective.

Pacing catheter

For patients with recurrent ventricular tachycardia, a pacing catheter is sometimes inserted into the right ventricle and single, double, or multiple electrical stimuli are introduced to terminate the arrhythmia. The biggest risk with this procedure is that recurrent ventricular tachycardia may convert to ventricular fibrillation, an even more dangerous arrhythmia. Electrical cardioversion may also be applied directly to myocardial tissue through the electrodes of the pacing catheter. A shock of 0.25 joule may be delivered in an attempt to terminate ventricular tachycardia.

Ablation therapy

If the irritable focus in your patient's heart has been mapped through an electrophysiology study and programmed electrical stimulation, ablation therapy with a radiofrequency catheter may be the next treatment of choice. A physician uses this invasive procedure to eliminate alternate pathways in the heart that cause cardiac arrhythmias and interfere with normal conduction. During catheter-induced ablation, the physician maneuvers a catheter to the target heart tissue and delivers a burst of radiofrequency or laser energy. The resulting heat alters a small portion of the myocardial tissue and, in many cases, eliminates the source of the patient's ventricular tachycardia.

Surgery

In some patients, surgery may be required to treat persistent ventricular tachycardia. Common surgical techniques used include:
- ventriculotomy to remove an area of tissue
- cryosurgery to freeze irritable tissue
- encircling endocardial ventriculotomy to isolate the area where arrhythmias occur
- endocardial resection to remove the critical area of tissue.

Automatic implantable cardioverter-defibrillator

If your patient has survived at least one episode of cardiac arrest or experiences recurrent, sustained ventricular tachycardia, a physician may insert an automatic implantable cardioverter-defibrillator (AICD). This internal device can be programmed to monitor the heart rhythm, to treat arrhythmias with appropriate electrical therapy, and to store data on each episode for retrieval by the physician (see *Treating ventricular arrhythmias: Automatic implantable cardioverter-defibrillator,* page 104).

An AICD functions like an external defibrillator but is fully automatic. It also delivers less energy because the electrical charge is applied directly to the epicardial surface. The device is programmed to detect different ventricular arrhythmias, including PVCs, ventricular fibrillation, and ventricular tachycardia, and can respond to each with the appropriate therapy. If your patient's AICD is also

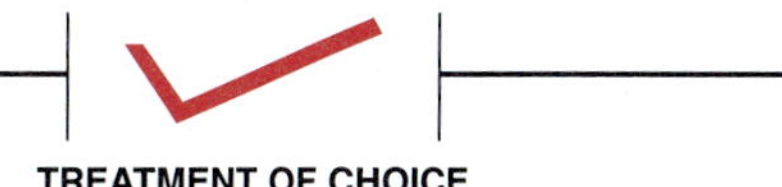

TREATMENT OF CHOICE

Antiarrhythmics and their effects

Use the table below to review the antiarrhythmic drugs commonly prescribed for ventricular tachycardia.

Drugs	Effects
Class Ia	
• quinidine • procainamide • disopyramide	• depress ectopic pacemaker rates, conduction, and excitability • cause reflex increase in sinoatrial (SA) node rate
Class Ib	
• lidocaine • tocainide • mexiletine • phenytoin	• suppress normal cardiac activity by blocking sodium channels
Class Ic	
• propafenone	• blocks sodium channels with weak beta-blocking activity • lowers excitability, conduction velocity, and automaticity in heart tissues
Class II	
• acebutolol • esmolol • propranolol	• block beta receptors • decrease heart rate • decrease inotropic effects
Class III	
• amiodarone • sotalol • bretylium	• block sodium, potassium, and calcium • slow SA node firing • slow atrioventricular (AV) node conduction time
Class IV	
• verapamil • adenosine	• block calcium channels • reduce heart rate • slow AV node conduction

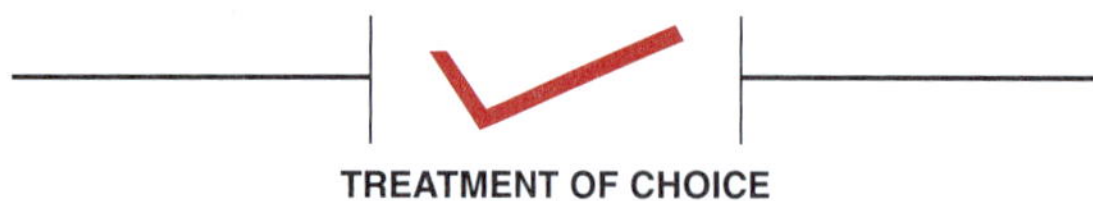

TREATMENT OF CHOICE

Treating ventricular arrhythmias: Automatic implantable cardioverter-defibrillator

Increasingly, physicians use automatic implantable cardioverter-defibrillators (AICDs) to treat ventricular arrhythmias. This fully automatic device, usually implanted in the patient's upper chest or abdomen, can be programmed to deliver an electrical shock directly to the myocardium.

An AICD is made up of defibrillator patches that attach to the patient's heart, endocardial sensing electrodes, and a subcutaneously implanted pulse generator. The sensing electrodes transmit data about the heart's electrical activity to the pulse generator, which is programmed to recognize ventricular arrhythmias. The generator then can terminate the arrhythmia by delivering rapid pacing impulses via the defibrillator patches.

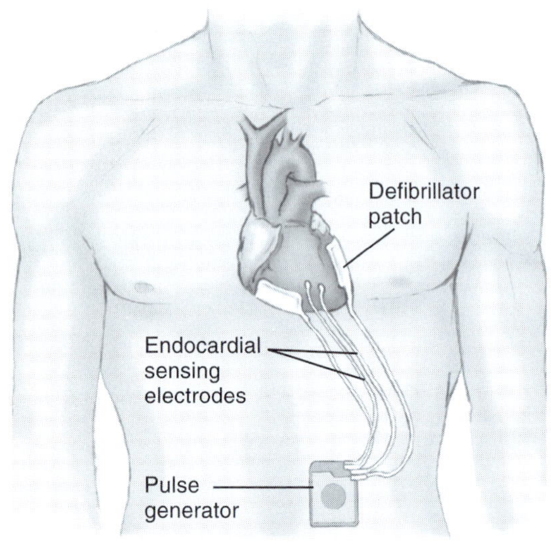

equipped as a pacing device, ventricular tachycardia may be terminated with rapid pacing pulses, which are painless to the patient.

Most AICDs have an electronic memory that stores various information, such as the number and types of treatments received, the success of each treatment, the patient's cardiac activity, and the status of the batteries and programmed settings of the device.

Complications

The complications of ventricular tachycardia range from mild, nonthreatening signs and symptoms to sudden cardiac death. Many patients experience decreased blood pressure with weak or absent pulses and a decreased level of consciousness. Unless treated immediately, your patient may become unconscious, and his cardiac rhythm may quickly deteriorate into ventricular fibrillation. If your patient with ventricular tachycardia has a pulse, early treatment generally includes electrical cardioversion and I.V. antiarrhythmic drugs. If your patient has no pulse, be prepared to initiate emergency resuscitation.

Nursing considerations

If your patient develops ventricular tachycardia, observe him carefully for the signs and symptoms of reduced CO, such as cool, clammy skin and decreased urine output. Also, look for the signs and symptoms of ventricular tachycardia, including dizziness or syncope, dyspnea, palpitations, chest pain, and anxiety.

Many times, ventricular tachycardia may lead to a situation requiring emergency treatment. If ventricular tachycardia occurs, your knowledge of emergency resuscitation equipment and procedures is crucial for the smooth, well-organized treatment of your patient.

If your patient with ventricular tachycardia doesn't maintain a pulse, begin emergency treatment immediately with cardiopulmonary resuscitation (CPR) and advanced cardiac life support. Establish and maintain a patent airway, and call for help. Besides CPR, emergency treatment may include I.V. access, frequent blood pressure readings, continuous pulse oximetry readings, and recurrent physical assessments. Be ready to prepare your patient for endotracheal intubation. Depending on his cardiac rhythm, he may require a 1-mg I.V. bolus of epinephrine every 3 to 5 minutes. Be prepared to assist in direct-current cardioversion or cardiac defibrillation, as indicated.

After your patient's ventricular tachycardia has been successfully treated, continue monitoring your patient's hemodynamic status, electrolyte balance, and ECG rhythm. Unless the conditions that originally caused the ventricular tachycardia are corrected, the arrhythmia may recur. Assess your patient's ECG for PVCs, prolonged QT intervals, and prominent U waves. Monitor your patient's laboratory values to detect abnormal acid-base or electrolyte levels. Immediately notify the physician of any abnormal findings.

Patient teaching

The sudden appearance of ventricular tachycardia can be emotionally devastating for your patient. He may feel helpless, frightened, or frustrated when faced with serious arrhythmias. Provide emotional support for your patient by explaining the cause of his arrhythmia and the procedures he'll undergo to control his condition. Also, give him time to ask questions and express his concerns.

Teach your patient about his arrhythmia, and explain the plan of treatment. Many patients and their families are poorly informed and have no idea what is happening when the condition occurs. Teach him and his family the dosage and any adverse effects of his prescribed drugs. Explain that he may have to initiate lifestyle changes and implement strategies for coping with a recurrence of the arrhythmia.

Ensure that your patient and his family understand the plan of treatment and have ample opportunity to ask questions and to participate in the decision making. Also, encourage family members to learn CPR, which could save your patient's life if the arrhythmia recurs after discharge.

Ventricular fibrillation

Ventricular fibrillation, the most common cause of sudden death in patients with underlying CAD, is responsible for about 90% of deaths after an MI.

This fatal arrhythmia results from a state of electrical chaos within the ventricles. In the normal heart, ventricular fibers contract and recover in unison. Ventricular depolarization produces the QRS complex on the ECG, and the mechanical contraction of the ventricles propels blood into the pulmonary artery and aorta. If the ventricles fibrillate, individual myocardial fibers quiver and twitch continuously at their own rate, without the coordinated activity necessary for effective ventricular contraction. Because of the disorganized electrical activity and absence of normal ventricular contractions and pumping action, circulation abruptly ceases. Sudden death occurs unless the arrhythmia is converted.

Pathophysiology

Although the exact cause of ventricular fibrillation isn't known, several cardiac disorders may contribute to this arrhythmia. Ventricular fibrillation most commonly occurs with CAD, an acute MI, and cardiomyopathy.

Ventricular fibrillation may occur spontaneously, without previous signs or symptoms of ventricular irritability or ischemia. An episode of ventricular fibrillation that develops without warning in a normal heart is called primary ventricular fibrillation. Primary ventricular fibrillation may also develop after an acute MI in patients who seem to have no complications. In some cases, ventricular fibrillation begins after a PVC or an episode of ventricular tachycardia. Secondary ventricular fibrillation is seen in patients with a history of heart failure or cardiogenic shock. Whereas primary ventricular fibrillation responds readily to defibrillation, secondary ventricular fibrillation is typically more difficult to treat.

Ventricular fibrillation is commonly the terminal event in various diseases. It may also occur because of the following:

- cardiac pacing
- cardiac catheterization
- cardiac surgery
- anesthesia
- toxic reaction to a drug
- hypoxia.

Accidental electrical shock or the electrical charge administered during cardioversion can precipitate ventricular fibrillation. Premature stimulation during the heart's vulnerable period can initiate ventricular fibrillation, especially in patients who have cardiac disease or damage to the heart's conduction system.

The heart is most vulnerable when the ven-

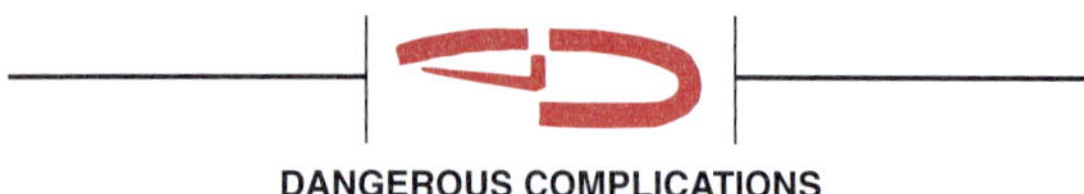

DANGEROUS COMPLICATIONS

Reviewing the cardiac effects of electrolyte imbalances

Electrolyte imbalances commonly result in ventricular arrhythmias. Use this table to review the cardiac effects of electrolyte imbalances that lead to these arrhythmias.

Electrolyte imbalance	Cardiac effect
hypokalemia	• increases myocardial excitability
hyperkalemia	• makes myocardium electrically unstable
hypocalcemia	• slows impulse conduction through atrioventricular junction and ventricles
hypercalcemia	• decreases myocardial automaticity and shortens systole
hypomagnesemia	• interferes with ventricular repolarization
hypermagnesemia	• interferes with conduction and repolarization

tricular fibers repolarize, shown on the ECG as a T wave. During this interval, some myocardial cells are only partially repolarized. If an electrical impulse enters the ventricles at this time, it may be conducted normally in fibers that are fully repolarized but not at all in fibers that are still in their refractory period. If a PVC occurs during this vulnerable period and falls on the T wave of the preceding complex, impulse reentry may develop, causing ventricular fibrillation.

Reentry phenomenon, a common cause of ventricular fibrillation, occurs when an impulse travels through an area of the myocardium, depolarizes it, and then reenters the same area to depolarize it again. With ventricular fibrillation, when an electrical impulse from a higher pacemaker in the conduction system reaches an unresponsive area within the ventricles, it traverses the area on both sides. The single impulse then becomes two. If these impulses reach another refractory area of tissue, they divide again, forming two more impulses. This chain reaction continues, forming a series of small electrical waves that travel in many directions simultaneously. The result is chaotic electrical activity in the ventricles, causing ventricular fibrillation.

Commonly, electrolyte imbalances disrupt the heart's conduction system. And these imbalances can result in ventricular fibrillation (see *Reviewing the cardiac effects of electrolyte imbalances*).

Ventricular fibrillation occasionally occurs as a reperfusion arrhythmia when blood is suddenly restored to a previously occluded coronary artery. This condition may occur during thrombolytic treatment for an MI, during coronary spasm relaxation, or during coronary angioplasty or bypass surgery. Reperfusion arrhythmias occur in up to 80% of patients with an MI being treated with thrombolytic drugs.

Ventricular fibrillation after an MI usually occurs during the first hour, but late ventricular arrhythmias can develop after 48 hours or more. When late ventricular fibrillation does develop, the patient's prognosis is poor. Late ventricular arrhythmias commonly impair left ventricular functioning and increase the risk of death.

If ventricular fibrillation occurs early in the course of an MI, the underlying cause may be increased excitability of myocardial tissue. Late ventricular fibrillation is most likely caused by the reentry phenomenon occurring at the edges of the infarcted myocardial tissue. Patients who develop late ventricular fibrillation tend to have electrically unstable myocardial tissue and may need long-term antiarrhythmic therapy to prevent sudden cardiac death.

Signs and symptoms

The sudden onset and dramatic signs and symptoms of ventricular fibrillation can be alarming to members of the health care team and to bystanders. The patient has no CO. And he rapidly loses consciousness and becomes unresponsive. You won't be able to palpate or auscultate a pulse, and the blood pressure is nonexistent. Respiratory arrest quickly follows the onset of ventricular fibrillation. Some patients develop seizures. The

Characteristics of ventricular fibrillation

Rate: can't be determined
Rhythm: can't be determined
P wave: can't be discerned; usually inverted
PR interval: none
QRS complex: can't be discerned

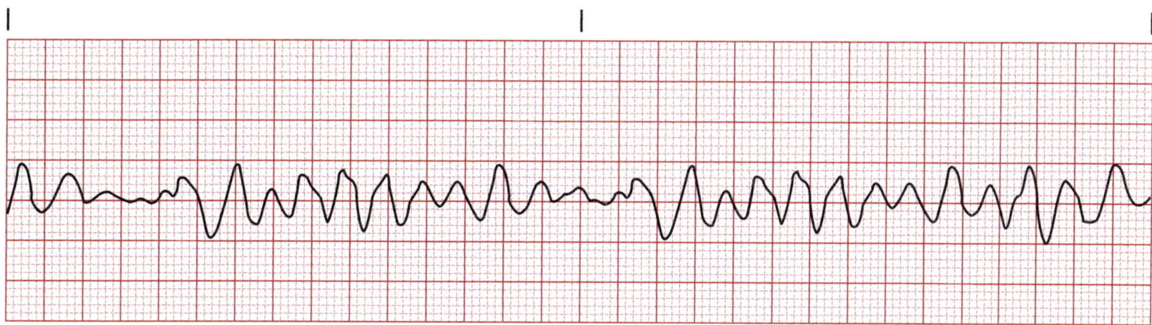

pupils dilate because of the lack of cerebral oxygenation. Cyanosis and death follow quickly unless the arrhythmia is treated effectively.

Because the arrhythmia may completely eliminate your patient's CO, several ECG characteristics may be absent. Usually, the rate of ventricular fibrillation can't be determined, and the rhythm is chaotic, with no recognizable P waves, QRS complexes, ST segments, or T waves (see *Characteristics of ventricular fibrillation*).

The disorganized electrical activity of ventricular fibrillation appears on the ECG as irregular, chaotic waveforms. During ventricular fibrillation, multiple ectopic foci in the ventricles fire rapidly and at random, producing no recognizable QRS complexes or atrial activity.

Nonconducting P waves may be present, but they typically aren't discernible. And R waves can't be distinguished. Thus, the PR interval is absent.

Ventricular fibrillation is classified by the amplitude of the waveform. Coarse ventricular fibrillation has a higher amplitude than fine ventricular fibrillation. The waveforms of fine ventricular fibrillation are sometimes barely noticeable and may closely resemble ventricular standstill, the absence of electrical activity (see *Distinguishing fine ventricular fibrillation from ventricular standstill,* page 108).

Treatment

Early recognition of ventricular fibrillation is crucial. Assess your patient immediately for decreased level of consciousness, absent pulses, and absent blood pressure. Keep in mind that as ventricular fibrillation progresses, myocardial tissue becomes more ischemic and less responsive to treatment. Your patient will have only a few minutes until brain death occurs.

Usually, the arrhythmia is treated with defibrillation. The physician may prescribe immediate administration of epinephrine or an antiarrhythmic drug in conjunction with defibrillation. Usually, emergency treatment also includes hyperventilating the patient and administering sodium bicarbonate for metabolic acidosis, a common complication of ventricular fibrillation. After the crisis has been successfully treated, the physician may order an electrophysiology study and an AICD to prevent a recurrence of the arrhythmia.

Defibrillation

Once ventricular fibrillation is confirmed, initiate CPR until a defibrillator is available. Early defibrillation is effective for converting ventricular fibrillation to a cardiac rhythm with significant myocardial

Distinguishing fine ventricular fibrillation from ventricular standstill

Ventricular standstill doesn't always appear as a flat line on the electrocardiogram (ECG) monitor. Sometimes, it can look just like fine ventricular fibrillation. The ECG baseline may be wavy because the patient has an atrial rhythm, and the resulting P waves appear to be fine ventricular fibrillation.

To correctly identify the patient's rhythm, perform a 12-lead ECG and examine at least two leads, including leads I and II or leads I and III.

Because these leads show P waves most clearly, you should be able to distinguish the P waves of ventricular standstill from the chaotic, irregular waves of fine ventricular fibrillation. If you still can't identify the rhythm, treat it as ventricular fibrillation.

impulses and contractions. Defibrillation is accomplished by passing a direct-current shock through the heart. The goal is to depolarize all myocardial cells at once and to terminate the chaotic electrical activity, allowing the SA node to resume pacing of the heart.

Ideally, defibrillation should be initiated by the first qualified person to reach the bedside. The sooner the shock is delivered, the greater the patient's chance of recovery. Defibrillation that isn't accomplished within 2 minutes of onset of the arrhythmia is less likely to be effective, especially in elderly patients.

During defibrillation, transthoracic resistance to the electrical current influences the amount of energy that actually reaches the patient's heart. The transthoracic resistance decreases by as much as 8% after each successive shock. The defibrillator must be set in the asynchronous mode to treat ventricular fibrillation. Because QRS waveforms are absent during ventricular fibrillation, the defibrillator won't deliver a shock in synchronous mode.

As resuscitation efforts continue, establish and maintain an I.V. access site, as appropriate, and administer supplemental oxygen. Assist with endotracheal intubation to establish an airway and provide oxygenation.

Epinephrine

The initial drug of choice for ventricular fibrillation is epinephrine, administered in conjunction with cardiac defibrillation. A physician may order a 1-mg I.V. push of epinephrine. Or he may administer the drug through the endotracheal tube. The endotracheal dosage should be calculated from a dilution of 1:10,000, which allows greater absorption of the drug through the pulmonary vasculature.

Epinephrine is used to increase myocardial excitability and to convert fine ventricular fibrillation to coarse fibrillation. Coarse fibrillation represents a higher level of electrical activity and is more responsive to defibrillation. After chest compressions are performed for 30 to 60 seconds to circulate the epinephrine, defibrillation with 360 joules should be attempted again. Epinephrine may be given every 3 to 5 minutes throughout the resuscitation effort.

Antiarrhythmic drugs

Depending on your patient's response, I.V. antiarrhythmic drugs such as lidocaine, procainamide, and bretylium may be used during the resuscitation effort, followed by chest compressions for 30 to 60 seconds to enhance the circulation of each drug. After administration of each drug, defibrillation with 360 joules should be attempted. If defibrillation successfully converts ventricular fibrillation to a more stable rhythm with palpable peripheral pulses, begin a continuous infusion of the last antiarrhythmic drug used.

If defibrillation is successful before the administration of drugs, expect to administer an I.V. bolus of lidocaine, followed by a continuous infusion. The standard lidocaine bolus is 1.5 mg/kg of body weight. The continuous infusion is typically started at 2 to 4 mg/minute, as prescibed.

Hyperventilation and sodium bicarbonate

Regardless of how short the episode, ventricular fibrillation produces metabolic acidosis. Lactic acid accumulates in the body because of the lack of perfusion to the tissues during circulatory arrest. Decreased ventilation during CPR also contributes to acidosis. Untreated acidosis, whether respiratory or metabolic, is hazardous because it reduces the threshold for recurrent ventricular fibrillation.

During resuscitation, the preferred method for controlling acidosis is having the patient hyperventilate. Although sodium bicarbonate is sometimes given as an I.V. push to treat metabolic acidosis, keep in mind that large doses can cause rebound alkalosis. Be aware that sodium bicarbonate administration will be based on your patient's arterial blood gas (ABG) results.

Electrophysiology studies

After your patient's condition becomes stable, he may undergo electrophysiology studies to determine the origin of the ventricular fibrillation. During an electrophysiology study, a physician inserts multielectrode catheters into a large vein and guides them to various locations inside the heart to record the heart's electrical activity. Simultaneous recordings are made from these intracardiac catheters and from body-surface electrodes.

If your patient receives programmed electrical stimulation, the physician may use the pacing electrodes on the catheters to stimulate the heart and induce the arrhythmia. The same electrodes also may be used to defibrillate the heart internally if the arrhythmia were to occur spontaneously during the procedure. If your patient is being treated with antiarrhythmic drugs, the electrophysiology study may be repeated after the drugs have reached therapeutic levels. If ventricular fibrillation can't be reintroduced by electrical stimulation, the drug treatment was probably effective.

Automatic implantable cardioverter-defibrillator

If your patient has survived at least one episode of cardiac arrest or has recurrent ventricular fibrillation, an AICD may be the treatment of choice. As with an AICD used to treat ventricular tachycardia, this device can be programmed to monitor the heart rhythm, to treat arrhythmias with appropriate electrical therapy, and to store data on each episode for a physician to review.

Complications

Because ventricular fibrillation is a life-threatening arrhythmia, emergency treatment with defibrillation is essential for your patient's survival. After ventricular fibrillation is converted to a more stable rhythm, patients typically require immediate treatment for complications such as cerebral damage due to hypoxia, acidosis, an MI, heart failure, and respiratory arrest.

Some patients who survive ventricular fibrillation suffer permanent organ damage caused by ischemia. If your patient's brain is denied oxygen for more than 3 minutes, CNS damage and coma may result. The kidneys, which are sensitive to ischemia, may fail after your patient has been resuscitated. Also, an MI may occur if the arrhythmia reduces blood flow through the coronary arteries.

Usually, a patient will remain at risk for recurrence of the arrhythmia. To prevent sudden death, a physician may order long-term therapy—such as antiarrhythmic drugs, electrophysiology studies, and the insertion of an AICD.

Nursing considerations

Usually, you will perform emergency measures, such as immediate defibrillation, when beginning treatment for ventricular fibrillation. Familiarize yourself with your unit's emergency supplies, including code carts, defibrillators, and airway equipment. Also, obtain advanced cardiopulmonary life-support training. Because you may be the first health care provider at your patient's bedside in an emergency, be prepared to provide defibrillation (see *Defibrillation: Step by step,* page 110).

Recovery from ventricular fibrillation may be a lengthy ordeal for your patient. After your patient's ventricular fibrillation has converted to a more stable rhythm, he may need airway support; careful monitoring of heart rate, rhythm, and vital signs; administration of complex drug therapy; and monitoring for complications such as heart failure, an acute MI, and worsening myocardial injury.

Check with the physician about follow-up tests to help diagnose the cause of the arrhythmia. Diagnostic tests may include repeat ECGs and laboratory tests to uncover electrolyte imbalances or an MI. Your patient may also require tests to determine whether substance abuse, hypothermia, a toxic reaction to a drug, or heart disease may have caused his arrhythmia.

Patient teaching

Provide emotional support to your patient and his family during and after treatment for the arrhythmia. Teach him about his treatment, the invasive monitoring devices, and any complicated

Defibrillation: Step by step

If your patient experiences life-threatening ventricular fibrillation during cardiopulmonary resuscitation (CPR), you may need to perform defibrillation following these steps:

1. Attach the electrodes to your patient's chest.

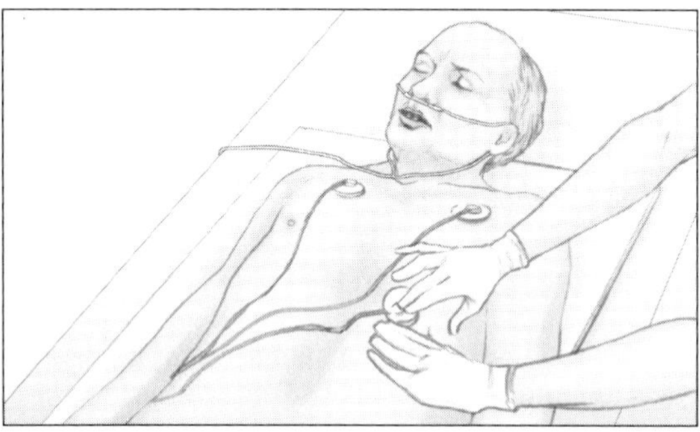

2. Assess his cardiac rhythm.
3. If defibrillation is indicated, apply conductive gel or paste to the defibrillator paddles or apply conductive gel pads to your patient's chest, as shown.

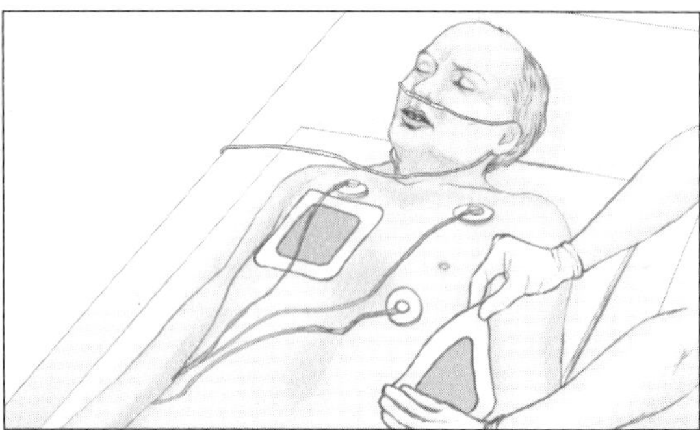

4. Turn on the defibrillator and set the energy level to 200 joules unless otherwise indicated.

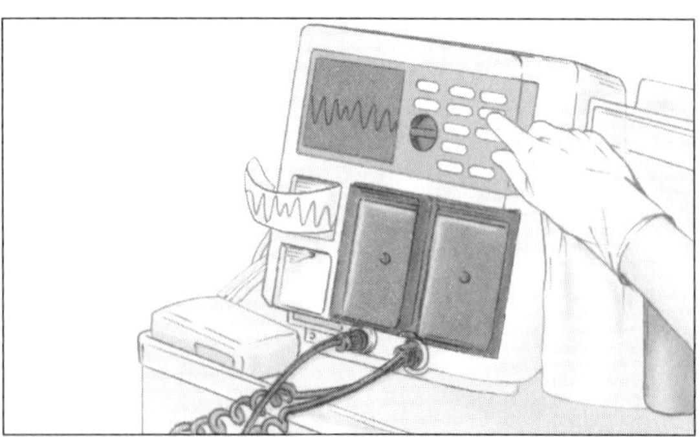

5. Charge the capacitors.
6. If you're not using an automatic unit, apply the paddles to your patient's chest with about 25 pounds of pressure per paddle.

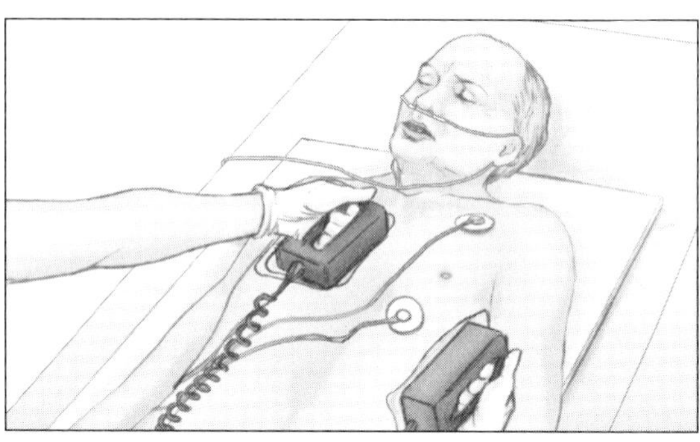

7. Check that no one else is touching the patient or the bed. Indicate that you're ready to shock the patient by loudly stating, "All clear." Then deliver the shock.
8. After delivering the shock, reassess your patient's rhythm on the monitor.
9. Deliver the countershock by pressing both buttons on the paddles simultaneously or as indicated by the manufacturer's directions.
10. Continue to assess your patient's rhythm. Ask another health care provider to assess your patient's carotid or femoral pulse so that you can keep the paddles on the patient's chest.
11. If your patient needs a second shock, increase the energy level to 300 joules unless otherwise indicated. Again, make sure no one is touching your patient or the bed before you deliver the shock.
12. After delivering the second shock, reassess your patient's rhythm. If he requires a third shock, increase the energy level to 360 joules.
13. After the third shock, continue to assess your patient's status, including his blood pressure, pulses, and pupillary response. If his ventricular fibrillation continues or if he has no pulse, resume CPR.

medical tests he may undergo. Also, provide your patient's family with regular reports on his status and prognosis.

During your patient's hospital stay, teach him about ventricular fibrillation and cardiac disease. Also, his continued survival may depend on compliance with antiarrhythmic drug therapy, lifestyle modifications, and follow-up with his physician. So be sure to teach him the actions, adverse effects, dosages, and interactions of his drugs. Also, tell him about the importance of adhering to physical-activity guidelines and dietary constraints. And explain when he should contact his physician and when he should call an ambulance.

Accelerated idioventricular rhythm

Accelerated idioventricular rhythm occurs when an ectopic focus in the ventricles assumes control of the heart and paces at a rate between 40 and 100 bpm. This arrhythmia occurs when the ventricular pacemaker takes over as an ectopic pacemaker for the heart. The term *idioventricular* means that the ventricles fire impulses on their own, without stimulation from a higher pacemaker. In the case of an accelerated rhythm, the ventricular cells fire at a rate above their intrinsic rate.

Usually, the onset of accelerated idioventricular rhythm is gradual, and unlike other ventricular arrhythmias, accelerated idioventricular rhythm is typically benign. In most cases, it doesn't compromise cardiac function or progress to more dangerous arrhythmias. The arrhythmia is usually transient, and in many patients, it disappears spontaneously within 30 cardiac cycles. The rhythm may terminate gradually as the dominant SA impulse accelerates or as the ventricular pacemaker slows.

Pathophysiology

Accelerated idioventricular rhythm commonly begins with either escape beats or fusion beats. Escape beats occur when the higher pacemakers fail to generate impulses and a ventricular beat escapes to pace the heart. Fusion beats are produced when impulses from two different foci meet in the ventricles and depolarize them simultaneously. This usually involves an impulse from above the ventricles and an ectopic ventricular impulse. The presence of fusion beats indicates AV dissociation, meaning that pacemaker sites in the atria and ventricles are firing independently of one another.

Determining your patient's heart rate will help you make the important distinction between accelerated idioventricular rhythm and ventricular tachycardia. A ventricular rhythm with a rate of 60 to 100 bpm is usually considered accelerated idioventricular rhythm, whereas a ventricular rhythm over 120 bpm is considered ventricular tachycardia. However, ventricular tachycardia may be slower than 120 bpm and accelerated idioventricular rhythm may exceed 100 bpm. As you interpret ventricular arrhythmias, remember the following guidelines:

- Accelerated idioventricular rhythm commonly begins with a fusion or escape beat, whereas ventricular tachycardia usually begins with a PVC.
- The onset of ventricular tachycardia is generally abrupt, but accelerated idioventricular rhythm usually begins gradually.
- Accelerated idioventricular rhythm is usually brief and terminates gradually, but ventricular tachycardia is more sustained and ends abruptly.

Many factors may contribute to accelerated idioventricular rhythm. The most common causes are a toxic reaction to digoxin, an MI, coronary reperfusion, and thrombolytic therapy.

Digoxin is the treatment of choice for chronic heart failure and atrial or junctional arrhythmias. However, nearly one-third of patients who take digoxin develop a toxic reaction, and cardiac arrhythmias are usually the first sign. Almost any arrhythmia can follow such a reaction, including accelerated idioventricular rhythm.

Digoxin slows atrial conduction by inhibiting myocardial-cell transport of sodium and potassium. Major effects on the myocardium include the following:

- slowed firing rate of the SA node
- depressed AV conduction
- prolonged refractory period in the AV node.

Many patients taking digoxin have other medical conditions, such as hypertension, diabetes, or renal insufficiency, that can affect the rate of drug metabolism and excretion. Your patient can experience the signs and symptoms of a toxic reaction even with normal blood digoxin levels.

About 20% of patients with an acute MI develop accelerated idioventricular rhythm. An MI occurs when blood flow through a coronary artery is blocked, causing ischemic injury and cell death in myocardial tissue. The usual causes are coronary artery thrombosis and prolonged coronary artery spasms.

Patients who have an inferior-wall or anterior-wall MI are most vulnerable to this rhythm disturbance. An anterior-wall MI usually results from blockage of the left anterior descending coronary artery. Because this artery supplies blood to the ventricular septum, its occlusion can produce ischemia of the left and right bundle branches, resulting in AV block. This occlusion slows electrical impulses from the atria and provides an opportunity for ectopic ventricular cells to pace the heart. Accelerated idioventricular rhythm is commonly the result.

An inferior-wall MI usually results from occlusion of the right coronary artery. Cardiac anatomy differs slightly in each patient, but branches from the right coronary artery usually supply blood to the AV junction and the bundle of His. In about 55% of patients, the right coronary artery also has a branch to the SA node and atria. Occlusion near this branch of the right coronary artery commonly results in sinus or AV block. The occlusion leads to decreased impulses from the higher pacemakers, allowing the ventricles to briefly control the heart with episodes of accelerated idioventricular rhythm.

Accelerated idioventricular rhythm can also develop as a reperfusion arrhythmia. Reperfusion arrhythmias occur when blood flow is suddenly restored to an occluded coronary artery. Reperfusion arrhythmias can occur after surgical bypass of an obstructed coronary vessel or after coronary angioplasty.

Most MIs result from coronary artery thrombosis. Commonly, a physician may use thrombolytic therapy to dissolve the clot, restore blood flow, and salvage myocardial tissue damaged by ischemia. The development of arrhythmias after thrombolytic therapy indicates coronary reperfusion. In fact, accelerated idioventricular rhythm occurs in over 50% of patients with successful reperfusion.

Signs and symptoms

A patient may not experience any signs or symptoms from the arrhythmia, especially if he has no apical-radial pulse deficit. And accelerated idioventricular rhythm doesn't always deteriorate into a more serious ventricular arrhythmia. As long as the heart rate remains normal, the arrhythmia may continue without hemodynamic compromise.

If a patient has signs and symptoms, they're usually mild and rarely more serious than occasional palpitations and dizziness. However, some patients may experience signs and symptoms of hypotension, angina, or heart failure that result from reduced CO and myocardial ischemia.

If your patient has accelerated idioventricular rhythm, his CO may decrease because the ventricles don't contract simultaneously. Patients with valvular heart disease, compromised peripheral circulation, and other cardiac problems are particularly likely to experience the signs and symptoms of reduced CO with accelerated idioventricular rhythm.

On a patient's ECG, the ventricular rate of accelerated idioventricular rhythm usually is 60 to 100 bpm. The atrial rate can't be determined because the atria don't depolarize in a normal manner. And the rhythm is usually regular (see *Characteristics of accelerated idioventricular rhythm*).

P waves may be present, but they are usually buried in the QRS complexes and are unrelated to ventricular activity. Usually, the PR interval isn't measurable. The R-R interval is fairly regular, but it may vary slightly.

As in most ventricular arrhythmias, the QRS complexes provide the most obvious clues. With accelerated idioventricular rhythm, they usually are wide and bizarre, with a duration of 0.12 second or more.

Treatment

Usually, accelerated idioventricular rhythm is benign, with a spontaneous onset and disappearance. If your patient requires treatment, a physician may prescribe atropine to treat it directly. Or he may treat the cause of the arrhythmia, such as a toxic reaction to digoxin.

Atropine

Atropine, the drug of choice to restore normal sinus rhythm, increases the sinus rate by blocking the actions of acetylcholine at receptors in the smooth muscle of the SA node. Increased sinus-node discharge usually allows the heart's normal pacemaker, the SA node, to override the ectopic ventricular site. The usual dosage of atropine for

Characteristics of accelerated idioventricular rhythm

Rate: 60 to 100 beats per minute
Rhythm: usually regular
P wave: none
PR interval: none
QRS complex: ≥ 0.12 second; wide and bizarre

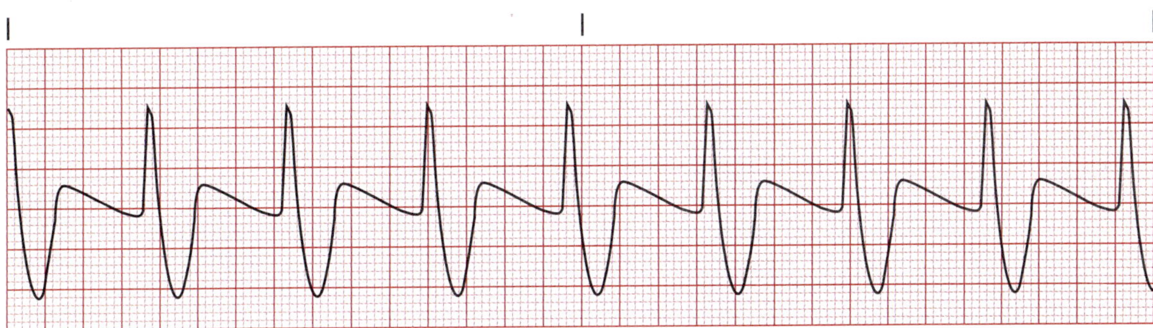

adults is 0.5 to 1 mg as an I.V. push, repeated as often as needed every 5 minutes to a total of 2 mg.

Monitor your patient for tachycardia when using atropine. Remember that low doses of this drug may actually depress the SA node. Other adverse effects of atropine include urinary hesitancy, urine retention, dry mucous membranes and skin, and decreased bronchial secretions.

If your patient has had an acute MI, use atropine with caution. The increase in heart rate caused by atropine may intensify the heart's oxygen demand and lead to ischemia. If your patient has glaucoma, atropine is contraindicated because it dilates the pupil and can cause severe eye pain. Elderly patients are especially sensitive to the adverse effects of atropine.

Digoxin dose adjustment

Normally, therapeutic blood levels of digoxin are 0.5 to 2 ng/ml. Increased digoxin levels may cause accelerated idioventricular arrhythmia as well as more serious arrhythmias and conditions, such as PVCs and heart block. If a toxic reaction to digoxin is the underlying cause of your patient's accelerated idioventricular rhythm, the physician may decide to stop the drug immediately. However, if your patient's arrhythmia isn't life threatening, the physician may simply resume digoxin at a lower dose and a less frequent interval.

Complications

Usually, complications of accelerated idioventricular rhythm result from underlying cardiac or systemic problems. The rhythm itself doesn't have serious consequences, except on rare occasions when it's accompanied by ventricular tachycardia. Nevertheless, you should investigate your patient's cardiac health status. Observe him for the signs and symptoms of decreased CO and ischemia and for the development of other arrhythmias on the ECG monitor.

Nursing considerations

If your patient has episodes of accelerated idioventricular rhythm, monitor his cardiac rhythm and perform a baseline physical assessment. Observe your patient for these signs and symptoms of decreased CO:
- dyspnea
- hypotension
- weakness

- cool, clammy skin
- dizziness or syncope
- chest pain.

Patient teaching

Tell your patient that treatment for accelerated idioventricular rhythm usually focuses on the underlying cause of the arrhythmia, such as an MI, reperfusion, or a toxic reaction to digoxin. If he is scheduled to undergo diagnostic testing to determine the cause of his arrhythmia, explain the tests and procedures. Also, explain the underlying conditions for which he's being tested.

Maintain a calm, quiet environment for your patient. And ease his anxiety by providing information about the ECG monitor, I.V. drugs, laboratory tests, and other procedures. Teach him about his arrhythmia and the signs and symptoms that may indicate an underlying condition. Also, encourage him to participate in his own health care by keeping follow-up appointments after discharge.

Ventricular escape rhythm

Ventricular escape rhythm, also called idioventricular rhythm, occurs when the cardiac conduction system fails to produce or conduct impulses in a normal manner and a ventricular pacemaker assumes control of the heart. For example, the heart's higher pacemakers may fail to initiate a rhythm, or impulses may be blocked beyond the AV node and unable to reach the ventricles. Ventricular escape rhythm is a normal protective mechanism of the conduction system designed to prevent complete cardiac standstill.

Pathophysiology

In the healthy heart, a cardiac impulse arises from special pacemaker cells in the SA node and is conducted through the internodal pathways to the AV node. The impulse slows at the AV node to allow sufficient time for blood from the atria to fill the ventricles before ventricular contraction occurs. The impulse then passes through the bundle of His, through the right and left bundle branches, and into the branching network of the Purkinje fibers.

Cells of the bundle of His and the Purkinje fibers have the fastest conduction velocity in the heart. The rapid spread of the impulse throughout these structures allows the ventricles to depolarize and contract almost simultaneously, providing efficient pumping action. If the sinus and junctional pacemakers fail to generate impulses, the bundle of His and the Purkinje fibers are able to pace the heart at an intrinsic rate of 15 to 40 bpm. Ventricular escape rhythm is generated when the Purkinje fibers assume the role of pacemaker.

Ventricular escape rhythm is most common in patients who have advanced heart disease or a severely damaged heart. This rhythm commonly precedes complete failure of the heart's electrical system. Other causes of ventricular escape rhythm may include a toxic reaction to a drug, myocardial ischemia, electrolyte imbalance, and hypoxia.

Many drugs used to treat arrhythmias actually contribute to rhythm disturbances such as ventricular escape rhythm. About 15% of patients who are taking an antiarrhythmic experience conduction disturbances caused by their drug.

Digoxin, commonly used to treat heart failure and arrhythmias, can cause ventricular escape rhythm. Digoxin inhibits the active transport of sodium and potassium across the cell membrane and has major effects on the myocardium, including:

- slowed firing of the SA node
- depressed AV nodal conduction
- prolonged refractory period of the AV node.

Depression of the pacemakers higher up in the conduction system may result in serious conduction block and bradycardia, leaving only the ventricular pacemakers to control the patient's heart rate. Cardiac arrhythmias are the first sign of a toxic reaction to digoxin in more than 50% of patients. Toxic levels of digoxin can cause almost any arrhythmia or conduction disturbance. Other drugs, such as quinidine, amiodarone, and calcium channel blockers, may enhance the effects of digoxin and increase your patient's risk of PVCs. Hypokalemia also increases the potency of digoxin.

Quinidine, used to manage a wide variety of atrial and ventricular arrhythmias, may cause ventricular escape rhythm. Quinidine decreases myocardial excitability and slows conduction ve-

locity. High blood levels of this drug may prolong conduction time in the SA and AV nodes to such an extent that a ventricular pacemaker takes control of the heart to prevent cardiac arrest. Your patient may experience the following signs and symptoms of a toxic reaction to quinidine:
- widened QRS complexes
- prolonged PR or QT intervals
- hypotension
- frequent ventricular ectopic beats.

Myocardial ischemia also may lead to severe conduction disturbances and ventricular escape rhythm. Ischemia may result from coronary artery occlusion, as in an MI, or from blood flow that is inadequate to meet the heart's metabolic needs. If ischemia is prolonged or severe, metabolism of the cardiac tissue changes from aerobic to anaerobic. Basic biochemical energy processes are unable to preserve cellular boundaries. And the affected areas of myocardial tissue can no longer produce or conduct electrical impulses.

Although the muscle layers of the myocardium are readily affected by ischemia, conduction tissue is more resistant because of its relatively low oxygen consumption and high levels of glycogen. Purkinje fiber cells survive longer than the surrounding muscle because of their proximity to oxygenated blood in the ventricular cavity. These ventricular conduction cells are able to pace the heart at a slow rate even after other parts of the conduction system fail.

Signs and symptoms

If your patient develops ventricular escape rhythm, you may see immediate signs of decreased CO because of the slow heart rate and loss of atrial kick. If the heart rate drops to between 15 and 40 bpm, decreased cerebral perfusion and myocardial ischemia are likely to follow. Your patient may experience the following signs and symptoms of decreased CO:
- dizziness or syncope
- anxiety
- confusion
- weakness
- cool, clammy skin
- hypotension
- chest pain
- dyspnea.

Your patient's signs and symptoms depend on the status of his underlying ventricular function, the presence of valvular heart disease, and the status of his peripheral circulation. The signs and symptoms of decreased CO may occur from the loss of atrial kick. If the ventricles are controlling the heart during ventricular escape rhythm, atrial and ventricular contractions are unsynchronized, and stroke volume decreases, resulting in a loss of blood flow to the coronary arteries and major organs.

On your patient's ECG, the ventricular rate is 20 to 40 bpm. The ventricular rhythm is fairly regular, although it may accelerate for a few cardiac cycles (see *Characteristics of ventricular escape rhythm,* page 116).

Usually, P waves are absent with ventricular escape rhythm because the atria don't depolarize normally. But if P waves do appear, they have no relationship to the QRS complexes. PR intervals aren't measurable. And typically, the R-R intervals are constant but may vary.

Because ventricular depolarization doesn't follow normal conduction pathways, QRS complexes are wide and bizarre, with a duration of 0.12 second or more. Also, the escape focus may shift to another part of the ventricle and generate QRS complexes with different contours and rates.

Treatment

If the bizarre, widened QRS complexes of ventricular escape rhythm appear on the cardiac monitor, your patient's heart may not be producing effective contractions. A rhythm with pulseless electrical activity may have occurred. Because ventricular escape rhythm may be life threatening, a physician usually prescribes immediate treatment for the arrhythmia.

Typically, a physician will insert a temporary electronic pacemaker. He may also prescribe drug therapy. Any treatment for this arrhythmia is directed at increasing the patient's heart rate.

Pacemaker

Typically, the primary treatment for ventricular escape rhythm is a temporary electronic pacemaker. The pacemaker provides an artificial stimulus to the heart muscle when initiation or con-

Characteristics of ventricular escape rhythm

Rate: 20 to 40 beats per minute
Rhythm: usually regular
P wave: none
PR interval: none
QRS complex: $\geq$ 0.12 second; wide and bizarre

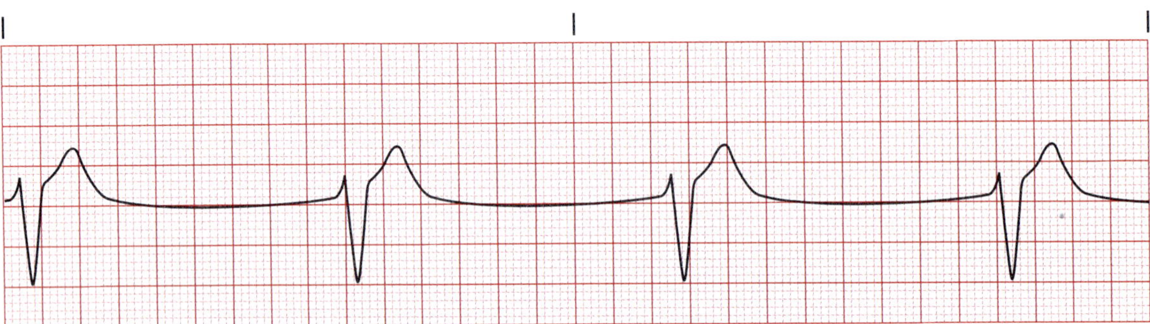

duction of impulses is defective. By increasing the heart rate, a pacemaker helps maintain adequate CO (see *How a temporary pacemaker controls ventricular escape rhythm*).

Drug therapy

Typically, a physician may prescribe I.V. isoproterenol for ventricular escape rhythm. This drug stimulates $beta_1$ and $beta_2$ receptors to increase the heart's rate and contractility. It's used to enhance the pacemaker function of the SA node and to improve AV conduction. Isoproterenol is usually given at 5 µg/minute using a solution prepared by diluting 10 ml of 1:5,000 solution in 500 ml of dextrose 5% in water.

Isoproterenol can cause rapid heart rates and other potentially dangerous adverse effects, so monitor your patient closely during administration of the drug. Because isoproterenol increases myocardial oxygen consumption, observe the cardiac monitor for ectopic arrhythmias and changes that indicate ischemia. Additional adverse effects include the following:

- headache
- flushed skin
- angina
- nausea
- dizziness
- diaphoresis
- weakness.

A physician also may prescribe atropine to treat ventricular escape rhythm. Atropine increases the heart rate by blocking the actions of acetylcholine at receptor sites in the smooth muscle of the SA node. The usual dose of atropine is a 0.5-mg to 1-mg I.V. push, repeated as often as needed every 5 minutes to a total of 2 mg.

During treatment with atropine, your patient will require monitoring for tachycardia. And as you know, low doses (less than 0.5 mg) may actually slow the heart. Other adverse effects of atropine include urinary hesitancy, urine retention, dry mucous membranes and skin, and decreased bronchial secretions. Because atropine usually increases the heart rate, it may also intensify your patient's myocardial oxygen demand. Remember to use atropine with caution in very young and elderly patients because they are especially sensitive to the drug's adverse effects.

Lidocaine, a drug commonly used to treat ventricular arrhythmias, shouldn't be given to patients with ventricular escape rhythm unless ventricular tachycardia is present. Because lidocaine suppresses depolarization of the ventricles, use of this drug may decrease ventricular activity and completely stop your patient's heart.

Complications

The hemodynamic effects of ventricular escape rhythm depend on the heart's ability to maintain normal CO. If this arrhythmia persists, serious consequences usually occur. Your patient may develop syncope, shock, myocardial ischemia, and heart failure. The imminent danger with ventricular escape rhythm is complete ventricular standstill. Therefore, the immediate goals of treatment are to increase the patient's heart rate and alleviate the signs and symptoms of the arrhythmia.

Most patients don't tolerate ventricular escape rhythm long enough to develop chronic complications. In most cases, the rhythm is either treated effectively with a pacemaker and drugs or quickly deteriorates into ventricular standstill. Chronic complications may result from the cardiac conditions that contributed to the patient's ventricular escape rhythm, including valvular heart disease, heart failure, and an MI.

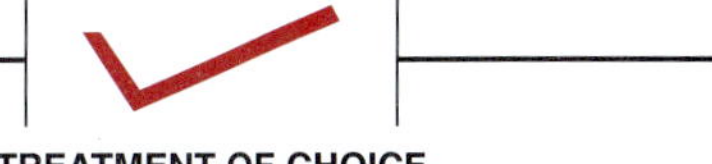

TREATMENT OF CHOICE

How a temporary pacemaker controls ventricular escape rhythm

A temporary electronic pacemaker is made up of a pulse generator and a catheter, which contains a lead wire with a bipolar endocardial sensing electrode. A physician inserts the catheter into the patient's heart through the right subclavian vein and guides it down through the tricuspid valve to the endocardium of the right ventricle.

Once the catheter is in place, the sensing portions of the lead wire transmit information about the patient's heart rhythm to the circuitry of the pulse generator. The pulse generator, in turn, discharges electrical impulses back through the lead wire to the right ventricle, thus pacing the heart.

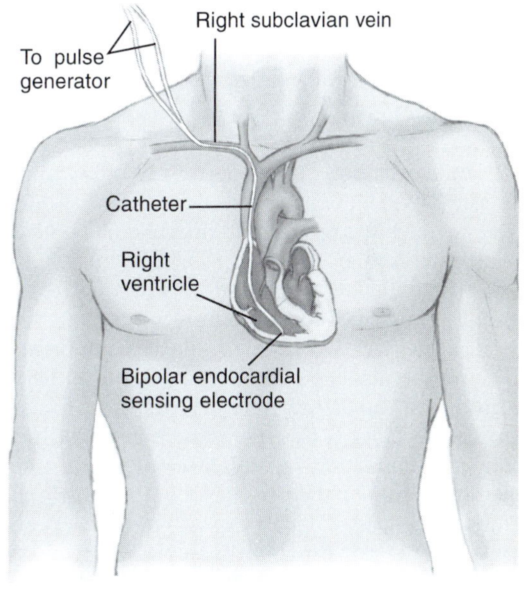

Nursing considerations

Continuously monitor your patient's heart rate and rhythm. Check his apical heart rate and other vital signs frequently, and complete a baseline physical assessment early in the course of treatment. Establish at least one but preferably two sites of I.V. access. If hypoxemia develops, monitor your patient's oxygen saturation continuously or repeat ABG levels as indicated. To treat mild hypoxemia, use a nasal cannula to deliver oxygen at 1 to 2 L/minute, as prescribed.

Maintain a calm environment for your patient. Pain, anxiety, and stress can increase his myocardial oxygen demand. Don't use sedatives to treat these problems because they may lower the patient's blood pressure and exacerbate bradycardia.

Patient teaching

Your patient will probably feel frightened and overwhelmed by his signs and symptoms and the interventions, which may include laboratory tests, ECG monitoring, and I.V. drugs. Provide clear explanations of all procedures to help ease his fears. Include the patient's family and caregivers in your teaching. In particular, you should teach your patient and his family the doses, action, and adverse effects of his prescribed drugs and the signs and symptoms of ventricular escape rhythm, such as slow pulse, hypotension, dizziness, and weakness. Also, make sure your

patient knows the following:
- how to check his own pulse and blood pressure
- when to contact his physician
- when to call an ambulance.

Ventricular standstill

If the ventricles don't receive adequate electrical stimulation, they may cease to contract. The resulting arrhythmia is ventricular standstill, also called asystole or cardiac arrest. *Ventricular standstill* is commonly defined as the complete absence of electrical activity in the myocardium. This arrhythmia differs from pulseless electrical activity because, with ventricular standstill, there's usually no electrical activity in the heart to be picked up by the ECG monitor.

The patient with ventricular standstill faces a grim prognosis. Treatment is rarely successful. This arrhythmia eventually appears in all dying patients and commonly represents a confirmation of death, rather than an arrhythmia requiring treatment.

Pathophysiology

Ventricular standstill may result from many different conditions that cause insufficient blood flow to the ventricles. Ventricular standstill can be divided into two categories: primary and secondary.

In primary ventricular standstill, the heart's electrical system fails to generate impulses that reach the ventricles. This is usually a result of myocardial ischemia and sclerotic degeneration of the SA node or the AV conducting system. Primary ventricular standstill usually is preceded by a bradyarrhythmia caused by sinus arrest or complete heart block. Typically, primary ventricular standstill indicates a problem within the heart and is the most serious form of the arrhythmia. Common causes of ventricular standstill include:
- cardiogenic shock
- advanced left ventricular heart failure
- an MI
- ineffective cardiac contractility
- ruptured ventricular aneurysm
- valvular heart disease
- electrolyte imbalances.

If severe ischemia occurs in the heart, pacemaker cells fail because they can't transport the ions necessary to control the transmembrane action potential. During an MI, an ischemic event that occurs over several hours, occlusion of the right coronary artery may result in malfunction of the SA and AV nodes. Extensive infarction may also cause severe bundle branch block, damaging the conduction system in the ventricles. Without adequate formation or conduction of electrical impulses, the ventricles can't contract and ventricular standstill may result.

Secondary ventricular standstill occurs when the heart's electrical system fails because of factors outside the myocardium. Noncardiac causes may include severe hypoxemia, acidosis, hemorrhage, enhanced vagal tone, electrical shock, hypothermia, and cocaine overdose. Although many disorders can lead to secondary ventricular standstill, the arrhythmia typically results from a condition that causes severe tissue hypoxia and acidosis.

The electrical shock from lightening can depolarize the myofibrils of the myocardial pacemakers, resulting in cardiac arrest. After a short time, the stunned ventricles may begin to contract again, either spontaneously or after CPR.

Hypothermia is another special circumstance in which ventricular standstill may occur as a physiologic response to decreased body temperature. Hypothermic patients may tolerate the arrhythmia for a relatively long time because of the decrease in metabolism that prevents tissue damage. Usually, hypothermia is treated with rapid rewarming and CPR. Remember, a patient with hypothermia may only appear clinically dead because of depressed cerebral blood flow and oxygen requirements.

Signs and symptoms

Ventricular standstill usually occurs suddenly, although the patient may experience faintness immediately before the heart stops. The patient loses consciousness within a few seconds and becomes pulseless, with absent or ineffective respirations. Agonal respiratory effort may continue only briefly. If ventricular standstill is preceded by a bradyarrhythmia such as AV block, your patient may display the signs and symptoms of decreased CO until he totally loses consciousness. Early signs and symptoms of decreased CO include:
- dizziness
- hypotension
- confusion
- weakness

Characteristics of ventricular standstill

Rate: none
Rhythm: none
P wave: none
PR interval: none
QRS complex: none

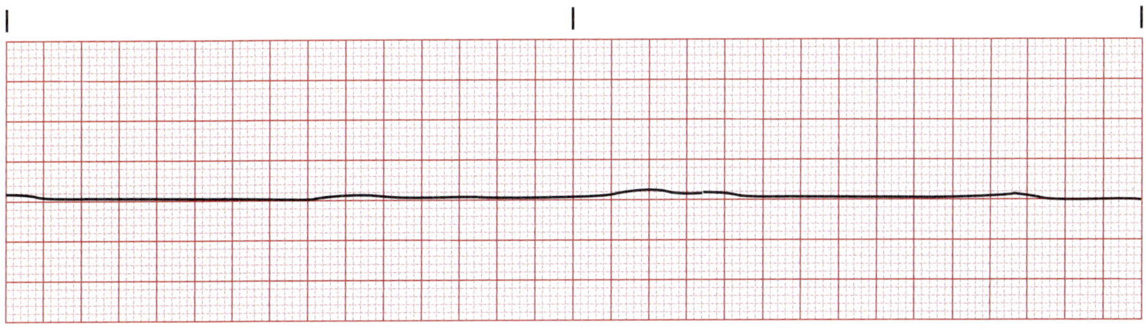

- cool, clammy skin
- chest pain
- dyspnea
- anxiety.

For your patient to have any chance of survival, his ventricular standstill must be recognized and treated immediately with appropriate resuscitative measures.

With ventricular standstill, your patient's ECG will show an absence of electrical activity. The heart rate can't be determined because there is no heartbeat. And the rhythm is nonexistent. Ventricular standstill appears as a straight line on the cardiac monitor (see *Characteristics of ventricular standstill*).

If complete heart block is present, the patient may have random P waves resulting from electrical activity in the atria that doesn't conduct to the ventricles.

However, the PR interval is not measurable because ventricular standstill produces no R waves. Also, the arrhythmia doesn't produce any QRS complexes.

Ventricular standstill has no pacemaker. However, fine ventricular fibrillation sometimes is mistaken for ventricular standstill. With fine ventricular fibrillation, electrical impulses do originate in the ventricles. Distinguishing the two arrhythmias is important because ventricular fibrillation may respond readily to treatment with defibrillation.

To rule out ventricular fibrillation, check your patient's rhythm in at least two different leads on the ECG monitor. QRS complexes may become apparent only if your patient is having a low-voltage ventricular tachycardia or coarse ventricular fibrillation.

Treatment

Because of the arrhythmia's seriousness, ventricular standstill always requires emergency treatment. And the first step in the treatment is quick assessment of the patient and the monitoring device. The flat line on your patient's ECG monitor may indicate ventricular standstill and full cardiac arrest. However, it also may indicate poor electrode contact. So check your patient for improper electrode placement and problems with his cardiac monitor. If he's unresponsive, open his airway, call for help, and begin CPR.

The goals of treatment are to maintain circulation to the patient's vital organs and to establish an airway. Your patient needs endotracheal intubation, high concentrations of oxygen, and immediate I.V. access. Typically, defibrillation isn't used to treat ventricular standstill unless fine ventricular fibrillation is suspected.

Even with early resuscitation and correct treatment, few patients fully recover from ventricular standstill. Resuscitation is most likely to be successful when ventricular standstill is caused by an event that can be corrected immediately, such as choking. Even then, the airway must be established quickly.

Depending on the patient's condition, a physician also may implement other emergency treatments to resuscitate the patient. Common treatments include transcutaneous pacing and drug therapy.

Transcutaneous pacing

Your patient may receive transcutaneous pacing, a noninvasive form of pacing commonly used as an emergency intervention because it can be initiated rapidly. Transcutaneous pacing provides pulses of electrical energy to the ventricles to stimulate ventricular contractions. This electrical energy is delivered to the heart through pacing electrodes placed on the patient's skin.

Drug therapy

The physician may prescribe epinephrine, a cardiac stimulant, for ventricular standstill. Usually, epinephrine is prescribed as a 1-mg I.V. push that may be repeated every 3 to 5 minutes. This drug is sometimes given through the endotracheal tube, where it's readily absorbed through the pulmonary vasculature. And the dose of epinephrine is increased as CPR continues.

A physician also may prescribe atropine, although the drug's effectiveness is diminished when ventricular standstill results from prolonged ischemia and mechanical injury to the myocardium. Atropine is given at 1 mg as an I.V. push every 3 to 5 minutes, up to a total of 0.04 mg/kg of body weight.

If your patient has preexisting hyperkalemia, the physician may prescribe sodium bicarbonate. Usually, this drug is administered by I.V. push at 1 mEq/kg. However, give this drug cautiously because administering it during CPR may cause rebound alkalosis.

Complications

Typically, few patients recover after the heart completely stops from ventricular standstill. Prompt treatment with CPR and transcutaneous pacing may increase your patient's chances of survival. However, a patient who does survive an episode of ventricular standstill may have severe complications because of decreased circulation to vital organs.

If the arrhythmia denies your patient's brain oxygen for more than 3 minutes, he may experience CNS damage. Because of oxygen deprivation, many survivors of ventricular standstill remain in a comatose state after reestablishing a normal sinus rhythm.

Your patient's heart may undergo infarction resulting from reduced blood flow through the coronary arteries. He also may develop chronic renal failure after resuscitation from cardiac arrest.

Nursing considerations

The success of resuscitating your patient with ventricular standstill depends on several factors, including:

- the setting in which the arrhythmia occurs
- the cause of his arrhythmia
- his health before the arrhythmia began.

Although ventricular standstill has the lowest survival rate of any cardiac arrhythmia, your patient has a better chance of survival if he receives CPR immediately after the arrhythmia begins. If the cause of the arrhythmia is easily reversible, as with an airway obstruction, your patient's chances of survival improve even more.

Other correctable underlying conditions include electrolyte imbalances, toxic reactions to drugs, and severe metabolic disturbances. While treating your patient for ventricular standstill, recall his clinical status before the arrhythmia. Remember that a patient with advanced cardiac disease and noncardiac problems, such as renal failure, pneumonia, sepsis, diabetes mellitus, and cancer, may not be successfully resuscitated, regardless of how quickly you begin resuscitative treatment. However, despite this grim prognosis, continue to treat your patient with ventricular standstill as though he'll survive.

If your patient survives an episode of ventricular standstill, his recovery may be a lengthy ordeal. As necessary, provide airway support. Carefully monitor his heart rate and vital signs to detect complications such as heart failure and an MI. Also, administer drug therapy, as prescribed.

Patient teaching

If your patient's ventricular standstill resulted from noncardiac causes such as renal failure, acute CNS disease, and uncontrolled infection, his treatment after resuscitation depends on the underlying disease. However, patients with such conditions have a survival rate of less than 10% after an in-hospital episode of ventricular standstill.

If your patient is successfully resuscitated, teach him about his disease and its treatment during his hospital stay. His continued survival may depend on his compliance with antiarrhythmic drug therapy and regular follow-up with his physician. Teach him about the doses, actions, adverse effects, and interactions of his drugs and the importance of following physical-activity guidelines and diet constraints, as prescribed. Also, make sure he knows the following:

- how to check his pulse and blood pressure
- when to contact his physician
- when to call an ambulance.

Your patient and his family will need emotional support. Help ease their fears and concerns by providing information about supportive therapies, invasive monitoring, and complicated procedures he may undergo. Encourage family members to learn CPR. Also, provide the family with regular reports on your patient's condition and prognosis. Whenever possible, family members should be allowed at the patient's bedside.

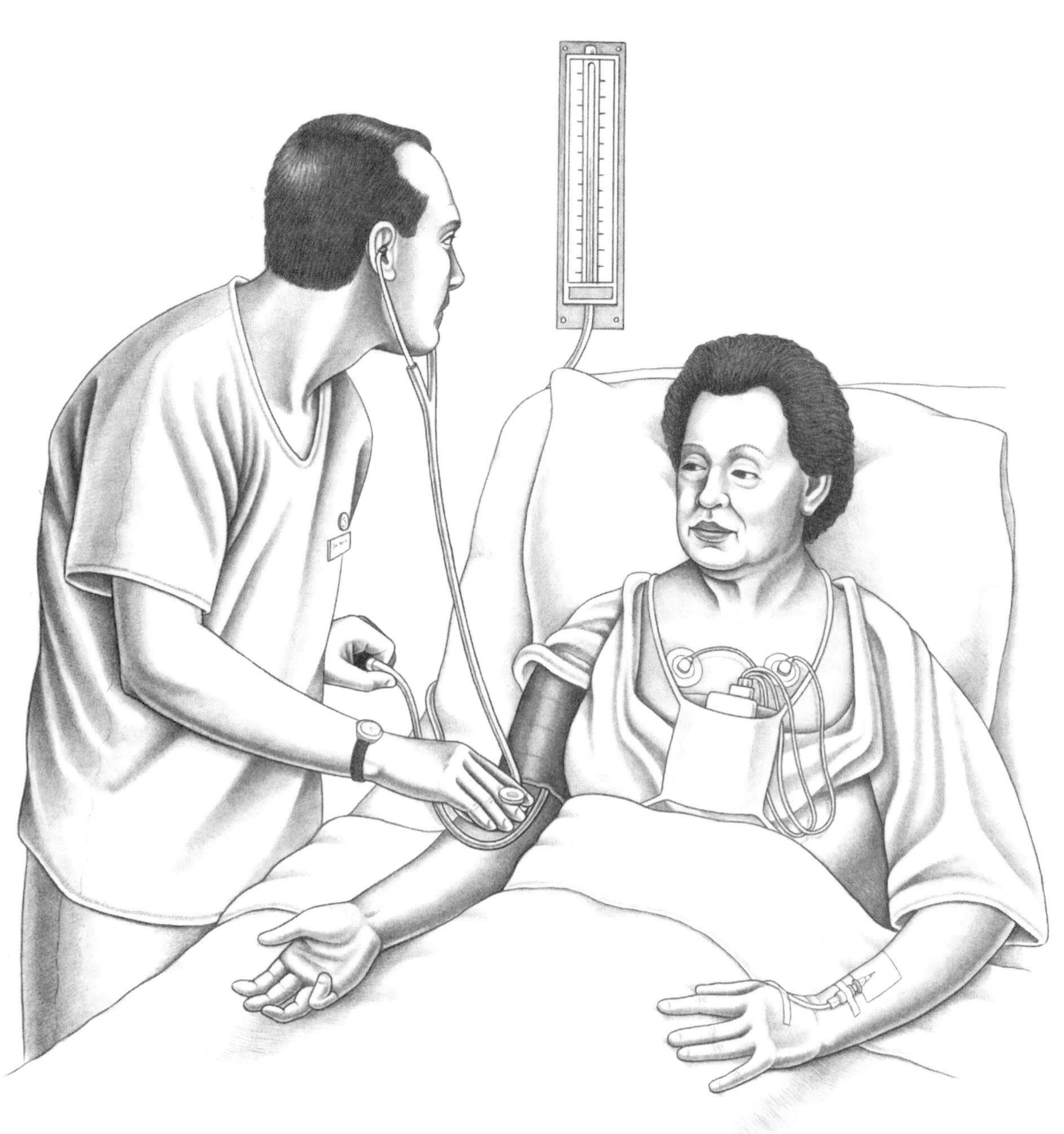

7

Atrioventricular Blocks

Atrioventricular (AV) blocks cover a wide range—from a mere delay in impulse conduction through the AV node to a complete blockage of impulse conduction down to the ventricles. And the range of implications for patients is just as wide.

Someone with the mildest form of AV block may not even know she has it. Or if she does know, the problem may be fairly easy to control. Someone with the most serious form, however, is at risk for seizures, coma, and death.

Unfortunately, if left untreated, any AV block can eventually cause serious complications because the less serious types can progress to the more serious types. That's why you need to know how to recognize all four types of AV block—first degree, second degree type I, second degree type II, and third degree—and how and when to respond appropriately.

First-degree atrioventricular block

The least serious of the AV blocks, first-degree AV block occurs when the AV junction delays the transmission of impulses from the atria to the ventricles longer than normal. Because transmission is only delayed and not completely blocked, first-degree AV block is really a conduction delay rather than a true arrhythmia.

Pathophysiology

The most common causes of first-degree AV block include AV node ischemia, vagal stimulation, a toxic reaction to certain drugs, and electrolyte imbalances.

Atrioventricular node ischemia

Normally, the AV node receives oxygenated blood from the right coronary artery. But if this artery becomes partially occluded or spastic (such as during an episode of angina) or if it becomes totally occluded (as with an acute inferior-wall myocardial infarction [MI]), the AV node can become ischemic, resulting in first-degree AV block.

Vagal stimulation

First-degree AV block may result from increased vagal tone. In the sinoatrial (SA) node, the AV node, and the atria, the supply of vagal fibers is dense. And because the vagus nerve innervates the gastrointestinal (GI) system, the vagal fibers in the heart can be stimulated during a GI event such as vomiting, gagging, or straining during a bowel movement.

If the vagus nerve is stimulated, the parasympathetic nervous system springs into action, releasing the neurotransmitter acetylcholine. Acetylcholine activates the cholinergic receptors, producing a cardiac inhibitory effect that decreases the speed of impulse conduction through the AV node.

Drug toxicity

First-degree AV block may result from the toxic effects of drugs prescribed for cardiovascular disease, such as digoxin, beta-blockers, and calcium channel blockers. First-degree AV block can also result from toxic blood levels of a tricyclic antidepressant.

Digoxin

Digoxin promotes the accumulation of calcium within heart cells, which can lead to first-degree AV block by slowing conduction through the AV node. This drug also can cause many other arrhythmias, such as ventricular fibrillation and ventricular tachycardia. And these arrhythmias can occur in conjunction with first-degree AV block, further complicating it.

Beta-blockers and calcium channel blockers

A toxic reaction to a beta-blocker or a calcium channel blocker can cause hypoglycemia and hyperkalemia. Both of these imbalances can alter myocardial conductivity, resulting in first-degree AV block.

Tricyclic antidepressants

In some patients, first-degree AV block may result from toxic blood levels of a tricyclic antidepressant. Within 2 hours of ingesting a tricyclic antidepressant, a patient can develop other conduction abnormalities, such as ventricular tachycardia, a widened QRS complex, a prolonged QT interval, and both second-degree and third-degree AV blocks. Because tricyclic antidepressants have a long half-life, cardiovascular reactions can occur long after your patient has stopped taking them.

Electrolyte imbalances

Various electrolyte imbalances, whether caused by a toxic reaction to a drug or some other condition, may alter myocardial conductivity and cause first-degree AV block. In particular, first-degree AV block may occur in patients who have abnormal blood levels of potassium, calcium, and magnesium.

Hypokalemia and hyperkalemia

Normally, a patient's blood potassium level is 3.5 to 5 mEq/L. When her blood potassium level becomes abnormally low or high, her myocardial conductivity may become altered, leading to first-degree AV block.

Hypokalemia commonly results from diuretic therapy. Other common causes of hypokalemia include conditions that increase GI losses of potassium, including vomiting, nasogastric suction, and diarrhea. Also, the metabolic alkalosis that accompanies these fluid losses can contribute to hypokalemia.

Hyperkalemia may occur in a patient taking a drug such as an angiotensin-converting enzyme inhibitor, a potassium sparing diuretic, a beta-blocker, heparin, or digoxin. Renal insufficiency and renal failure can lead to hyperkalemia. Another common but generally overlooked cause of hyperkalemia is the use of potassium supplements.

Hypocalcemia and hypercalcemia

If your patient has first-degree AV block, assess her blood calcium level. Normally, it should be 9 to 10.5 mg/dL. If your patient's level is abnormally low or high, either hypocalcemia or hypercalcemia may be the cause of her AV block.

Common causes of hypocalcemia include hypoparathyroidism and massive blood transfusions (more than 6 units in 24 hours). Hypercalcemia may result from hyperthyroidism and the use of thiazide diuretics.

Hypomagnesemia and hypermagnesemia

Normally, a patient's magnesium level is 1.2 to 2 mEq/L. If your patient has an abnormally low or high magnesium level, hypomagnesemia or hypermagnesemia may be causing her first-degree AV block, either directly or indirectly.

Typically, hypomagnesemia indirectly causes first-degree AV block by enhancing the toxic effect of a digitalis glycoside. Hypomagnesemia commonly occurs in critically ill patients and in those with diarrhea, a history of alcoholism, and poor nutrition. Hypomagnesemia also may result from the use of a diuretic. And the condition is commonly accompanied by hypokalemia.

Hypermagnesemia may cause your patient's first-degree AV block directly, by altering myocardial conductivity, or indirectly, by binding with calcium and increasing blood calcium levels within the heart cells. Common causes of hypermagnesemia include the use of magnesium salts, laxatives that contain magnesium, and antacids. Hypermagnesemia may also result from magnesium loss in muscle tissue, which is commonly caused by crushing injuries, soft-tissue trauma, and burns.

Characteristics of first-degree atrioventricular block

Rate: depends on underlying rhythm
Rhythm: regular or irregular
P wave: smooth, rounded, upright
PR interval: > 0.2 second
QRS complex: < 0.12 second

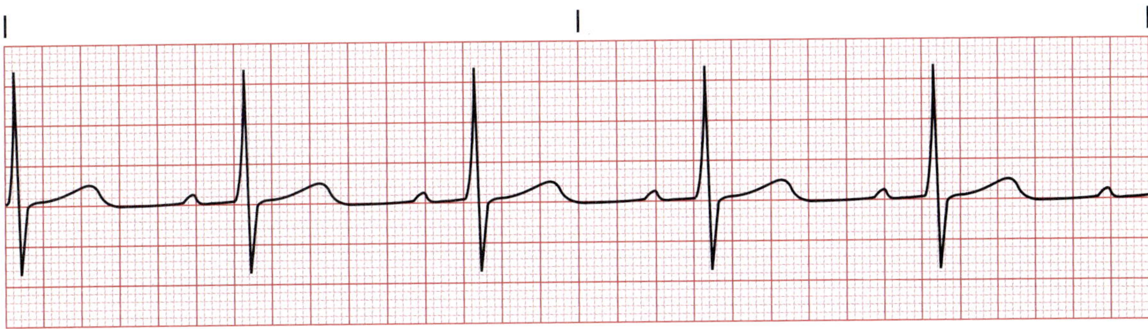

Signs and symptoms

Most patients with a first-degree AV block are asymptomatic. However, an underlying arrhythmia may cause your patient to experience signs and symptoms. For example, if your patient has first-degree AV block with sinus tachycardia or sinus bradycardia, she may experience chest pain and dyspnea and have a decreased level of consciousness.

Typically, with first-degree AV block, the only abnormality on your patient's electrocardiogram (ECG) is a PR interval greater than 0.2 second. The P waves appear normal, occur regularly, and are followed by a QRS complex. The QRS complex has a normal duration unless the patient has an underlying intraventricular conduction defect or a bundle branch block (see *Characteristics of first-degree atrioventricular block*).

With first-degree AV block, your patient's heart rate depends on her underlying rhythm. Usually, her rhythm will be regular, unless she also has a sinus arrhythmia. For example, her underlying sinus rhythm may be bradycardic (less than 60 beats per minute [bpm]), normal (60 to 100 bpm), or tachycardic (greater than 100 bpm). If your patient has such a sinus arrhythmia, her heart rate increases when she inhales and decreases when she exhales.

If your patient has an underlying tachycardia, her P waves may be embedded in the T wave of the preceding complex. And the faster her heart rate, the more likely her P waves will be embedded in the T wave.

Treatment

Because patients with first-degree AV block usually are asymptomatic, they typically don't require treatment for the conduction delay. However, if your patient experiences the signs and symptoms of first-degree AV block, the physician may treat it with atropine, dopamine, or a pacemaker. The physician also may focus treatment on correcting the underlying cause of the arrhythmia.

Atropine

First-degree AV block may occur with underlying bradycardia. In cases of vagal stimulation, both the SA and AV nodes can be affected by the release of acetylcholine. The SA node may slow impulse generation, producing sinus bradycardia, which alone can be profound. And impulse transmission through the AV node may become so delayed that it produces extremely prolonged PR intervals, adding first-degree AV block to the sinus bradycardia.

If your patient has a PR interval greater than 0.5 second, the physician may prescribe atropine to accelerate conduction through the AV node. A physician also may prescribe the drug for a patient who is at risk for first-degree AV block progressing to second-degree and third-degree AV block, which may occur if your patient experiences an acute MI. Typically, you'll administer 0.5 to 1 mg of atropine I.V. every 3 to 5 minutes to a total dose of 0.03 mg/kg.

Dopamine

If your patient with first-degree AV block also has low blood pressure caused by bradycardia, the physician may prescribe dopamine. Typically, you'll mix one or two ampules of the drug (400 mg per ampule) in 250 ml of dextrose 5% in water (D_5W), yielding a concentration of 1,600 or 3,200 µg/ml. The initial rate of infusion is usually 1 to 5 µg/kg/minute; the maintenance infusion rate is 2 to 10 µg/minute.

Pacemaker

Because most patients don't experience the signs and symptoms of first-degree AV block, a physician may not insert a permanent pacemaker unless the arrhythmia progresses to second-degree and third-degree AV block. However, if drug therapy is unsuccessful in a symptomatic patient with bradycardia and first-degree AV block, the physician may insert a temporary pacemaker.

A transcutaneous pacemaker can be applied quickly and conveniently at the bedside without special equipment. However, transcutaneous pacing requires a significantly higher current output than transvenous pacing. This increased current may cause chest-wall discomfort and skin burns. And the procedure can be extremely painful, in many cases requiring the use of I.V. analgesics and sedatives such as short-acting benzodiazepines.

With transcutaneous pacing, the heart is stimulated by two cutaneous electrodes: one to the left of the sternum and centered as close as possible on the point of maximal impulse and the other to the left of the thoracic spinal column and directly behind the anterior electrode. These electrodes deliver an electrical impulse that's conducted through the chest wall to stimulate the myocardium (see *Positioning the electrodes for transcutaneous pacing*).

Activate the device as prescribed by the physician, usually at a rate of 60 to 80 bpm. You may have to increase the output slowly until capture is achieved. You'll recognize capture when a pacer spike followed by a wide QRS complex is evident on your patient's ECG.

Underlying causes

If the cause of your patient's first-degree AV block is known, a physician may treat it to alleviate the arrhythmia. Commonly, a physician may treat first-degree AV block by treating a patient for a toxic reaction to a drug or an electrolyte imbalance.

Drug toxicity

The treatment for first-degree AV block resulting from a toxic reaction to digoxin depends on the extent of your patient's hemodynamic stability. If she remains hemodynamically stable, potassium and magnesium therapy, in conjunction with volume replacement, may correct the toxic reaction within a few hours.

If your patient has a severe reaction, a physician may prescribe I.V. digoxin immune FAB, which binds to free digoxin, creating an inactive compound that's excreted in the urine. Digoxin immune FAB begins to take effect in minutes and completely reverses the toxic effects within 30 minutes.

Each vial of digoxin immune FAB contains 38 mg, which should be reconstituted with 4 ml of sterile water and then diluted with 0.9% sodium chloride solution and administered I.V. over 15 to 30 minutes. Each vial of digoxin immune FAB binds 0.6 mg of digoxin. Usually, three to five vials are enough to reverse the toxic effects. And a patient's blood digoxin levels typically rise dramatically after this therapy.

For a toxic reaction to a beta-blocker, a physician may prescribe an infusion of 500 to 1,000 ml of 0.9% sodium chloride solution. A physician also may prescribe an epinephrine infusion at 2 to 100 µg/minute before, after, or in conjunction with glucagon, an antihypoglycemic.

For symptomatic hypotension caused by a toxic reaction to a calcium channel blocker, a physician may prescribe 500 to 1,000 ml of 0.9% sodium chloride solution. The next best treatment for your patient who fails to respond to the fluid therapy is 5 to 10 ml of I.V. calcium chloride.

If your patient has overdosed on tricyclic antidepressants, the physician may order activated charcoal for gastric decontamination. Gastric lavage is usually used if the patient is unconscious.

Positioning the electrodes for transcutaneous pacing

Transcutaneous pacing is commonly prescribed to treat symptomatic bradycardia, which may result from an atrioventricular block, and to maintain a patient's heart rate during an emergency. To perform transcutaneous pacing, place the two electrodes in the following positions:

- left of the sternum, centered as close as possible on the point of maximal impulse
- left of the thoracic spinal column, directly behind the anterior electrode.

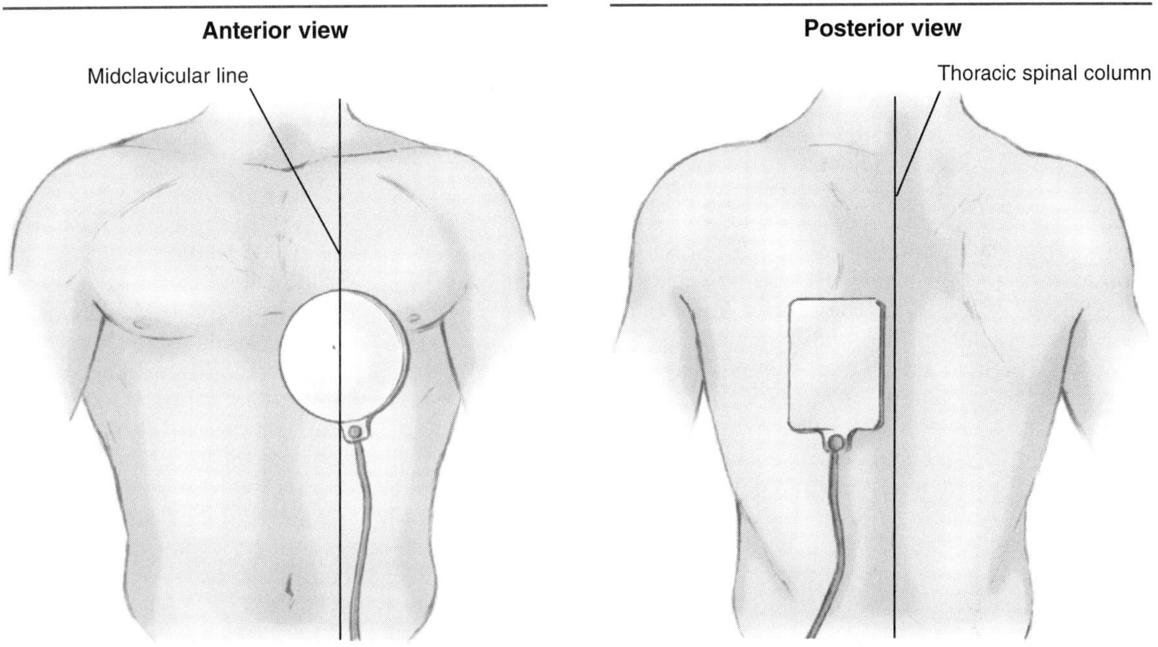

Electrolyte imbalances

If your patient has hypokalemia, you'll typically give 10 mEq of potassium chloride diluted in 50 to 100 ml of D_5W over a minimum of 30 minutes. This dose can be repeated, as prescribed.

If administering potassium chloride, reassess your patient's blood potassium level every hour until it measures 4 to 4.5 mEq/L. With hypokalemia, the physician may prescribe as much as 5 to 10 mEq/hour. The physician also may prescribe oral potassium supplements to treat less acute cases of hypokalemia.

If your patient has elevated blood potassium levels, the physician may prescribe I.V. calcium or an infusion of hypertonic 0.9% sodium chloride solution. This treatment will help correct the conduction defects caused by hyperkalemia. Insulin and glucose can be used to shift potassium from the extracellular to the intracellular compartments, which helps reduce the toxic effects of elevated blood potassium levels. The physician may prescribe I.V. furosemide to enhance potassium excretion by the kidneys. An exchange agent such as sodium polystyrene sulfonate effectively removes potassium. Sodium polystyrene sulfonate liquid is usually given with sorbitol to enhance potassium loss in the bowel. A 25-g dose may remove 12.5 to 25 mEq of potassium, but the onset of action takes 1 to 2 hours.

If your patient's first-degree AV block results from hypocalcemia, be sure to check her most current albumin level. Calcium binds to protein, so the calcium level will be falsely low if your patient's blood albumin level is below normal. If your patient with first-degree AV block has hypocalcemia, the physician may prescribe up to 90 mg of elemental calcium I.V., or one ampule of 10% calcium gluconate diluted in at least 100 ml of D_5W, infused over 10 minutes.

Be prepared to follow the initial dose with a continuous infusion of 0.5 to 2 mg/kg of elemental calcium mixed in 1,000 ml of D_5W infused over the next 6 hours.

Oral doses of calcium may be prescribed at 1 to 1.5 g/day. Oral calcium comes in various forms. The elemental calcium content varies with the calcium salt preparation; for example, calcium carbonate is 40% elemental calcium. So your patient's oral dose will need to be adjusted according to the amount of elemental calcium provided in each product.

Hypercalcemia commonly requires correction by hydration with 1 to 2 L of 0.9% sodium chloride solution, along with 80 to 100 mg of I.V. furosemide every 1 to 2 hours until normal calcium levels are achieved. This fluid and diuretic combination therapy decreases calcium reabsorption in the loop of Henle.

For hypomagnesemia, the physician may prescribe 1 to 2 g of magnesium sulfate diluted in 50 to 100 ml of D_5W infused over 15 to 60 minutes. Typically, magnesium sulfate is given as an infusion of 0.5 to 1 g/hour for 24 hours, as indicated, after the initial bolus.

Treatment for hypermagnesemia may include 10 ml of a 10% calcium gluconate solution, glucose and insulin, and forced diuresis with large volumes of 0.9% sodium chloride solution.

Complications

Usually, first-degree AV block itself doesn't cause any acute complications. It can, however, progress to second-degree and third-degree AV block, especially in a susceptible patient, such as one who has had an acute MI. And a patient typically may experience complications that, although associated with first-degree AV block, actually result from the underlying cause of the arrhythmia.

If an acute MI has caused first-degree AV block, watch for acute complications, such as ventricular tachycardia, ventricular fibrillation, cardiogenic shock, worsening heart failure, pericarditis, cardiac tamponade, and ruptured papillary muscle.

If a toxic reaction to digoxin has caused first-degree AV block, complications may include fatigue, blurred vision, color perception disturbances, weakness, nausea, vomiting, and abdominal pain. A toxic reaction to digoxin can lead to many arrhythmias besides first-degree AV block, including atrial tachycardia, atrial fibrillation, junctional tachycardia, premature ventricular contractions (PVCs), ventricular tachycardia, and ventricular fibrillation.

First-degree AV block commonly results from a toxic reaction to a beta-blocker or a calcium channel blocker, which depresses myocardial contractility, reduces heart rate, and alters mental status. Many patients develop hypotension, lethargy, coma, and seizures. And your patient's first-degree AV block may progress to second-degree and third-degree AV block and cardiac arrest.

If a toxic reaction to a tricyclic antidepressant has caused first-degree AV block, your patient may have widened QRS complexes and ventricular arrhythmias. Because of the extreme cardiotoxic effects of these drugs, high blood levels can also lead to seizures, coma, and death.

If an electrolyte imbalance has caused first-degree AV block, complications usually result from the effects of the imbalance on other body systems. Most of these imbalances involve cardiac complications besides first-degree AV block and also affect the neuromuscular and GI systems. Hypokalemia can cause skeletal muscle weakness and GI problems such as paralytic ileus and constipation. Hyperkalemia can lead to numbness, weakness, flaccid paralysis, ventricular fibrillation, and cardiac arrest.

If hypercalcemia causes first-degree AV block, your patient may experience complications such as a decreased level of consciousness, flaccidity, nausea, vomiting, and constipation. Hypercalcemia can enhance the toxic effects of digoxin, cause muscle tremors and seizures, and decrease myocardial contractility, leading to cardiac arrest.

Hypomagnesemia can produce first-degree AV block and other conduction disturbances, such as widening of the QRS complex. Other potential complications of hypomagnesemia include lethargy, coma, and impaired respirations.

Nursing considerations

If your patient develops first-degree AV block, document it with an ECG tracing. Measure and document the PR interval. Determine whether the underlying sinus rhythm is a normal sinus rhythm, sinus tachycardia, or sinus bradycardia. Also, assess your patient's vital signs immediately and evaluate her for any changes that indicate hemodynamic instability.

Because bradycardia can quickly lead to hemodynamic instability, assess your patient immediately for signs and symptoms such as chest pain, dyspnea, and decreased level of consciousness. Also, assess her for hypotension, progressively worsening heart failure, and the development of an acute MI. If any of these signs and symptoms is present, notify the physician immediately and be prepared to administer atropine, as prescribed. Establish I.V. access immediately. And start infusing D_5W, 0.9% sodium chloride solution, or other fluids to keep the vein open. Begin supplemental oxygen at 4 to 6 L/minute by nasal cannula, as prescribed.

First-degree AV block commonly results from myocardial ischemia, injury, or infarction, specifically in the AV junctional area. Assess your patient for the signs and symptoms of myocardial ischemia, injury, and infarction, including diaphoresis, indigestion, nausea, vomiting, dyspnea, hypotension, and pain in the chest, shoulder, arm, neck, and jaw.

The pain caused by ischemia and an infarction requires immediate attention. If your patient is normotensive, give her one tablet of sublingual nitroglycerin every 5 minutes, as prescribed, up to three doses or until her pain is relieved.

If nitroglycerin relieves the pain, the patient is probably experiencing angina. However, remember that other conditions, such as esophageal spasm, also respond to nitrates.

If nitroglycerin doesn't alleviate your patient's pain, she may be experiencing an acute MI. As ordered, administer 1 to 3 mg of morphine I.V. over 1 to 5 minutes, repeating doses until the pain has been relieved. Usually, nitroglycerin is administered I.V. at 10 to 20 μg/minute and increased by 5 to 10 μg/minute every 5 to 10 minutes.

Obtain a 12-lead ECG as soon as possible, and watch for the development of Q waves or changes in ST segments and T waves in all 12 leads. Because first-degree AV block can be caused by partial occlusion, total occlusion, and spasm of the right coronary artery, look specifically for the development of Q waves, elevation of the ST segment, and inversion of the T wave in leads II, III, and aV_F.

If your patient's first-degree AV block results from injury to the AV node, observe her ECG for progressively worsening conduction delays. Commonly, these delays result from valvular heart disease and heart surgery. If the PR interval becomes extremely prolonged or if your patient develops second-degree or third-degree AV block, the physician may insert a permanent pacemaker, depending on how well your patient tolerates the block. Assess your patient's clinical response to the arrhythmia. Note her level of consciousness, steadiness of gait, vital signs, and activity tolerance.

For a toxic reaction to digoxin, assess your patient for concurrent arrhythmias and their related signs and symptoms. Administer digoxin immune FAB, as prescribed.

If a toxic reaction to a beta-blocker has caused your patient's first-degree AV block, assess her laboratory values, especially her blood potassium levels. Also, assess her ECG for the signs and symptoms of the arrhythmia.

If a toxic reaction to a calcium channel blocker has caused your patient's first-degree AV block, assess her for the signs and symptoms of other related arrhythmias, such as bradycardia. Because calcium channel blockers may cause liver or kidney dysfunction, the physician may order a blood chemistry profile or blood electrolyte levels to determine whether an imbalance is causing your patient's arrhythmia. So be prepared to obtain a specimen for blood testing (see *Blood testing: Correct venipuncture technique,* page 130).

Pay close attention to your patient's arterial blood gas (ABG) levels. Remember that an increase of 0.1 in arterial pH reflects decreased blood potassium levels by approximately 0.4 mEq/L. Other causes of hypokalemia include dialysis treatments, problems in renal regulation of potassium, and excess mineralocorticoid levels, which can result from Cushing's syndrome, hyperaldosteronism, and corticosteroid use.

The rapid fluid shifts that occur after accidental and surgical traumas can also induce a hypokalemic state. In patients with multiple injuries, hypokalemia usually starts within 1 hour and may resolve within 24 hours after the trauma.

If your patient has hypokalemia, assess her for possible causes of fluid loss. Also, assess her ABG levels for metabolic alkalosis. Then, correct volume depletion and replace potassium orally or I.V., as prescribed.

If your patient with first-degree AV block has hyperkalemia, assess her drug history. Find out if she's taking a prescribed potassium supplement. Note whether she takes an over-the-counter nu-

Blood testing: Correct venipuncture technique

If a physician suspects that your patient's arrhythmia results from a toxic reaction to a drug, you may need to draw a specimen for a blood test. To perform the venipuncture, align the needle with the vein and insert it at a 30-degree angle with the bevel side up, as shown. Remember, improper technique can result in hemolysis, which may lead to inaccurate results.

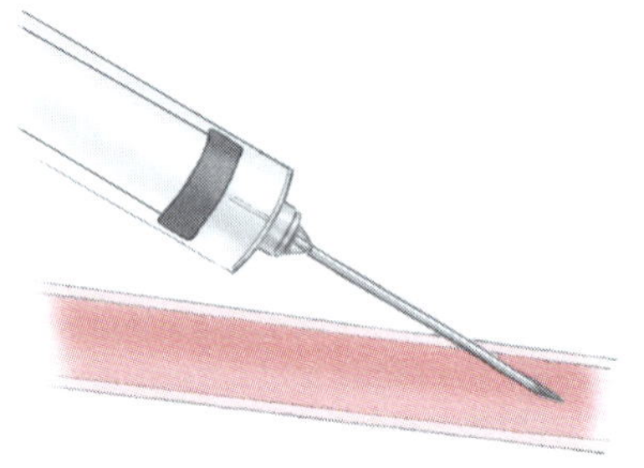

tritional supplement with added potassium. Also, withhold potassium supplements until you consult with the physician.

Assess your patient for any condition that may stimulate the vagus nerve, such as vomiting, gagging, straining during a bowel movement, and forceful coughing. If you suspect that vagal stimulation is causing your patient's first-degree AV block, notify the physician of your assessment. You may alleviate the arrhythmia by administering an antiemetic, laxative, enema, or cough suppressant, as prescribed.

Second-degree atrioventricular block type I

Second-degree AV block is classified as either a type I block (also called Mobitz I or Wenckebach block) or a type II block. In both types, the SA node produces impulses normally, but the AV node fails to send one or more of these impulses through to the ventricles. However, second-degree AV block type I produces a different rhythm than second-degree AV block type II.

Pathophysiology

Second-degree AV block type I typically results from an abnormally long refractory period in the cells of the AV junction. As you know, impulses generated by the SA node typically are slowed as they pass through the AV junction. However, with second-degree AV block type I, the AV junction holds the impulses for varying lengths of time with each cardiac cycle.

The gradually increasing impulse delay appears on the ECG as a specific pattern: the AV node progressively slows its transmission time with each cardiac cycle, producing PR intervals that grow longer and longer. As the conduction delay increases, the P wave moves closer and closer to the T wave of the preceding cycle. The conduction delay continues to progress until the atrial contraction disrupts the refractory time of the preceding cardiac cycle. This pattern appears on the ECG as a P wave so close to the T wave of the preceding complex that it isn't followed by a QRS complex of its own. As the conduction system recovers from the disruption in the refractory period, the ECG pattern begins again.

Second-degree AV block type I may result from many of the same conditions that can cause first-degree AV block, including AV node ischemia, vagal stimulation, a toxic reaction to a drug, and an electrolyte imbalance. Second-degree AV block type I also may result as a complication of cardiac surgery and certain cardiovascular diseases.

Atrioventricular node ischemia

Second-degree AV block type I most commonly results from ischemia in the AV junctional area. Normally, the AV node receives oxygenated blood from the right coronary artery. If this artery is partially occluded or in spasm—such as during an episode of angina—the AV junction can become ischemic, causing a transient second-degree AV block type I. If the artery becomes totally occluded—such as in an acute inferior-wall MI—second-degree AV block type I may last 72 to 96 hours.

Vagal stimulation

Second-degree AV block type I commonly accompanies increased vagal tone. As you know, stimulation of the vagus nerve can occur during GI events such as vomiting, gagging, and straining during a bowel movement. If the vagus nerve is stimulated, the parasympathetic nervous system springs into action, releasing the neurotransmitter acetylcholine. Acetylcholine activates cholinergic receptors, producing a cardiac inhibitory effect, which slows conduction through the AV node and can cause a second-degree AV block rhythm.

Drug toxicity

As with first-degree AV block, second-degree AV block type I may result from the toxic effects of drugs prescribed for cardiovascular diseases, such as digoxin, beta-blockers, and calcium channel blockers.

With a toxic reaction to digoxin, impulse conduction may be overly depressed, resulting in a second-degree AV block type I. And if your patient has decreased renal function, she may develop a toxic reaction even with therapeutic blood digoxin levels.

In patients who are taking a beta-blocker or a calcium channel blocker, second-degree AV block type I may occur as an adverse effect of drug therapy. In such patients, the benefit of using drug therapy to terminate supraventricular tachycardia or a ventricular arrhythmia may outweigh the risk of developing second-degree AV block type I, which is commonly benign and asymptomatic. For such a patient, observe her ECG tracing and document changes in the length of the PR interval. The physician may decide not to treat the arrhythmia until your patient's PR interval becomes progressively longer or until she experiences adverse signs and symptoms such as bradycardia and hypotension.

Second-degree AV block type I also may occur in patients who've overdosed on tricyclic antidepressants. These drugs inhibit fast sodium channels, and they slow phase 0 depolarization and the onset of cardiac contraction. This slowing of conduction can cause AV blocks as well as other serious arrhythmias.

Electrolyte imbalances

Normal cardiac function depends on ion currents across myocardial cell membranes. Action potential generation, impulse conduction, and myocardial contraction are all vulnerable to altered blood electrolyte levels. And as with first-degree AV block, second-degree AV block type I can result from hypokalemia, hyperkalemia, hypocalcemia, hypercalcemia, and hypermagnesemia, any of which may decrease conduction velocity in the AV node. Also, hyperkalemia, hypercalcemia, and hypomagnesemia can enhance the toxic effect of a digitalis glycoside.

Cardiovascular surgery

The AV node can be damaged during any type of heart surgery. In particular, a transient second-degree AV block rhythm may occur after cardiothoracic surgery because the heart's conduction system is irritable from ischemic changes until the myocardium fully recovers.

Cardiovascular diseases

Because of its location just above the tricuspid valve in the lower part of the atrial septum, the AV node can be injured by many heart and valve diseases, resulting in second-degree AV block type I and other AV blocks. Diseases that can affect the AV node include valvular heart diseases, rheumatic heart disease, endocarditis, cardiomyopathies, myocarditis, and congenital heart disease.

Signs and symptoms

Patients with second-degree AV block type I usually tolerate the arrhythmia well and don't experience any signs or symptoms. However, if your patient's ventricular rate drops significantly, she may experience the signs and symptoms of decreased cardiac output (CO), including chest pain, dyspnea, and decreased level of consciousness.

On an ECG, the hallmark of second-degree AV block type I is the repetitive cycle of progressively prolonged PR intervals followed by a P wave that isn't followed by a QRS complex. This cycle is called group beating (see *Characteristics of second-degree atrioventricular block type I*, page 132).

If you see an ECG with clusters of beats followed by pauses, suspect second-degree AV block type I. Typically, the pattern contains two, three, and four cardiac cycles with progressively prolonged PR intervals, although the pattern can include as many as 20 cardiac cycles with very slow progression of the PR interval before the pause.

Because impulses originate in the SA node, the P waves appear normal and occur at regular intervals. In cycles in which the P wave is followed by a QRS complex, the QRS is of normal duration unless the patient has an underlying intraventricular conduction defect or bundle branch block.

The R-R intervals are irregular and fall into a pattern with the PR intervals: the PR intervals progressively lengthen while the R-R intervals progressively shorten. Usually, the PR interval lengthens most significantly between the first and second cardiac cycles. After the first two cycles,

Characteristics of second-degree atrioventricular block type I

Atrial rate: 60 to 100 beats per minute
Ventricular rate: slower than atrial rate
Rhythm: irregular
P wave: smooth, rounded, upright; some not followed by QRS complex
PR interval: > 0.2 second; progressively lengthens until P wave doesn't conduct QRS complex, then pattern starts over
QRS complex: < 0.12 second

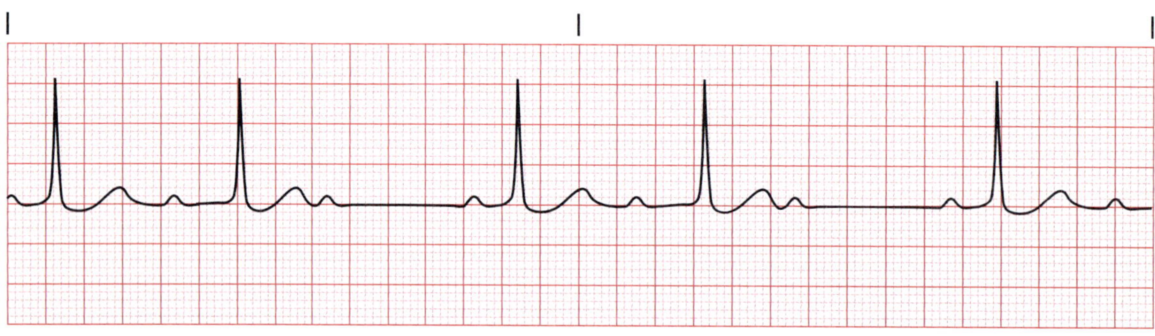

the PR interval continues to lengthen, but not to the same degree.

Second-degree AV block type I can be easily confused with other arrhythmias that cause pauses, such as nonconducted premature atrial contractions and SA exit block. The key difference is that the other arrhythmias lack progressively prolonged PR intervals.

Treatment

Second-degree AV block type I usually isn't a serious arrhythmia and doesn't require treatment. However, if your patient experiences signs and symptoms with the arrhythmia, the physician may order atropine, dopamine, epinephrine, or a pacemaker. As with first-degree AV block, the physician may also seek to alleviate second-degree AV block type I by treating its underlying cause.

Atropine

If your patient experiences the signs and symptoms of second-degree AV block type I, they probably result from underlying bradycardia. And if your patient's ventricular rate falls below 60 bpm, the physician may prescribe atropine to accelerate conduction through the AV node. Usually, atropine is prescribed only for patients who are symptomatic and at risk for having their second-degree AV block type I progress to second-degree AV block type II and third-degree AV block. Such a progression commonly occurs after an acute MI. As prescribed, 0.5 to 1 mg of atropine usually is administered I.V. every 3 to 5 minutes to a total dose of 0.03 mg/kg.

Dopamine

If your patient develops hypotension, which may result from underlying bradycardia, the physician may also order dopamine, a potent vasoconstrictor. As ordered, mix the contents of one or two ampules of dopamine (400 mg per ampule) in 250 ml of D_5W, yielding a concentration of 1,600 to 3,200 µg/ml. Usually, the initial rate of infusion is 1 to 5 µg/kg/minute, with a final dose of 5 to 20 µg/kg/minute. During the infusion, assess your patient's blood pressure as often as every 5 minutes. Also, titrate the dopamine infusion quickly, based on her response to therapy.

Epinephrine

If your patient experiences severe signs and symptoms of second-degree AV block type I, the physician may prescribe an epinephrine infusion instead of dopamine. Typically, you'll give 1 mg of the drug (1 ml of a 1:1,000 solution) added to 500 ml of 0.9% sodium chloride solution or D_5W. Usually, an initial infusion is 2 to 10 µg/minute.

Pacemaker

If drug therapy is unsuccessful in the symptomatic patient with bradycardia and second-degree AV block type I, the physician may use a temporary pacemaker, which may be either transcutaneous or transvenous. A transcutaneous pacemaker has several advantages. It can be initiated quickly and conveniently at the bedside and requires no special equipment such as a fluoroscope, which is required for transvenous pacing. However, transcutaneous pacing can be extremely painful. Your patient may require I.V. analgesics and sedatives such as short-acting benzodiazepines.

If your patient can't tolerate transcutaneous pacing, the physician may insert a transvenous pacemaker. With this procedure, the physician inserts a pacing catheter with a lead wire through a large vein into the right ventricle. Fluoroscopy commonly guides this process. If you are assisting in the procedure, be prepared to attach a pulse generator to the other end of the lead wire.

For either the transcutaneous or the transvenous approach to cardiac pacing, the physician usually activates the device at a rate of about 80 bpm. Then, the output is slowly increased until capture is achieved. Capture is evident when a pacer spike is followed by a wide QRS complex.

Underlying causes

As with first-degree AV block, a physician may alleviate second-degree AV block type I by treating the arrhythmia's underlying cause, which may be a toxic reaction to a drug or an electrolyte imbalance.

Drug toxicity

If a toxic reaction to digoxin has caused your patient's second-degree AV block type I and her condition is stable, potassium and magnesium therapy in conjunction with volume replacement may correct the toxic effects in a few hours. However, for a severe toxic reaction, the physician may prescribe digoxin immune FAB. Each vial of digoxin immune FAB binds 0.6 mg of digoxin. And, usually, three to five vials are enough to reverse the toxic effects.

If your patient's arrhythmia results from a toxic reaction to a beta-blocker, the physician may prescribe a bolus of 500 to 1,000 ml of 0.9% sodium chloride solution to treat hyperkalemia, a possible effect of the toxic reaction. The physician may prescribe 1 to 5 mg of glucagon for a hypoglycemic reaction. He also may prescribe an epinephrine infusion of 2 to 100 µg/minute before, after, or in conjunction with glucagon administration.

Usually, a physician treats tricyclic antidepressant overdose using gastric decontamination with activated charcoal. If your patient's condition is unstable, the physician may prescribe I.V. alkalinization therapy. Alkalinization decreases the nonprotein-bound form of the tricyclic molecule. For alkalinization, the physician may order 1 mEq/kg of sodium bicarbonate infused over 1 to 2 minutes. Your patient will probably receive an infusion of two ampules (50 to 100 mEq) of sodium bicarbonate in 0.9% sodium chloride solution at 150 to 200 ml/hour until her arterial pH reaches 7.5 to 7.55.

Electrolyte imbalances

For hypokalemia, treatment usually is focused on correcting volume depletion and replacing potassium, which can be administered I.V. or orally. Usually, a physician prescribes potassium I.V. as 10 mEq of potassium chloride diluted in 50 to 100 ml of D_5W, given over 1 hour. This dose can be repeated, as prescribed. When administering potassium chloride, recheck your patient's blood potassium level every 4 hours, as prescribed, or until the blood potassium level measures 4 to 4.5 mEq/L.

The physician also may prescribe an exchange agent such as sodium polystyrene sulfonate to remove potassium from the body. Typically, this drug is given with sorbitol to enhance potassium loss in the bowel. A 25-g dose removes 12.5 to 25 mEq of potassium.

For hypocalcemia, a physician typically prescribes 10 ml of 10% calcium gluconate or 10% calcium chloride administered I.V. at 1 to 2 ml/minute. If your patient's hypocalcemia is severe, the physician may order a constant infusion of elemental calcium at 15 to 20 mg/kg every 4 to 8 hours, at a rate of 15 to 20 mg/minute or less.

If your patient's second-degree AV block type I results from hypercalcemia, the physician may order 1 to 2 L of 0.9% sodium chloride solution to hydrate the patient and 80 to 100 mg of furosemide administered every 1 to 2 hours I.V. to decrease calcium reabsorption in the loop of Henle.

For hypomagnesemia, a physician usually prescribes 1 to 2 g of magnesium sulfate diluted in 50 to 100 ml of D_5W and administered over 15 to 60 minutes. This initial dose is followed by an infusion of 0.5 to 1 g/hour for 24 hours.

Treatment for hypermagnesemia may include 10 ml of a 10% calcium gluconate solution, glucose and insulin, and forced diuresis with large volumes of 0.9% sodium chloride solution.

Complications

Second-degree AV block type I itself doesn't usually cause complications. It can, however, progress to second-degree AV block type II and third-degree AV block, especially after an acute MI. Any complications that occur in conjunction with second-degree AV block type I typically result from the underlying cause of the arrhythmia.

If your patient's second-degree AV block type I results from a toxic reaction to digoxin, acute complications include the involvement of the CNS and GI system. Your patient may experience such signs and symptoms as blurred vision, halos, poor color perception, fatigue, weakness, nausea, vomiting, and abdominal pain. A toxic reaction to digoxin can also lead to other arrhythmias in addition to second-degree AV block type I, including PVCs, ventricular tachycardia, ventricular fibrillation, atrial tachycardia, junctional tachycardia, and atrial fibrillation.

If a toxic reaction to a beta-blocker or a calcium channel blocker has caused second-degree AV block type I, acute complications of the reaction usually result from decreased myocardial contractility, which, in turn, may cause a declining heart rate and altered mental status. Your patient may develop hypotension, lethargy, coma, and seizures. Her arrhythmia also may progress to second-degree AV block type II and third-degree AV block, which can eventually lead to cardiac arrest.

If second-degree AV block type I results from an underlying disease that damages the heart and valves, such as rheumatic heart disease, endocarditis, cardiomyopathy, myocarditis, or congenital heart disease, the complications of the arrhythmia depend on which disease process is at work. For example, inflammatory heart diseases can lead to other arrhythmias, such as atrial arrhythmias, ventricular arrhythmias, second-degree AV block type II, and third-degree AV block.

Nursing considerations

If your patient develops second-degree AV block type I, document the arrhythmia with an ECG tracing. Calculate her atrial and ventricular rates. And determine whether her ventricular rate is bradycardic. Also, assess your patient's vital signs immediately and evaluate her for any changes that indicate hemodynamic instability.

If your patient develops bradycardia with a ventricular rate slower than 60 bpm, immediately assess her for the signs and symptoms of decreased CO, such as chest pain, dyspnea, and decreased level of consciousness. If any of these signs or symptoms occur, notify the physician immediately. Be prepared to administer 0.5 to 1 mg of atropine I.V. every 3 to 5 minutes to a total dose of 0.03 mg/kg, as prescribed.

If your patient isn't bradycardic but is experiencing signs and symptoms, such as a change in mental status, hypotension, and cool, clammy skin, assess her immediately for evidence of an acute MI. Second-degree AV block type I commonly results from ischemia and injury to the AV junction. Assess your patient for such signs and symptoms as diaphoresis, indigestion, nausea, vomiting, hypotension, dyspnea, and pain in the chest, shoulder, arm, neck, and jaw.

If an acute MI causes second-degree AV block type I, observe your patient for emergent acute complications. These can include other serious arrhythmias and conditions, such as ventricular tachycardia and ventricular fibrillation, cardiogenic shock, heart failure, pericarditis, cardiac tamponade, and ruptured papillary muscle.

If your patient exhibits the signs and symptoms of any of these arrhythmias and conditions, establish I.V. access immediately and start fluids such as D_5W and 0.9% sodium chloride solution to keep the vein open. Administer oxygen at 4 to 6 L/minute by nasal cannula, as indicated. The pain caused by ischemia and an infarction requires immediate attention. If your patient is normotensive, give her one tablet of nitroglycerin every 5 minutes up to three times, as ordered. If nitroglycerin relieves the pain, your patient is probably experiencing angina.

Conditions such as esophageal spasm may also respond to nitrates. If nitroglycerin doesn't alleviate the pain, your patient may be experiencing an MI. As prescribed, administer 1 to 3 mg of morphine over 1 to 5 minutes, repeating doses as necessary until the pain is relieved. For an MI, nitroglycerin is usually infused I.V. at 10 to 20 μg/minute and increased by 5 to 10 μg/minute every 5 to 10 minutes.

Assess your patient's drug history carefully to determine whether she's taking commonly prescribed cardiac drugs such as digoxin, a beta-blocker, or a calcium channel blocker. If she is, discuss changing the dose or discontinuing the drug with the physician.

If a toxic reaction to a calcium channel blocker has caused your patient's arrhythmia, assess her for the signs and symptoms of other related arrhythmias. Because such a toxic reaction is associated with hyperglycemia, assess your patient's blood glucose level.

If your patient has hypokalemia, assess her for possible causes of fluid loss. Also, assess her ABG levels for metabolic alkalosis.

If your patient has hyperkalemia, assess her drug history to see whether she is taking oral potassium supplements. If necessary, withhold the drug until you can consult with the physician.

In a patient who has overdosed on tricyclic antidepressants, second-degree AV block type I is a very mild cardiac sign and usually requires no specific intervention. Be aware, however, that within 2 hours of ingesting tricyclic antidepressants, your patient may experience other serious arrhythmias and conduction defects, such as ventricular tachycardia, second-degree AV block type II, third-degree AV block, a widened QRS complex, and a prolonged QT interval.

If second-degree AV block type I results from increased vagal tone, assess your patient for factors that may be stimulating the vagus nerve, such as vomiting, gagging, straining during a bowel movement, and forceful coughing. Administer a preventive drug such as an antiemetic, a laxative, or a cough suppressant, as indicated.

Second-degree atrioventricular block type II

Like second-degree AV block type I, second-degree AV block type II (also called Mobitz II block) occurs because the AV node fails to send one or more electrical impulses through to the ventricles. However, unlike second-degree AV block type I, second-degree AV block type II can rapidly progress to third-degree AV block and ventricular standstill. Thus, second-degree type II block is a lethal arrhythmia.

Pathophysiology

Second-degree AV block type II results from many of the same factors that cause first-degree AV block and second-degree AV block type I. The most common causes are myocardial ischemia and injury that extends to the conduction system. Other causes include vagal stimulation, a toxic reaction to a drug, an electrolyte imbalance, certain cardiovascular diseases, and cardiac surgery.

Myocardial ischemia and injury

An occlusion or spasm of the right coronary artery affects the inferior wall of the left ventricle and can cause myocardial ischemia, injury, and infarction. An interruption of blood flow through this artery also affects the SA node, AV node, bundle of His, and left posterior bundle branch. Interrupted blood flow commonly causes arrhythmias such as first-degree AV block, second-degree AV block type I, and second-degree AV block type II.

The left anterior descending coronary artery supplies blood to the right bundle branch, left anterior bundle branch, and anterior wall of the left ventricle. If damage to this artery leads to angina and an acute anterior-wall MI, second-degree AV block type II usually develops. In such an instance, the patient usually has a poor prognosis.

Vagal stimulation

Second-degree AV block type II sometimes results from increased vagal tone. As you know, the vagus nerve can be stimulated by a GI event such as vomiting, gagging, and straining during a bowel movement. This stimulation causes the parasympathetic nervous system to spring into action, releasing the neurotransmitter acetylcholine. Acetylcholine activates cholinergic receptors, producing a cardiac inhibitory effect. In some patients, acetylcholine release can lead to blocked impulses at the bundle of His and the bundle branches, resulting in second-degree AV block type II.

Drug toxicity

Second-degree AV block type II may result from the toxic effects of drugs prescribed for cardiovascular diseases such as digoxin, beta-blockers, and calcium channel blockers. However, whereas first-degree AV block and second-degree AV block type I may occur when these drugs merely delay impulse conduction, second-degree AV block type II occurs when these drugs block conduction.

As with less severe AV blocks, second-degree AV block type II may result from tricyclic antidepressant overdose. Tricyclic antidepressants inhibit fast sodium channels and slow phase 0 depolarization in the bundle of His and Purkinje fibers, thus slowing impulse conduction.

Electrolyte imbalances

Second-degree AV block type II commonly results from various electrolyte imbalances. Hypokalemia, hyperkalemia, hypocalcemia, hypercalcemia, and hypermagnesemia can affect conduction velocity in the AV junction and ventricles, leading to the arrhythmia. And in some patients, hyperkalemia, hypercalcemia, and hypomagnesemia may cause the arrhythmia indirectly by instigating a toxic reaction to a digitalis glycoside.

Cardiovascular diseases and surgery

The AV junction and ventricular conduction systems can be injured by many heart and valve diseases, resulting in second-degree AV block type II. These diseases include valvular heart disease, rheumatic heart disease, endocarditis, cardiomyopathies, myocarditis, and congenital heart disease. Second-degree AV block type II commonly occurs in older patients as the conduction system undergoes degenerative changes. Also, the major cardiac conduction areas can be damaged during heart surgery, leading to a transient second-degree AV block type II postoperatively.

Signs and symptoms

Whether a patient who experiences second-degree AV block type II exhibits signs and symptoms depends on her ventricular rate and how well she tolerates the arrhythmia. Typically, she may experience the signs and symptoms of the arrhythmia when her ventricular rate drops to 40 bpm or less.

Your patient with second-degree AV block type II also may experience the signs and symptoms of bradycardia that typically result from decreased CO. These signs and symptoms include dizziness, light-headedness, decreased level of consciousness, nausea, anxiety, dyspnea, and chest pain.

On your patient's ECG, you'll see more P waves than QRS complexes. The corresponding QRS complexes may be either narrow or wide, depending on the level of the block. If the block occurs at the bundle of His, the QRS complex is narrow, measuring less than 0.12 second. More commonly, if the block occurs within the bundle branches, the QRS complex is wide, measuring 0.12 second or more. In either case, the R-R interval is regular (see *Characteristics of second-degree atrioventricular block type II*).

The atrial and ventricular rates are different. The atrial rate usually is a normal sinus rhythm, 60 to 100 bpm. The ventricular rate usually is one-half to one-fourth the atrial rate, depending on the number of P waves blocked before each QRS complex.

The ECG usually shows a pattern of two, three, four, or more P waves before each QRS complex. Usually, the number of P waves before each QRS complex is constant. If two P waves appear before each QRS complex, the arrhythmia is second-degree AV block type II with 2:1 conduction; if three P waves, second-degree AV block type II with 3:1 conduction; if four P waves, second-degree AV block type II with 4:1 conduction.

If the number of P waves before each QRS complex varies, the arrhythmia is called variable second-degree AV block type II. Second-degree AV block type II with a 3:1 or higher conduction ratio is also called a high-grade block (see *Understanding variable second-degree atrioventricular type II blocks,* page 138).

Second-degree AV block type II may also slow impulse transmission at the AV node. On your pa-

Characteristics of second-degree atrioventricular block type II

Atrial rate: 60 to 100 beats per minute
Ventricular rate: one-half, one-third, or one-fourth of atrial rate
Rhythm: regular, if atrial beats are consistently conducted to ventricles
P wave: smooth, rounded, upright; some not followed by QRS complex
PR interval: > 0.2 second
QRS complex: < 0.12 second

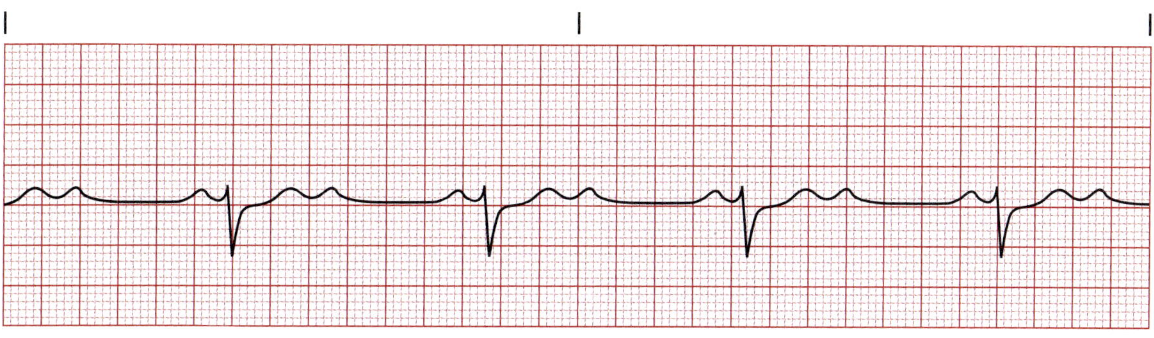

tient's ECG, you can identify this condition by examining all of the cycles in which P waves are followed by QRS complexes.

First, check to make sure these PR intervals are constant. Then check their lengths. If impulse transmission is slowed at the AV node, the PR intervals will be prolonged, which results from second-degree AV block type II alone, not second-degree AV block type II with a first-degree AV block.

Treatment

Second-degree AV block type II can quickly lead to third-degree AV block and even ventricular standstill. With second-degree AV block type II, your patient's ventricular rate may be as low as 20 bpm. This dangerous bradycardia requires a fast response. You may need to begin cardiopulmonary resuscitation (CPR), depending on your patient's signs and symptoms. A physician may treat the arrhythmia directly using atropine, emergency pacing, dopamine, epinephrine, or isoproterenol. He also may initiate treatment for the underlying cause of the arrhythmia.

Atropine

For your patient with second-degree AV block type II, the physician may order 0.5 to 1 mg of atropine to be given every 3 to 5 minutes up to a total dose of 0.03 to 0.04 mg/kg. Atropine increases the sinus rate and conduction through the AV node. However, if the problem is at the level of the bundle of His and bundle branches, atropine usually isn't effective. In fact, it may cause harm by further slowing the ventricular rate.

Pacemaker

If drug therapy with atropine is unsuccessful, your patient may require emergency pacing. Typically, the physician may order a transcutaneous pacemaker until a transvenous pacemaker can be inserted. During transcutaneous pacing, two pacing electrodes are attached to the patient, anteriorly and posteriorly, which supply current directly through the skin to pace the heart.

Dopamine

After atropine has been administered and emergency pacing initiated, the physician may prescribe dopamine to treat hypotension, which commonly

Understanding variable second-degree atrioventricular type II blocks

If the ratio of P waves to QRS complexes varies in a patient with second-degree atrioventricular block, her arrhythmia has progressed to a serious state. Typically, the patient will have regular, constant P-P intervals, but her R-R intervals will vary as the ratio of P waves to QRS complexes fluctuates between 3:1 and 4:1.

3:1 second-degree atrioventricular type II block

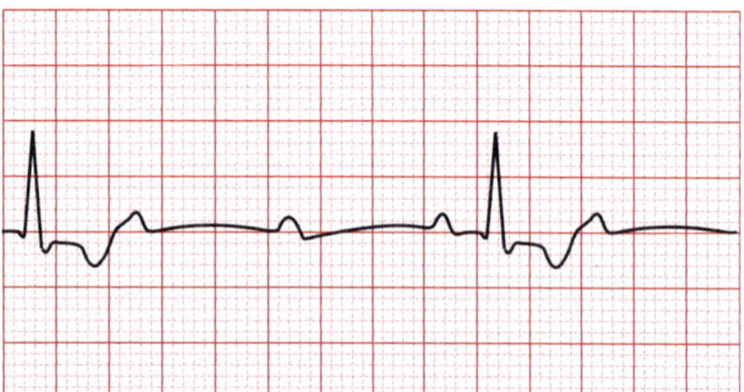

4:1 second-degree atrioventricular type II block

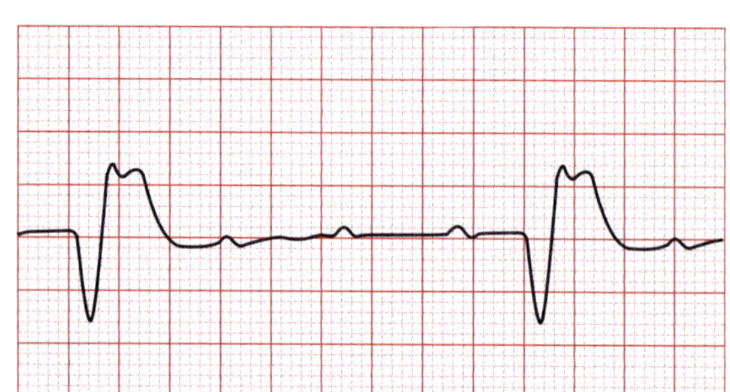

occurs with second-degree AV block type II. Usually, you'll give dopamine I.V. at 1 to 5 µg/kg/minute and then increase the dose to 5 to 20 µg/kg/minute, until blood pressure has returned to your patient's baseline level.

Epinephrine

Administer epinephrine at 2 to 10 µg/kg/minute for symptomatic bradycardia, as prescribed. The usual concentration is 1 mg in 500 ml of D_5W.

Isoproterenol

If the patient still has significant bradycardia despite the use of atropine, pacing, dopamine, and epinephrine, the physician may prescribe isoproterenol. An isoproterenol infusion is commonly started at 2 µg/minute and titrated up to 10 µg/minute until the patient achieves a heart rate of at least 60 bpm.

Underlying causes

As with other AV blocks, a physician may attempt to alleviate second-degree AV block type II by treating the underlying cause. Common causes of the arrhythmia include a toxic reaction to a drug and an electrolyte imbalance. And the treatment for these underlying conditions is similar to the treatment for other AV blocks.

Drug toxicity

Drugs that commonly cause toxic reactions and second-degree AV block type II include digoxin, beta-blockers, and calcium channel blockers. If your patient's arrhythmia results from a toxic reaction to digoxin, the physician may prescribe digoxin immune FAB as 38 mg (one vial) reconstituted with 4 ml of sterile water and then diluted with 0.9% sodium chloride solution, given I.V. over 15 to 30 minutes. If your patient's condition is stable, the physician also may prescribe potassium and magnesium therapy, in conjunction with volume replacement, which usually corrects the toxic effects within a few hours.

A toxic reaction to a beta-blocker may cause hypoglycemia or hyperkalemia. Assess your patient's blood glucose and blood potassium levels. Also, assess her for related arrhythmias and their signs and symptoms. Prepare to administer a bolus of 500 to 1,000 ml of 0.9% sodium chloride solution. If your patient doesn't respond to the the treatment, the physician may prescribe 1 to 5 mg of I.V. glucagon. He may also prescribe an epinephrine infusion at 2 to 100 µg/minute before, after, or in conjunction with glucagon.

If your patient's arrhythmia results from a toxic reaction to a calcium channel blocker, assess her for related arrhythmias and their signs and symptoms. If your patient is hypotensive, the physician may prescribe 500 to 1,000 ml of 0.9% sodium chloride solution. If your patient fails to respond to fluid therapy, the physician may prescribe 5 to 10 ml of I.V. calcium chloride.

If your patient develops refractory second-degree AV block type II from a tricyclic antidepressant overdose, the arrhythmia can be life threatening. Within 2 hours of ingestion, your patient also may experience many other serious arrhythmias and conduction defects, such as ventricular tachycardia, a widened QRS complex, prolonged QT intervals, and third-degree AV block.

If your patient is unconscious, be prepared to perform gastric lavage (see *Gastric lavage: Confirming proper tube placement,* page 140). If her condition is unstable, the physician may prescribe alkalinization therapy, which decreases the nonprotein-bound form of the tricyclic molecule. To perform alkalinization, administer 1 mEq/kg of sodium bicarbonate over 1 to 2 minutes. This procedure is commonly followed by an infusion of two ampules (50 to 100 mEq) of sodium bicarbonate in 0.9% sodium chloride solution at 150 to 200 ml/hour until your patient's arterial pH reaches 7.5 to 7.55.

Electrolyte imbalances

If your patient has hypokalemia, administer potassium replacement supplements I.V. or orally, as prescribed. Usually, you'll give I.V. potassium as 10 mEq of potassium chloride diluted in 50 to 100 ml of D_5W and infused over 1 hour or longer. This dose can be repeated as necessary. Check your patient's blood potassium level every hour until it measures 4 to 4.5 mEq/L. Typically, oral potassium is used to treat less acute cases of hypokalemia.

If your patient has hyperkalemia, anticipate the use of calcium or an infusion of hypertonic 0.9% sodium chloride solution, which reverses the conduction defects of hyperkalemia. The physician may prescribe insulin with glucose to reduce the toxic effects of potassium. The physician may also prescribe furosemide to enhance potassium excretion by the kidneys.

For the patient with hypocalcemia, administer 10 to 20 ml of 10% calcium gluconate or 10% calcium chloride at 1 to 2 ml/minute I.V., as prescribed. If hypocalcemia is severe, prepare a constant infusion at a rate of 15 to 20 mg/minute.

Hypercalcemia commonly requires correction by hydrating the patient with 1 to 2 L of 0.9% sodium chloride solution and by giving her 80 to 100 mg of furosemide I.V. every 1 to 2 hours, as needed, until her blood calcium levels are corrected.

Hypomagnesemia can contribute to your patient's second-degree AV block type II by enhancing the toxic effects of a digitalis glycoside. To treat hypomagnesemia, a physician may prescribe 1 to 2 g of magnesium sulfate, which must be diluted in 50 to 100 ml of D_5W, administered over 15 to 60 minutes.

Treatment for hypermagnesemia may include 10 ml of a 10% calcium gluconate solution, glucose and insulin, and forced diuresis with large volumes of 0.9% sodium chloride solution.

Complications

Without immediate treatment, second-degree AV block type II can be lethal. It can progress to third-degree AV block and ventricular standstill as well as profound bradycardia. The bradycardia can significantly reduce CO, leading to an acute MI, heart failure, and decreased level of consciousness.

Other acute complications of second-degree AV block type II may result from the underlying cause of the arrhythmia. If an acute MI has caused second-degree AV block type II to develop, be alert for acute complications from this disease process, which may include arrhythmias such as ventricular tachycardia and ventricular fibrillation. Other complications include cardiogenic shock, heart failure, pericarditis, cardiac tamponade, and ruptured papillary muscle.

If a toxic reaction to digoxin has caused second-degree AV block type II, the patient may experience acute complications of the CNS and the GI system. Also, a toxic reaction to digoxin can lead to arrhythmias besides second-degree AV block type II, including PVCs, ventricular tachycardia, ventricular fibrillation, atrial tachycardia, junctional tachycardia, and atrial fibrillation.

If a toxic reaction to a beta-blocker or a calcium channel blocker has caused second-degree AV

Gastric lavage: Confirming proper tube placement

Before performing gastric lavage, assess your patient for proper tube placement. Inject 15 to 30 cc of air into the tube as you auscultate the abdomen about 3 inches below the xiphoid process, as shown.

If you have difficulty injecting air, the tube may be kinked or coiled in the esophagus. If you hear a swoosh or gurgling sound, use the syringe to gently aspirate gastric secretions. Successful aspiration confirms the tube placement in the stomach. If you can't aspirate secretions, advance the tube and try again. If you still can't confirm the proper tube placement, the patient will be sent for X-rays.

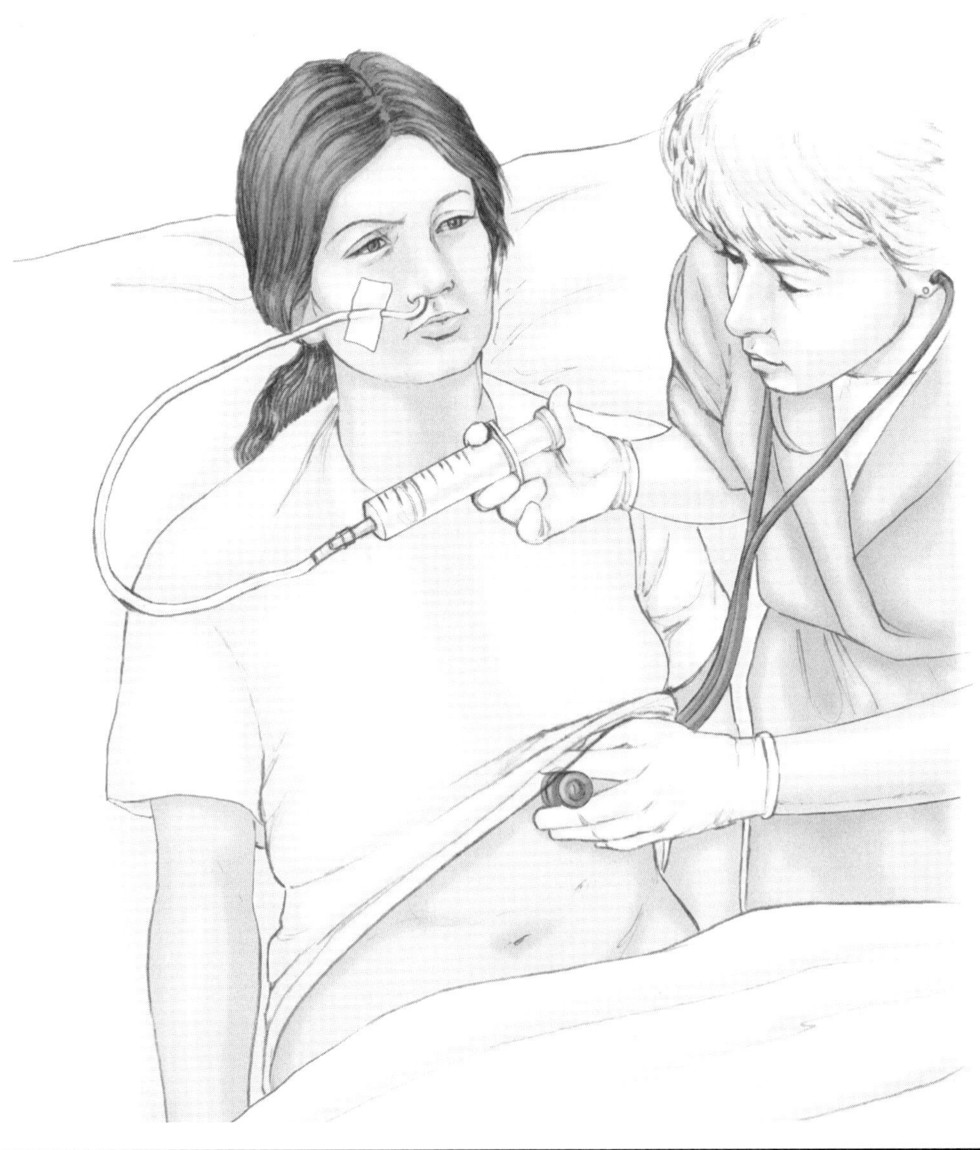

block type II, conditions such as depressed myocardial contractility, declining heart rate, and altered mental status may lead to acute complications. Many patients develop hypotension, lethargy, coma, and seizures. Such patients are at risk for progression to third-degree AV block, which can cause cardiac arrest.

If an overdose of a tricyclic antidepressant results in second-degree AV block type II, complications may include widened QRS complexes, ventricular arrhythmias, seizures, coma, and death.

If an electrolyte imbalance results in second-degree AV block type II, the imbalance also may affect other body systems. Many such acute complications involve the neuromuscular and GI systems. For example, if second-degree AV block type II results from hypercalcemia, complications can include decreased level of consciousness, flaccidity, nausea, vomiting, and constipation. Hypercalcemia can also enhance the toxic effects of a digitalis glycoside.

Nursing considerations

If you suspect that your patient has second-degree AV block type II, immediately assess her to determine how well she's tolerating the arrhythmia. Document the arrhythmia with an ECG tracing. And calculate her atrial and ventricular rates and determine the conduction ratio between her P waves and QRS complexes. If the ratio of P waves to QRS complexes increases or if the ratio varies, report this finding to the physician immediately.

If your patient is pulseless and has no spontaneous respirations, call for help and begin CPR immediately. If your patient has a pulse and is breathing, assess her for the signs and symptoms of decreased CO. Also, assess her for hypotension, decreased level of consciousness, chest pain, and dyspnea.

If your patient displays any of these serious signs and symptoms, be prepared to intervene. Begin by securing her airway and administering supplemental oxygen. For a patient who isn't in respiratory distress, a physician usually prescribes oxygen at a rate of 2 L/minute by nasal cannula. If the patient is in mild respiratory distress, flow rates of 4 to 6 L/minute may be indicated. For your patient in severe distress, you may have to provide 60% to 100% oxygen. Use a high-flow face mask, partial rebreather mask, nonrebreather mask, or endotracheal intubation with mechanical ventilation (see *Administering supplemental oxygen,* page 142).

While securing the airway and starting oxygen administration, be sure your patient is attached to a continuous cardiac monitor, pulse oximeter, and automatic blood pressure monitor. Also, obtain a 12-lead ECG tracing. Be prepared to start I.V. access. The physician may prescribe 0.9% sodium chloride solution or D_5W to keep the vein open.

Angina and an acute MI can cause second-degree AV block type II. Alternatively, second-degree AV block type II can compromise coronary circulation enough to cause angina and an acute MI. Determining which event came first can be difficult. In either case, react quickly to salvage myocardial tissue. Quickly scan all 12 ECG leads for any acute changes, such as the development of Q waves and changes in ST segments and T waves. Involvement of the inferior wall produces acute changes in leads II, III, and aV_F. And anterior-wall involvement appears in leads V_1 through V_4.

Assess your patient for the signs and symptoms of angina and an MI, including diaphoresis, indigestion, nausea, vomiting, hypotension, dyspnea, and pain in the chest, shoulder, arm, neck, and jaw. If your patient is experiencing any of these signs and symptoms, establish I.V. access immediately and start fluids such as D_5W or 0.9% sodium chloride solution to keep the vein open. Begin oxygen at 4 to 6 L/minute by nasal cannula.

The pain caused by myocardial ischemia or an MI requires immediate attention. If your patient is normotensive, give her sublingual nitroglycerin, one tablet every 5 minutes for up to three doses, as prescribed. If nitroglycerin relieves the pain, your patient is probably experiencing angina, although other conditions such as esophageal spasm can respond to nitrates as well. If nitroglycerin fails to alleviate the pain, your patient may be experiencing an acute MI. You may have to administer 1 to 3 mg of morphine over 1 to 5 minutes, repeating doses until the pain is relieved.

Assess your patient for movements that can stimulate the vagus nerve, such as vomiting, gagging, straining during a bowel movement, and forceful coughing. As necessary, alleviate vagal stimulation by administering an antiemetic, a laxative, an enema, or a cough suppressant, as indicated.

If your patient is receiving dopamine, watch for nausea and vomiting, which are common adverse

Administering supplemental oxygen

If your patient with an atrioventricular block requires supplemental oxygen, you can administer it via nasal cannula, a face mask, or an endotracheal tube. Typically, you'll give low concentrations of oxygen via a nasal cannula and higher concentrations of oxygen via a face mask or an endotracheal tube. If your patient with an endotracheal tube suffers respiratory arrest or has inefficient respirations, you may need to ventilate her with a handheld resuscitation bag, as shown.

Nasal cannula

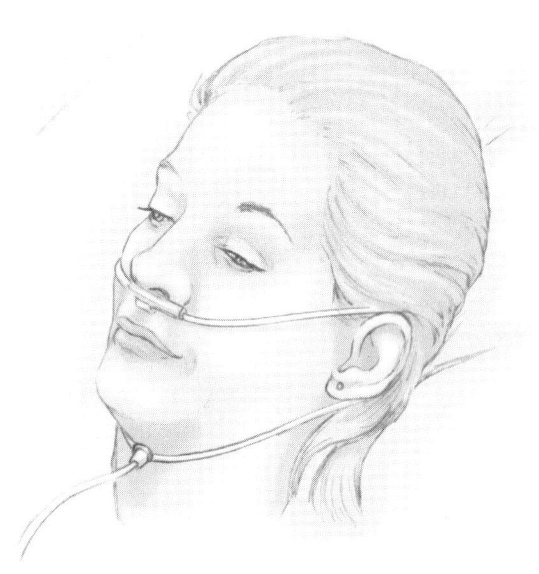

Face mask

Endotracheal intubation

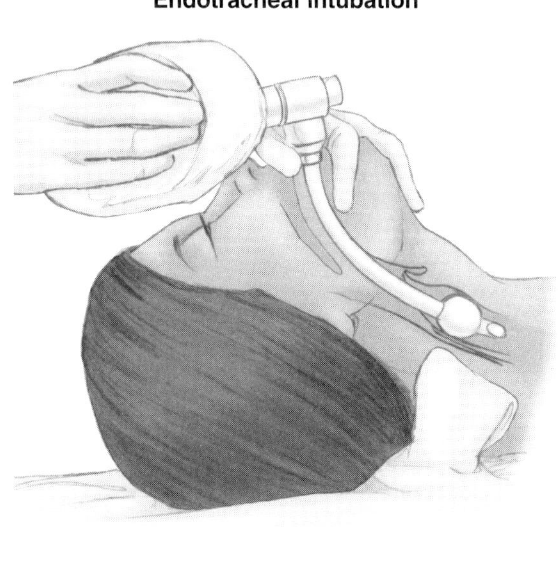

effects at higher levels of infusion. Dopamine infiltration can produce tissue necrosis. If infiltration develops, move the infusion to a different I.V. site. Try to maintain the original I.V. access until the physician has examined the patient. Usually, a physician prescribes 5 to 10 mg of phentolamine diluted in 10 to 15 ml of 0.9% sodium chloride solution and injected subcutaneously into the area surrounding the infiltration. Observe the site frequently over the next 3 to 4 hours for signs of tissue necrosis and vasculitis. If the antidote is successful, tissue blanching usually resolves within the first hour.

Assess your patient's drug history. A toxic reaction to a beta-blocker may precipitate a hypoglycemic reaction or hyperkalemia. Assess your patient's blood glucose and blood potassium levels. Also, assess her for any concurrent arrhythmias and their signs and symptoms.

If she is taking a commonly prescribed calcium channel blocker such as nifedipine, verapamil, or diltiazem, discuss changing the dose or discontinuing the drug with the physician.

A toxic reaction to a calcium channel blocker may cause hyperglycemia. Be prepared to perform a bedside blood glucose test, as ordered.

Review your patient's laboratory test results carefully. Give careful attention to blood levels of potassium, calcium, and magnesium.

If your patient develops second-degree AV block type II as a result of hyperkalemia, assess her drug history to see whether she's still receiving oral or I.V. potassium supplements. If so, withhold the supplement until you consult with the physician.

If your patient has hypokalemia, assess her for possible causes of fluid loss. Also, assess her ABG levels for metabolic alkalosis.

If second-degree AV block type II results from injury to the atrial or ventricular conduction system, focus on preparing your patient for the insertion of a permanent pacemaker.

Third-degree atrioventricular block

Third-degree AV block, also called complete heart block and AV dissociation, is the most serious of the heart blocks: it can rapidly progress to ventricular standstill and death. This arrhythmia typically occurs after a progression from first-degree and second-degree AV block.

Pathophysiology

A third-degree AV block may develop in the AV node, the bundle of His, or the bundle branches. When such a block develops in the AV node, impulses travel normally from the atria into the AV node, but they can't exit. When a block develops in the bundle of His or the bundle branches, the impulses can travel through the AV node normally, but they can't reach the ventricles.

Because impulse transmission is blocked between the atria and the ventricles, the ventricles depend on another part of the conduction system to pace them. Typically, this alternate pacemaker is located immediately below the site of impulse blockage.

If impulse transmission is blocked at the AV node, the bundle of His takes over as the ventricular pacemaker. If the blockage occurs at the bundle of His, a small portion of the bundle may retain automaticity and pace the ventricles.

More commonly, the bundle branches assume the role of pacemaker for the ventricles. If one of the branches—right, left anterior, or left posterior—is blocked, the remaining branches typically take over as the pacemaker. If all three branches are blocked, the Purkinje fibers take control. And if the Purkinje fibers can't compensate for the blockage, ventricular standstill occurs.

If the AV node takes over the pacing of the ventricles, it produces a junctional escape rhythm. The AV node fires at a regular rate of 40 to 60 bpm and operates independently from the SA node.

If the bundle branches or Purkinje fibers take control of pacing the ventricles, they produce a ventricular escape rhythm. These areas fire at a regular rate of 20 to 40 bpm, also completely independent of the SA node.

Third-degree AV block can be caused by ischemia, injury, or an MI that extends to the conduction system. Also, the arrhythmia commonly results from a spasm, partial occlusion, or total occlusion of a coronary artery, which can precipitate myocardial ischemia, injury, or an MI. Other causes of this arrhythmia include vagal stimulation, a toxic reaction to a drug, an electrolyte imbalance, a cardiovascular disease, and cardiac surgery.

Myocardial ischemia and injury

Usually, the right coronary artery supplies oxygenated blood to the inferior wall of the left ventricle, the SA node, and the AV node. The artery also supplies oxygenated blood to the bundle of His and the left posterior bundle branch. If any condition reduces this arterial blood flow, ischemia, injury, or an MI of the left ventricular part of the conduction system may result and, in turn, cause third-degree AV block.

The left anterior descending coronary artery supplies blood to the right bundle branch, left anterior bundle branch, and anterior wall of the left ventricle. If a problem with this artery leads to angina and an acute anterior-wall MI, your patient may experience third-degree AV block. If third-degree AV block results from an anterior-wall MI, the patient has a poor prognosis because this type of arrhythmia usually signifies substantial myocardial damage.

Vagal stimulation

As with other AV blocks, third-degree AV block may result from increased vagal tone. As you know, if the vagus nerve is stimulated, the parasympathetic nervous system springs into action, releasing the neurotransmitter acetylcholine. Acetylcholine activates cholinergic receptors, producing a cardiac inhibitory effect. In some patients, vagal stimulation can lead to blocked impulses at the bundle of His and within the bundle branches.

Drug toxicity

As with other AV blocks, third-degree AV block may result from the toxic effects of drugs prescribed for cardiovascular diseases, such as digoxin, calcium channel blockers, and beta-blockers.

Digoxin increases vagal tone, which depresses impulse conduction through the AV node. The AV node's receptiveness to multiple stimuli is reduced, allowing fewer impulses to reach the ventricles.

Beta-blockers and calcium channel blockers slow conduction through the AV junction and ventricles. Typically, a physician may prescribe them to treat another arrhythmia, such as supraventricular tachycardia. However, toxic levels of these drugs can cause AV junction and ventricular conduction problems, resulting in third-degree AV block.

Third-degree AV block may result from an overdose of tricyclic antidepressants. As you know, these drugs inhibit fast sodium channels and slow phase 0 depolarization in myocardial cells.

Electrolyte imbalances

Electrolyte imbalances that affect the AV junction and ventricular conduction system can result in third-degree AV block. Cardiac function depends on ion currents across myocardial cell membranes. Action potential generation, impulse conduction, and myocardial contraction are all vulnerable to altered electrolyte levels.

In particular, hypokalemia, hyperkalemia, hypocalcemia, hypercalcemia, and hypermagnesemia can affect conduction velocity in the AV junction and ventricles, leading to third-degree AV block. And hyperkalemia, hypercalcemia, and hypomagnesemia can enhance the toxic effects of a digitalis glycoside, which can, in turn, cause the arrhythmia.

Cardiovascular diseases and surgery

Many diseases of the heart and valves can injure the AV junction and ventricular conduction systems, causing third-degree AV block. Such diseases include valvular heart diseases, rheumatic heart disease, endocarditis, cardiomyopathies, myocarditis, and congenital heart disease.

Cardiac conduction also can be damaged during heart surgery, causing a transient third-degree AV block that usually occurs postoperatively. Also, third-degree AV block commonly results from the degenerative changes of the conduction system that accompany aging.

Signs and symptoms

Whether a patient with third-degree AV block exhibits the signs and symptoms of the arrhythmia depends on her ventricular rate and how well she tolerates the arrhythmia. For example, if your patient has a junctional escape rhythm with an intrinsic ventricular response of 40 to 60 bpm, she may not have any signs or symptoms. However, if she has a ventricular escape rhythm with a rate of only 20 to 40 bpm, she'll probably experience

Characteristics of third-degree atrioventricular block

Atrial rate: 60 to 100 beats per minute (bpm)
Ventricular rate: 40 to 60 bpm if controlled by junctional focus; 20 to 40 bpm if controlled by ventricular focus
Rhythm: regular
P wave: smooth, rounded, upright; some not followed by QRS complex
PR interval: none; P waves have no relationship to QRS complexes
QRS complex: < 0.12 second if controlled by junctional focus; ≥ 0.12 second if controlled by ventricular focus

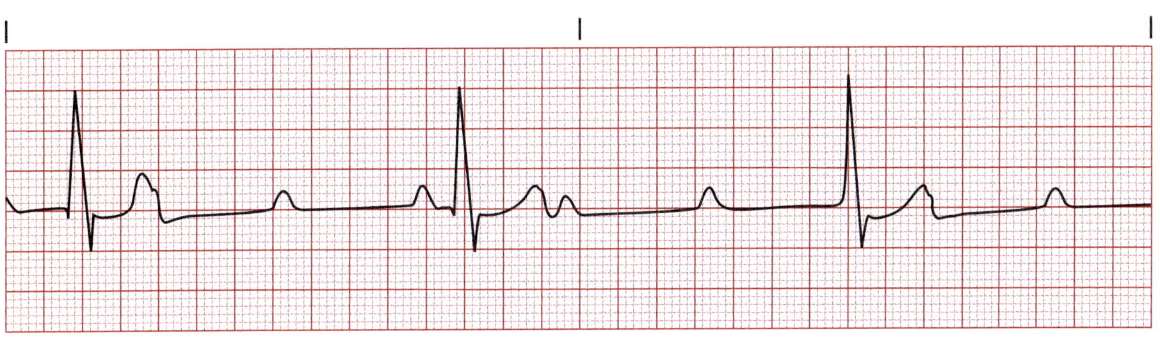

the signs and symptoms of profound bradycardia. These signs and symptoms may include decreased level of consciousness, dyspnea, and chest pain.

On your patient's ECG, the hallmark sign of third-degree AV block is the lack of relationship between the P waves and QRS complexes, which is why third-degree AV block is commonly called AV dissociation. The P waves appear normal and regular. But the tracing will have more P waves than QRS complexes. By using calipers to find all the P waves, you'll notice that some P waves are close to the QRS complex, others are far away, and some are merged into other parts of the cycle, such as the QRS complex, ST segment, and T wave (see *Characteristics of third-degree atrioventricular block*).

The QRS complexes may be normal or wide, depending on the level of the block and the level of the ventricular pacemaker. If the patient has a junctional escape rhythm—with the ventricular pacemaker at the AV node or the bundle of His—the QRS complex is narrow, measuring less than 0.12 second. If the patient has a ventricular escape rhythm—with the ventricular pacemaker at the level of the bundle branches or the Purkinje fibers—the QRS complex is wide, measuring 0.12 second or more.

Treatment

In many patients, the ventricular rate in third-degree AV block is markedly bradycardic. And third-degree AV block can quickly lead to ventricular standstill. Typically, this arrhythmia requires emergency treatment, beginning with emergency pacing, I.V. dopamine, and I.V. epinephrine. For profound bradycardia, the physician also may prescribe isoproterenol. And the physician may try to alleviate the arrhythmia by treating its underlying cause (see *Caring for a patient with third-degree atrioventricular block,* pages 146 and 147).

Pacemaker

Be prepared to start emergency pacing for your patient, as ordered. You can use a transcutaneous pacemaker until a transvenous pacemaker can be inserted. During transcutaneous pacing, two pacing electrodes are attached to the patient, one an-

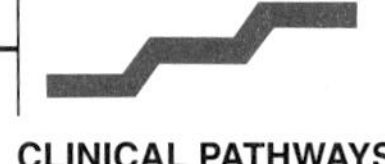

CLINICAL PATHWAYS

Caring for a patient with third-degree atrioventricular block

	History and physical examination	Diagnostic tests	Discharge planning
Day 1	• history of acute myocardial infarction, valvular heart disease, rheumatic heart disease, endocarditis, myocarditis, cardiomyopathy, congenital heart disease, open-heart surgery, or coronary artery bypass graft • history of precipitating factors such as toxic reaction to digoxin, calcium channel blocker, or beta-blocker; tricyclic antidepressant overdose; or electrolyte imbalances • physical assessment on admission • duration of arrhythmia • vital signs every 15 minutes, as necessary • urine output	• 12-lead electrocardiogram (ECG) • blood electrolyte levels • blood urea nitrogen (BUN) and creatinine levels • blood levels of drugs such as digoxin • arterial blood gas levels or pulse oximetry readings • chest X-ray	• Identify support systems. • Review adverse effects of drugs.
Day 2	• vital signs every 4 hours, as necessary • systems review every shift • fluid intake and output	• 12-lead ECG • laboratory tests, including complete blood count (CBC), chemistry profile, blood electrolyte levels, prothrombin time (PT), activated partial thromboplastin time, international normalized ratio (INR), and drug levels, as ordered • cardiac catheterization, if appropriate • routine urinalysis • pulse oximetry readings every 4 hours	• Identify patient's understanding of disease process. • Initiate review of arrhythmia management.
Day 3	• vital signs every 4–8 hours • systems review every shift • fluid intake and output • assessment of pacemaker insertion site	• 12-lead ECG • laboratory tests, including CBC, PT, INR, and electrolyte, BUN, and creatinine levels • chest X-ray to confirm placement of permanent pacemaker • pulse oximetry readings every shift	• Give patient contact number for transtelephonic monitoring and follow-up after permanent pacemaker insertion. • Arrange for follow-up appointments with laboratory to monitor PT and INR every week.
Day 4	• vital signs every shift • systems review every shift • assessment of pacemaker insertion site	• CBC, PT, INR, and pulse oximetry readings every day	• Review discharge instructions. • Answer patient's questions. • Provide resource options for continued needs. • Coordinate follow-up appointments with physician after discharge.

Drugs	Interventions	Patient teaching
• I.V. atropine 0.5–1 mg up to 3 mg, as prescribed • I.V. epinephrine 2–10 μg/min, as prescribed • I.V. dopamine 5–20 μg/min for hypotension, as prescribed • I.V. isoproterenol 10 μg/min, as prescribed, until heart rate reaches 60 beats per minute • local anesthetic for transvenous pacemaker insertion, as needed • I.V. fluid replacement, as prescribed	• Continuously monitor cardiac rhythm. • Ensure that emergency equipment and external pacemaker are readily available. • Initiate temporary transcutaneous pacemaker for emergency pacing, as needed. • Maintain bed rest. • Deliver oxygen with mechanical ventilation, if indicated.	• Explain all procedures and treatments to allay anxiety. • Orient patient to unit.
• I.V. atropine, epinephrine, dopamine, or isoproterenol, as prescribed • antianxiety drugs, as prescribed • I.V. fluid replacement, as prescribed	• Continuously monitor cardiac rhythm. • Ensure that emergency equipment and external pacemaker are readily available. • Prepare patient for cardiac catheterization, if indicated. • Obtain informed consent for permanent pacemaker, if indicated. • Avoid giving patient anything by mouth after midnight if she's scheduled for permanent pacemaker insertion. • Reassure patient. • Administer oxygen, as needed.	• Review basic cardiac anatomy and physiology. • Teach patient and family about causes of third-degree atrioventricular block. • Explain permanent pacemaker insertion to patient.
• I.V. atropine, epinephrine, dopamine, or isoproterenol, as prescribed • I.V. fluid replacement, as prescribed • oral analgesic for pacemaker incision pain, as needed	• Continuously monitor cardiac rhythm. • Examine rhythm strip for appropriate pacemaker function (presence of pacing artifact and appropriate capture). • Ensure that emergency equipment is readily available. • Encourage increased activity level. • Advance diet, as tolerated. • Administer oxygen, as needed.	• Instruct patient to avoid magnetic fields after pacemaker insertion. • Reinforce importance of regular transtelephonic monitoring to ensure proper pacemaker function. • Teach patient to take her pulse. • Discuss need for medical identification tag or bracelet. • Teach patient about risks and adverse effects of warfarin therapy. • Stress that patient must avoid injury while taking anticoagulant.
• oral analgesic for pacemaker incision pain, as needed	• Continuously monitor cardiac rhythm. • Examine rhythm strip for appropriate pacemaker function. • Ensure that emergency equipment is readily available. • Increase patient's activity, as tolerated. • Administer oxygen, as needed.	• Teach patient passive range-of-motion exercises for affected side after pacemaker insertion. • Initiate exercises, as ordered by physician. • Review and reinforce all prior teaching.

teriorly and one posteriorly. The anterior electrode is placed to the left of the sternum, at the point of maximal impulse. The posterior electrode is placed to the left of the spinal column, under the clavicle. Position the two electrodes so that they would connect through the patient's chest if you drew an imaginary line between them.

The heart is generally paced at a rate of 60 to 80 bpm. The physician adjusts the output until the electrical impulses elicit a captured beat. Check the ECG monitor for capture. Look for a pacemaker spike followed by a wide QRS complex. Also, check your patient's pulse to ensure that these paced beats are perfusing.

Transcutaneous pacemakers can be painful. Your patient is likely to feel the electrical impulses, which can cause her chest-wall muscle to contract. During this procedure, your patient may need sedation and analgesics.

Transcutaneous pacemakers should be used only briefly, until your patient's condition can be stabilized for insertion of a transvenous pacemaker. Transvenous pacemakers can be either temporary or permanent. The physician's choice depends on your patient's diagnosis and the cause of the third-degree AV block. If the physician determines that the block results from a toxic reaction to a drug, an electrolyte imbalance, or another short-term and easily correctable cause, he may insert a temporary pacemaker until the underlying cause can be resolved. If the physician determines that the arrhythmia results from a long-lasting condition, such as degeneration of the conduction system caused by aging, he'll probably decide to insert a permanent pacemaker.

Dopamine

After pacing has been started, administer dopamine, as prescribed, to treat the hypotension that may result from third-degree AV block. Usually, dopamine is given at a rate of 5 to 20 μg/kg/minute.

Epinephrine and isoproterenol

If your patient with third-degree AV block experiences profoundly symptomatic bradycardia, the physician may prescribe epinephrine at 2 to 10 μg/kg/minute. And if significant bradycardia remains despite the use of pacing, dopamine, and epinephrine, the physician also may prescribe isoproterenol. Usually, isoproterenol is titrated at 10 μg/minute until the patient's heart rate reaches 60 bpm.

Underlying causes

The physician may also attempt to alleviate third-degree AV block by treating its underlying cause. Like other AV blocks, third-degree AV block commonly results from a toxic reaction to a drug or an electrolyte imbalance.

Drug toxicity

The treatment of third-degree AV block that results from a toxic reaction to digoxin depends on your patient's hemodynamic stability. Because such a reaction commonly results from hypokalemia, hypomagnesemia, and dehydration, the physician may prescribe potassium and magnesium therapy in conjunction with volume replacement. However, if your patient has a severe toxic reaction to a digitalis glycoside, the physician may prescribe digoxin immune FAB to reduce the toxic effect more quickly.

For a toxic reaction to a beta-blocker, administer a bolus of 500 to 1,000 ml of 0.9% sodium chloride solution, as prescribed. If your patient doesn't respond to the extra fluid, you may need to administer 1 to 5 mg of glucagon, depending on her blood glucose level. The physician also may prescribe an epinephrine infusion at 2 to 100 μg/minute before, during, or after glucagon administration.

If your patient's arrhythmia results from a toxic reaction to a calcium channel blocker, assess her for other related arrhythmias and their signs and symptoms. If your patient is hypotensive, administer 500 to 1,000 ml of 0.9% sodium chloride solution, as prescribed.

Third-degree AV block that results from tricyclic antidepressant overdose can be life threatening. Within 2 hours of ingestion, patients also can experience many other serious arrhythmias and conduction defects, such as ventricular tachycardia, a widened QRS complex, and a prolonged QT interval.

To treat tricyclic antidepressant overdose, the physician may order gastric decontamination with activated charcoal. Gastric lavage is used if your patient is unconscious.

If your patient's condition is unstable, the physician may prescribe alkalinization therapy. To perform alkalization, administer 1 mEq/kg of sodium bicarbonate over 1 to 2 minutes. And administer two ampules (50 to 100 mEq) of sodium bicarbonate in 0.9% sodium chloride solution at 150 to 200 ml/hour until your patient's pH reaches 7.5 to 7.55, as prescribed.

Electrolyte imbalances

For hypokalemia, I.V. potassium is usually administered over 1 hour as 10 mEq of potassium chloride diluted in 50 to 100 ml of D_5W. A physician also may prescribe oral potassium to treat less acute cases of hypokalemia.

If your patient has hyperkalemia from a toxic reaction to a calcium channel blocker, anticipate an infusion of calcium or hypertonic 0.9% sodium chloride solution, which reverses the conduction defects of hyperkalemia. The physician may prescribe insulin with glucose to reduce the toxic effects of hyperkalemia. Also, the physician may prescribe furosemide to enhance potassium excretion by the kidneys.

For the patient with hypocalcemia, administer 10 to 20 ml of 10% calcium gluconate or 10% calcium chloride I.V. at a rate of 1 to 2 ml/minute, as prescribed. If hypocalcemia is severe, the physician may order a constant infusion of elemental calcium at a dose of 15 to 20 mg/kg every 4 to 8 hours at 15 to 20 mg/minute or less.

In many cases, hypercalcemia requires correction with 1 to 2 L of 0.9% sodium chloride solution to hydrate the patient and 80 to 100 mg of furosemide I.V. every 1 to 2 hours to promote diuresis.

Hypomagnesemia, commonly accompanied by hypokalemia, can be caused by decreased intake, which is common in critically ill patients and in patients with diarrhea, a history of alcoholism, and poor nutrition. For hypomagnesemia, administer 1 to 2 g of magnesium sulfate diluted in 50 to 100 ml of D_5W over 15 to 60 minutes, as prescribed. After the initial bolus, give your patient an infusion of 0.5 to 1 g/hour until normal levels are achieved.

Hypermagnesemia may require I.V. administration of 10 ml of a 10% calcium gluconate solution, glucose and insulin, and forced diuresis with large volumes of 0.9% sodium chloride solution.

Complications

Without prompt treatment, third-degree AV block can be lethal. It can cause profound bradycardia, which can, in turn, significantly reduce CO, leading to an acute MI and heart failure. Also, if left untreated, third-degree AV block can progress to ventricular standstill.

Most other acute complications of third-degree AV block result from the underlying cause of the arrhythmia. If an acute MI caused third-degree AV block, watch for acute complications from the infarction. Cardiac complications can include other arrhythmias, such as ventricular tachycardia and ventricular fibrillation. And other complications include cardiogenic shock, heart failure, pericarditis, cardiac tamponade, and ruptured papillary muscle.

If third-degree AV block results from the toxic effects of digoxin, acute complications may include blurred vision, halos, incorrect color perception, fatigue, weakness, nausea, vomiting, and abdominal pain.

If your patient's third-degree AV block results from a toxic reaction to a beta-blocker or calcium channel blocker, acute complications can result from depressed myocardial contractility, declining heart rate, and altered mental status. Your patient may develop hypotension, lethargy, coma, and seizures. In such patients, progression to refractory third-degree AV block can lead to cardiac arrest.

If your patient's third-degree AV block results from an electrolyte imbalance, she may experience complications as a result of the imbalance and its effect on other body systems. Most of these imbalances cause cardiac complications besides third-degree AV block and may involve your patient's neuromuscular and GI systems. For example, hypermagnesemia can also cause lethargy, coma, and impaired respirations.

If third-degree AV block results from an underlying disease process such as valvular heart disease, rheumatic heart disease, endocarditis, cardiomyopathy, myocarditis, or congenital heart disease, the arrhythmia's complications will depend on the disease process. Inflammatory heart diseases can lead to other arrhythmias, such as atrial and ventricular arrhythmias, which, in turn, can lead to heart failure. Structural disorders can also lead to ventricular arrhythmias and heart failure.

Nursing considerations

Correctly identifying third-degree AV block depends on verifying a lack of relationship between the P waves and QRS complexes. To do so, you must first carefully identify all P waves.

If you suspect third-degree AV block, react quickly. Document it immediately with an ECG tracing. Calculate your patient's atrial and ven-

Giving your patient emotional comfort

A sudden cardiac arrhythmia, especially one that's debilitating or life threatening, can be emotionally devastating to a patient. Anger, anxiety, fear, and depression commonly accompany the illness.

The emotional response varies greatly from patient to patient. Some feel guilty because they can't continue to work regularly. Others wonder if they're being punished for something they've done or neglected to do. Lying in bed while a cardiac monitor records every heartbeat gives a patient plenty of time to worry. And the sights and sounds of the typical cardiac unit may only increase her fears.

Although some patients adopt coping mechanisms on their own, you can help improve your patient's emotional state by maintaining a calm environment and providing frequent opportunities for her to discuss her fears and concerns. You may quell your patient's fears and ease her anxiety by increasing her knowledge of her condition. So teach her about her arrhythmia, her drug regimen, and her upcoming tests and procedures.

When talking to your patient, concentrate on her specific anxieties. She's probably concerned about one or more of these common fears:

- the threat of chronic illness and death
- impending lifestyle changes
- high-tech treatments she doesn't understand
- financial concerns, including possible job loss
- inadequate support systems after discharge.

To successfully manage her illness, your patient needs to be in control of her life. You can help restore her sense of control by encouraging her to plan daily activities to occupy her time, helping her to understand her illness, preparing her for the lifestyle changes she has to make, and involving her in planning her care.

tricular rates and determine the escape rhythm. Remember, third-degree AV block that occurs with a ventricular escape rhythm is more serious.

Assess your patient immediately to determine how well she's tolerating the bradycardia. If she is pulseless and lacks spontaneous respirations, call for help and initiate CPR. If the patient has a pulse and is breathing, assess her for the signs and symptoms of decreased CO. Also, assess her for hypotension, shock, and heart failure. Look for signs and symptoms such as decreased level of consciousness, chest pain, and dyspnea.

If your patient has any of these serious signs and symptoms, initiate appropriate treatment, as indicated. If necessary, secure your patient's airway and administer supplemental oxygen. For a patient who isn't in respiratory distress, the physician may prescribe supplemental oxygen at 2 L/minute by nasal cannula. For a patient in mild respiratory distress, the physician may prescribe 4 to 6 L/minute. For a patient in severe respiratory distress, the physician may use mask devices that deliver even higher oxygen concentrations, or your patient may require endotracheal intubation and mechanical ventilation.

Attach a continuous cardiac monitor, pulse oximeter, and automatic blood pressure machine to your patient. Also, as ordered, start an I.V. infusion of 0.9% sodium chloride solution to keep her vein open.

An acute MI and angina can cause third-degree AV block. Alternatively, third-degree AV block can compromise the coronary circulation enough to cause angina and an acute MI. You may not be able to tell which event came first. Evaluate all 12 leads of your patient's ECG, watching for any acute changes, such as the development of Q waves or alterations in ST segments and T waves.

Assess your patient for such signs and symptoms as diaphoresis, indigestion, nausea, vomiting, hypotension, dyspnea, and pain in the chest, shoulder, arm, neck, and jaw. If the patient has any of these signs and symptoms, establish I.V. access immediately and start fluids such as D_5W or 0.9% sodium chloride solution to keep the vein open. Administer oxygen at 4 to 6 L/minute by nasal cannula, as prescribed.

The pain caused by ischemia and an MI requires immediate attention. If your patient is normotensive, give one tablet of nitroglycerin every 5 minutes up to three times, as ordered. If nitroglycerin relieves your patient's pain, she's probably experiencing angina, although conditions such as esophageal spasm can also respond to nitrates.

If nitroglycerin fails to alleviate the pain, your patient may be experiencing an MI. Administer 1 to 3 mg of morphine over 1 to 5 minutes, repeating the doses, as prescribed or until the pain is relieved. Usually, nitroglycerin is administered I.V. at 10 to 20 μg/minute and can be increased by 5 to 10 μg/minute every 5 to 10 minutes.

Assess your patient for anything that could stimulate the vagus nerve, such as vomiting, gagging, forceful coughing, and straining during a bowel movement. If your patient experiences any of these conditions, take actions to alleviate them, such as administering an antiemetic, laxative, enema, or cough suppressant, as indicated.

If your patient is receiving dopamine, observe her for nausea and vomiting, which are common adverse effects of an excessive infusion rate. A dopamine infiltration can produce tissue necrosis. Treat such an infiltration immediately with phentolamine, as prescribed.

Assess your patient's drug history to determine whether she's taking digoxin, a beta-blocker, or a calcium channel blocker. If your patient takes any of these drugs, discuss changing the dose or discontinuing the drug with the physician.

If your patient has a toxic reaction to digoxin, remember that digoxin also has excitatory effects on atrial and ventricular fibers. Assess your patient for other arrhythmias such as premature atrial contractions, atrial tachycardia, junctional tachycardia, PVCs, and ventricular tachycardia.

If your patient has a toxic reaction to a beta-blocker, assess her blood glucose and potassium levels. Such a reaction may be associated with hypoglycemia or hyperkalemia.

If your patient with third-degree AV block has hyperkalemia, assess her drug history to see whether she's taking oral or I.V. potassium supplements. If so, withhold the drug until you have collaborated with the physician.

If your patient has hypokalemia, assess her for possible causes of fluid loss. Also, assess her ABG levels for metabolic alkalosis. As prescribed, correct the volume depletion and hypokalemia with oral or I.V. potassium supplements.

Hyperglycemia may result from a toxic reaction to a calcium channel blocker. Be prepared to perform a bedside blood glucose test, as ordered.

If third-degree AV block occurs because of injury to the atrial and ventricular conduction systems, which may be caused by heart disease, heart surgery, and degeneration related to aging, focus on preparing the patient for insertion of a permanent pacemaker. Explain the procedure to your patient and be sure informed consent has been obtained. Offer emotional support to calm her fears about the procedure and her condition (see *Giving your patient emotional comfort*).

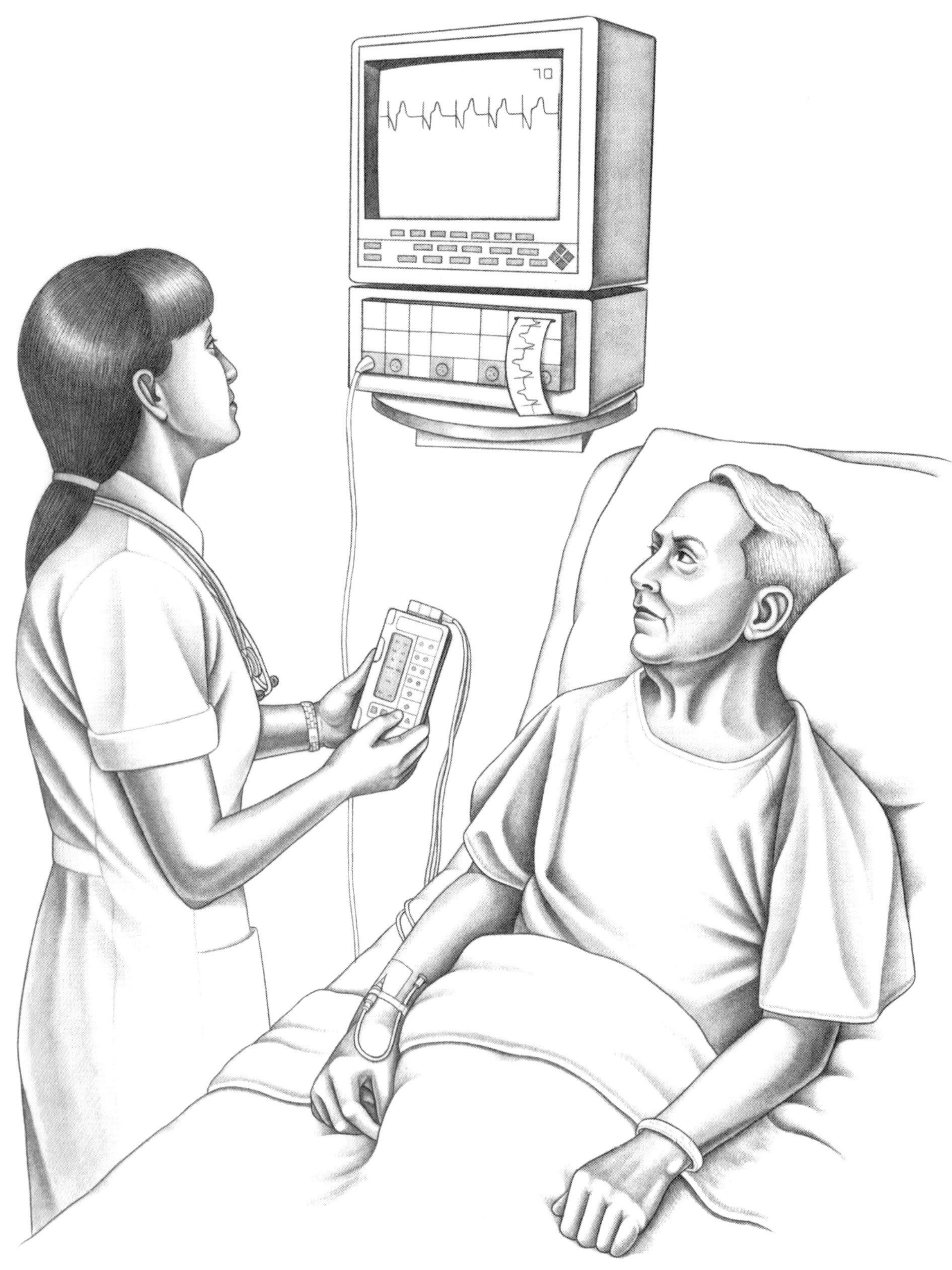
70

8

Pacemakers

In the United States each year, more than 136,000 patients receive permanently implanted pacemakers. And even more patients require temporary pacemakers. So no matter where you work, chances are that you'll care for someone who needs or already has a pacemaker.

To care for these patients, you must know the many features of pacemakers today as well as the medical conditions that make pacemakers necessary. Also, you must be able to read the electrocardiograms (ECGs) of patients with pacemakers so that you can recognize and respond to pacemaker malfunctions.

Types and characteristics of pacemakers

When a patient with an arrhythmia or heart disease can't maintain an adequate cardiac output (CO), a physician may order a pacemaker. This mechanical device emits an electrical stimulus to myocardial tissue, triggering depolarization and myocardial contractions—and boosting CO.

Pacemakers are either temporary or permanent. Typically, a physician orders a temporary pacemaker for brief periods during an emergency. The power source for this type of pacemaker is outside of the patient's body. A permanent pacemaker, on the other hand, is implanted in the patient's chest or abdominal wall to treat recurrent and persistent problems.

Both types have the same three main components: the pulse generator, the lead system, and the electrodes (see *Pacemaker close-up,* page 154).

Temporary pacemakers

Temporary pacemakers fall into two categories: transcutaneous pacemakers, which provide stimulus by way of external leads, and transvenous pacemakers, which provide stimulus by way of internal or epicardial leads.

Temporary transcutaneous pacemakers

Usually, temporary transcutaneous pacemakers are used for emergency pacing. Emergency medical technicians use portable, battery-powered transcutaneous pacemakers outside of the hospital. And hospital personnel use electrically powered transcutaneous pacemakers in acute care settings. Temporary transcutaneous pacing, also known as noninvasive pacing, is completely external and can be instituted by nurses.

Transcutaneous pacemakers can treat patients with various arrhythmias. In particular, patients with symptomatic bradycardia respond well to transcutaneous pacing, especially when they don't respond to atropine. Transcutaneous pacing also may be used to treat patients with pulseless electrical activity or asystole. And this noninvasive form of pacing may be used as an alternative to invasive pacing or as a standby treatment for the patient at risk for developing severe, symptomatic bradycardia (see *Using temporary transcutaneous pacing,* page 155).

Pacemaker close-up

Invasive temporary and permanent pacemakers have three basic components: the pulse generator, lead system, and electrodes.

The pulse generator contains the electronic components of the pacemaker and the power source, which is usually a lithium battery.

The leads carry the electric current from the pulse generator to the myocardium. Because they're insulated with silicone or polyurethane, the leads deliver electrical stimuli from the pulse generator to the heart cells without stimulating other body tissues.

Electrodes, the bare metal tips of the leads, make contact with the myocardium. The negative electrode discharges the impulse. The positive electrode completes the circuit. Electrodes can also detect electrical impulses from the heart and then transmit this information through the lead system and back to the pulse generator.

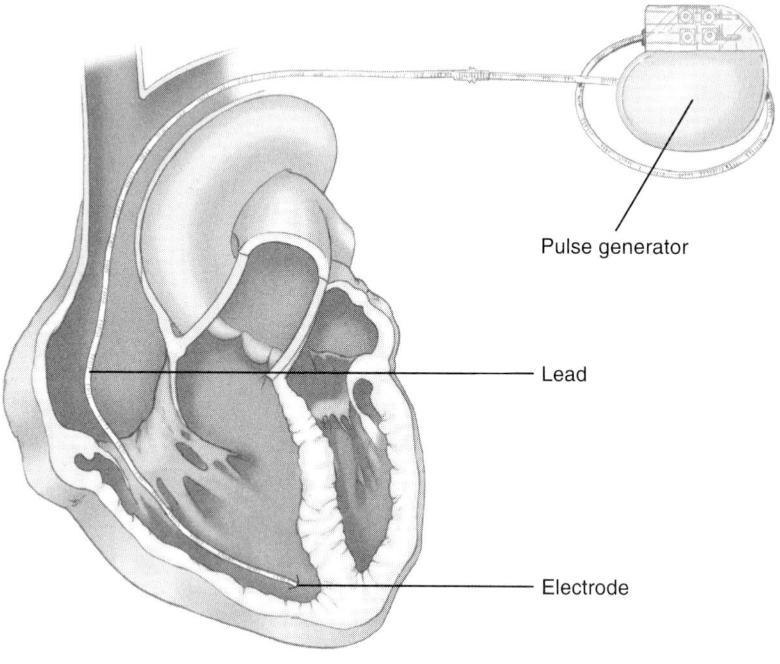

Usually, transcutaneous pacing systems have a pulse generator with a heart monitor and defibrillator. The leads and electrodes are completely external. The electrode pads, approximately the size of defibrillator pads, have conductive gel and an adhesive edge that adheres to the chest. Transcutaneous pacemaker electrodes can be single function (for pacing only) or multiple function (for monitoring, pacing, and defibrillation). Usually, transcutaneous pacemakers that have multiple-function electrodes require separate electrodes for ECG monitoring because the device can't both pace and monitor the heart rhythm from the same leads.

Because the transcutaneous pacing electrodes don't contact the heart directly, the pacemaker device produces a relatively high-voltage electrical impulse to depolarize the heart muscle. With each impulse generated, the patient feels the electrical stimulus as an unpleasant sensation or shock. The shock can cause skeletal muscles in the chest and abdominal wall to contract or twitch. Because of this discomfort, transcutaneous pacing is used for only brief periods. But this form of pacing allows

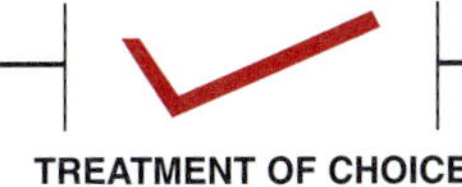

TREATMENT OF CHOICE

Using temporary transcutaneous pacing

If your patient develops symptomatic bradycardia, prepare to intervene with temporary transcutaneous pacing, using the following guidelines.

Preparing the patient

- Assess the underlying rhythm.
- Prepare the skin by trimming or shaving the chest hair, as necessary.
- Clean the skin with soap and water. Don't use alcohol, benzoin, or an antiperspirant.
- Dry the skin thoroughly and then gently abrade it.
- Apply the electrodes to the prepared skin surfaces. Don't cover dressings, incisions, wires, tubes, a long-term venous access port, a permanent pacemaker, or an implantable cardioverter-defibrillator with the electrodes.
- Seal the adhesive around the entire surface of each electrode.
- Don't put a nitroglycerin patch near the electrodes because stray electric current can cause sparking.

Initiating pacing

- Set the prescribed heart rate on the pacemaker and gradually increase the output from 0 milliamperes (mA) to the level at which you see capture for each pacing stimulus. Remember that most patients achieve capture at output levels of 50 to 90 mA, but that the level may vary depending on a patient's acid-base status and electrolyte levels.
- Familiarize yourself with your patient's rhythm-strip recording. The pacing spike may be followed by signal distortion that can appear to be a QRS complex but is only an artifact of the pacemaker. To distinguish a pacemaker artifact from a QRS complex, palpate the patient's pulse. His pulse won't be palpable with an artifact, but it will be with a QRS complex.
- During pacing, monitor your patient's skin color, mental status, urine output, and pulse oximetry readings.

nurses or paramedics to begin treatment early, before the physician arrives, ultimately improving the patient's chances of survival.

When a conscious patient is receiving transcutaneous pacing, institute comfort measures. Explain the procedure to the patient and warn him that he may feel an unpleasant sensation or shock. If indicated, obtain a prescription for an analgesic from the physician. Keep in mind that using the lowest voltage possible to maintain consistent capture will reduce the amount of discomfort. If your patient is anxious, administer sedation, as prescribed, and use distraction techniques, such as guided imagery, and relaxation exercises to reduce discomfort.

If the patient will need continued pacing, he should be switched to a temporary transvenous pacemaker or a permanent pacemaker.

Temporary transvenous pacemakers

As described, temporary transvenous pacemakers may have internal leads or epicardial leads. With a transvenous pacemaker with internal leads, a physician inserts the leads through the venous system, usually the cephalic, subclavian, or external jugular vein, into the right atrium, the right ventricle, or both. Typically, a physician inserts these leads using a balloon-tipped catheter. When the balloon passes the end of the introducer sheath, it's inflated. As with a pulmonary artery catheter, the balloon on the tip facilitates gentle forward movement of the lead catheter through the heart without damaging the tricuspid valve.

Insertion of the transvenous pacemaker internal leads can be performed at the patient's bedside or in the radiology department under fluoroscopy. An ECG may also be used to evaluate the location of the electrode.

With a transvenous pacemaker with epicardial leads, the physician attaches the leads to epicardial electrodes on the outer surface of the heart. This procedure requires cardiac surgery to attach the leads.

Both types of transvenous pacemaker leads—internal and epicardial—are attached externally to a pulse generator. And depending on the placement of the electrodes, the pacemaker device can be used for either single-chamber pacing or dual-chamber pacing.

Single-chamber pacing

With single-chamber pacing, a physician places electrodes to pace either the atria or the ventricles. Typically, a physician uses temporary transvenous single-chamber pacing for patients with symptomatic bradycardia, sick sinus syndrome with tachyarrhythmias and bradyarrhythmias, a drug overdose that places the patient at high risk for bradycardia or asystole, or a high degree of atrioventricular (AV) block, which places the patient at risk for asystole.

Dual-chamber pacing

With dual-chamber pacing, a physician places electrodes to pace both the atria and the ventricles. Temporary transvenous dual-chamber pacing may be used in patients who have more complex arrhythmias or who may need the extra stroke volume of an atrial contraction. If the patient needs temporary pacing before the insertion of a permanent pacemaker, a trial period with temporary transvenous dual-chamber pacing may help the physician evaluate whether the patient would benefit from a permanent dual-chamber or a permanent single-chamber device.

Temporary dual-chamber pacing with epicardial leads is commonly used after cardiac surgery. After open-heart surgery, most patients have epicardial electrodes loosely sutured to the outer surface of the heart. These electrodes are usually temporary. And they're placed to treat arrhythmias such as tachycardias and bradycardias that develop as a result of surgical damage or postoperative hypoxia and electrolyte imbalances.

With this form of temporary pacing, the physician places two electrodes on the atrial surface of the heart and two electrodes on the ventricular surface, allowing bipolar dual-chamber pacing. And he attaches leads to the electrodes, which extend out through the chest wall and are sutured to the skin. Typically, the atrial lead exits the right side of the chest, and the ventricular lead exits the left side.

Epicardial leads, normally attached to the pulse generator for pacing, can also be used to obtain an epicardial atrial ECG. By using alligator clips to connect the leads to the ECG electrodes, you can monitor electrical activity from the surface of the heart. This may prove helpful when an arrhythmia is difficult to interpret from a routine ECG tracing.

Permanent pacemakers

A permanent pacemaker has the same three main components as a temporary pacemaker. However, the pulse generator of a permanent pacemaker is surgically implanted through a small incision in the patient's chest or abdominal wall. This pulse generator is connected by an internal lead system either transvenously to electrodes within the heart's chambers or directly to epicardial electrodes on the surface of the heart.

Permanent pacemakers are rate-responsive, meaning they have a mechanism, usually a crystal in the pulse generator, that senses changes in the patient's activity level and generates impulses to pace the heart accordingly. For example, as the muscles of the chest wall contract with exercise, the crystal in the pulse generator begins to vibrate. And the pulse generator, in turn, increases the rate of firing according to the frequency of these vibrations.

Both the maximum rate of firing and the target heart rate can be programmed in the pacemaker. And these programmed rates can be adjusted, as necessary, to maximize the patient's response to activity. Also, some permanent pacemakers contain sensing mechanisms that respond to blood temperature, blood pH, and partial pressure of oxygen in arterial blood.

Single-chamber pacing

Permanent pacemakers used for single-chamber pacing have one lead, which a physician places to pace either the atria or the ventricles. The pacemaker's sensing and pacing abilities are restricted to the chamber in which the lead is placed (see *Recognizing single-chamber and dual-chamber pacing*).

Typically, a physician uses a permanent pacemaker for single-chamber atrial pacing in patients with a sinoatrial (SA) node arrhythmia. For this pacing to be effective, the patient must have an intact AV node and normal ventricular conduction.

A physician may use a permanent pacemaker

Recognizing single-chamber and dual-chamber pacing

Pacemakers produce characteristic electrocardiogram waveforms, depending on whether they pace the atria, the ventricles, or both. The colored asterisks on the waveforms identify the pacemaker impulses for these three types of pacing.

Atrial pacing

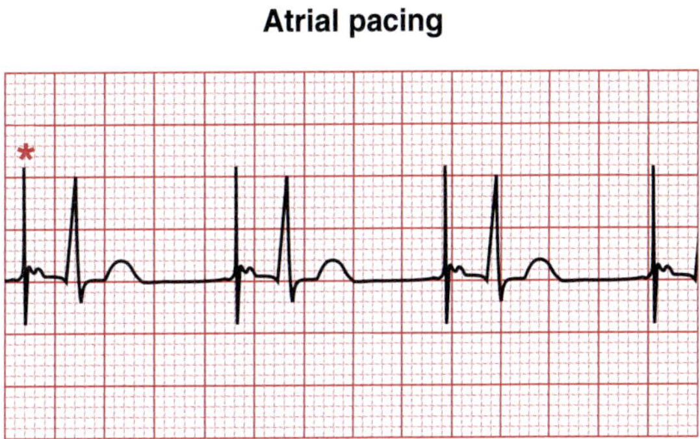

Ventricular pacing

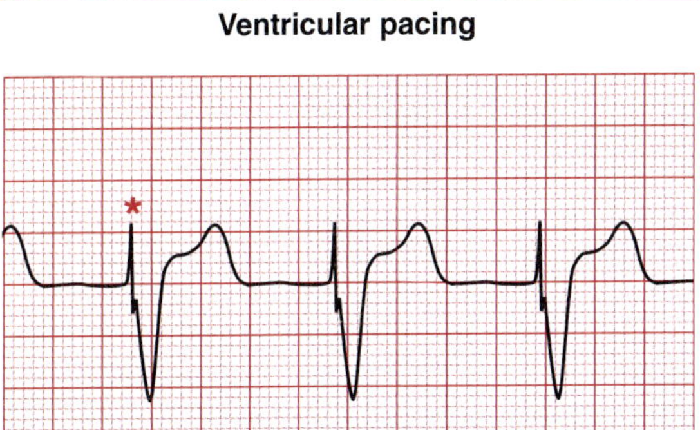

Dual-chamber pacing

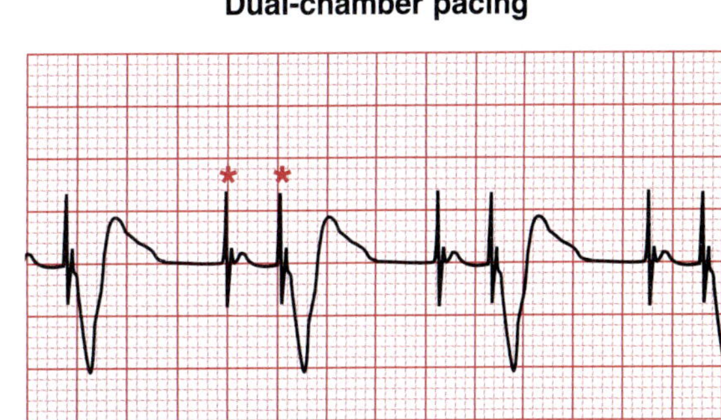

for single-chamber ventricular pacing in patients with an SA node arrhythmia and symptomatic bradycardia, second-degree AV block, third-degree AV block, bifascicular block, or trifascicular block. Also, a physician may use a single-chamber ventricular pacemaker in very elderly patients with a limited activity level and in patients with chronic atrial fibrillation. And some patients may require this type of pacemaker to prevent severe bradycardia or AV block from a drug regimen with a high risk of causing these arrhythmias.

Dual-chamber pacing

Permanent pacemakers used for dual-chamber pacing have two lead systems: one in the atria and one in the ventricles. The pacemaker senses and paces both the atria and the ventricles, while adapting automatically to the patient's underlying rhythm.

A physician may use permanent dual-chamber pacing for patients with SA node and AV node arrhythmias who don't have reliable intrinsic conduction to transmit electrical impulses through either heart chamber. If the patient's SA node is functional, a physician may use this type of pacing for patients with bifascicular or trifascicular block. Also, dual-chamber pacing may be used in patients with neurogenic syncope that's provoked by carotid sinus stimulation, ECG pauses of more than 3 seconds, or severe heart failure that results from hypertrophic or dilated cardiomyopathy.

Pacemaker modes

Pacemakers have two basic modes for pacing: asynchronous and synchronous. A physician determines the appropriate mode for pacing based on the patient's clinical condition, his hemodynamic status, and the performance of his SA node and AV conduction pathway.

Asynchronous pacing

In the asynchronous pacing mode, the pacemaker continuously discharges electrical impulses at a preset rate. This is the simplest form of pacing, but certain dangers limit its use. An asynchronous pacemaker doesn't sense the underlying electrical activity of the patient's heart. It fires regardless of the patient's own rate and rhythm. Thus, the pacemaker may compete with the patient's intrinsic rhythm, which could produce an arrhythmia. For example, if the pacemaker discharges an electrical impulse to the ventricle during the relative refractory period of an intrinsic heartbeat, the pacemaker impulse may cause R-on-T phenomenon, resulting in ventricular tachycardia or ventricular fibrillation.

Synchronous pacing

In the synchronous pacing mode, the electrodes that deliver the pacing stimulus can also sense electrical activity from the myocardium. When the pacemaker senses an impulse, it inhibits the pulse generator from discharging an impulse. The pacemaker is programmed to discharge an electrical impulse only if another impulse doesn't arise within a specific period of time, which is why this mode is also called demand pacing.

With dual-chamber synchronous pacing, sensing occurs in both chambers, and pacing may occur in either chamber, both chambers, or not at all. Sensing is based on the pacemaker settings and the underlying heart rhythm. The pacing capabilities of each pacemaker are preprogrammed, and you can identify them by the pacemaker's code.

Pacemaker code system

Pacemakers use a uniform code system to describe how they are programmed. This system has five letters that indicate the chamber paced, the chamber sensed, the response to sensing, the programmability, and antiarrhythmia function.

Chamber paced

The first letter in the pacemaker code refers to the chamber that's paced or the chamber in which the electrodes are placed. This letter can be *A* for atrial, *V* for ventricular, or *D* for dual-chamber pacing.

Chamber sensed

Sensing occurs if the pacemaker is programmed to detect electrical impulses at the electrodes. The electrodes then send a signal to the pulse generator that indicates electrical activity has occurred in the atrium, ventricle, or both chambers.

The second letter of the pacemaker code refers to the chamber that's sensed. Again, the code letters are *A* for atrial, *V* for ventricular, and *D* for dual-chamber sensing. Also, an *O* may be used to represent a pacemaker that isn't programmed to sense electrical activity in any chamber, such as in asynchronous pacing.

Response to sensing

The third letter of the pacemaker code refers to the way in which a pacemaker responds to a sensed impulse. This letter may be *I* for inhibited firing, *T* for triggered or tracking response to sensing, *D* for dual-chamber inhibition or dual mode of response, or *O* for no response.

With inhibited firing, which is the most common response to sensing, the pacemaker is programmed so that it doesn't fire impulses if it senses any intrinsic electrical activity in either the atria or the ventricles. The pacemaker impulse is synchronized to the intrinsic activity of the conduction system. And the device fires on demand only.

With a triggered response to sensing, the pacemaker is programmed so that the pulse generator fires after sensing an intrinsic electrical impulse in either the atria or the ventricles. A tracking response to sensing, a feature of newer pacemakers, means that the pacemaker is programmed so that the pulse generator fires at a preset interval after sensing an electrical impulse.

With dual-chamber inhibition or dual mode of response (inhibition and tracking), the pacemaker is programmed to react to intrinsic electrical impulses in both the atria and the ventricles.

Programmability

The fourth letter of the pacemaker code refers to the pacemaker's programmable features. This letter may be *P* for simple programmable features, *M* for multiple programmable features, *C* for communicating features, *R* for rate modulation features, or *O* for no programmable features.

Typically, a simple programmable feature is rate change. A slower pacing rate may be programmed for a patient who has intermittent bradyarrhythmia or sinus bradycardia with intermittent episodes of sinus arrest or AV block. A faster pacing rate may be programmed to increase a patient's CO or to prevent arrhythmias. An advantage of this simple programmable feature is the pacemaker's ability to mimic the circadian response with a slower rate when the patient is asleep and a faster rate when he's awake.

Multiple programmable features on a pacemaker may include controls for rate, CO, sensitivity, mode of pacing, hysteresis, refractory period, AV interval, and polarity. Such a pacemaker may also be programmed to regulate its energy output, pulse width, and voltage amplitude.

A pacemaker may have a feature that allows it to telemetrically communicate information to an external computer. Also, a pacemaker may be able to control the rate by increasing impulse firing using a special activity-sensing mechanism.

Antiarrhythmia function

The fifth letter of the pacemaker code refers to the antiarrhythmia function of a pacemaker. This letter may be *P* for a pacemaker that can provide rapid overdrive pacing, *S* for one that can discharge a defibrillation shock, *D* for one that can both provide rapid overdrive pacing and discharge defibrillation shocks, or *O* for one that doesn't have an antiarrhythmia function.

Pacemaker electrocardiograms

An ECG that's generated by an electronic pacemaker differs somewhat from one that's generated by the intrinsic activity of the heart. For example, the rate produced by a pacemaker may vary with the pacemaker's programming or with the patient's activity level. One pacemaker may function perfectly by pacing the heart at 72 beats per minute (bpm), while another type of pacemaker, pacing the heart at this same steady rate, may be malfunctioning.

Regularity of the rhythm isn't always helpful in determining the proper function of a pacemaker. An effective device may produce an irregular rhythm because natural heartbeats are interspersed with those produced by the pacemaker. Also, ventricular pacemaker complexes are initiated from within the ventricles. Such a QRS complex is broad and commonly resembles a premature QRS complex (see *How a pacemaker initiates ventricular depolarization*).

As you know, the pulse generator of an electronic pacemaker produces an electrical impulse to pace the heart. The impulse, in turn, produces an artifact that's visible on the ECG. This artifact

How a pacemaker initiates ventricular depolarization

When a pacemaker initiates an impulse in the right ventricle, the impulse must travel across the interventricular septum to depolarize the left ventricle.

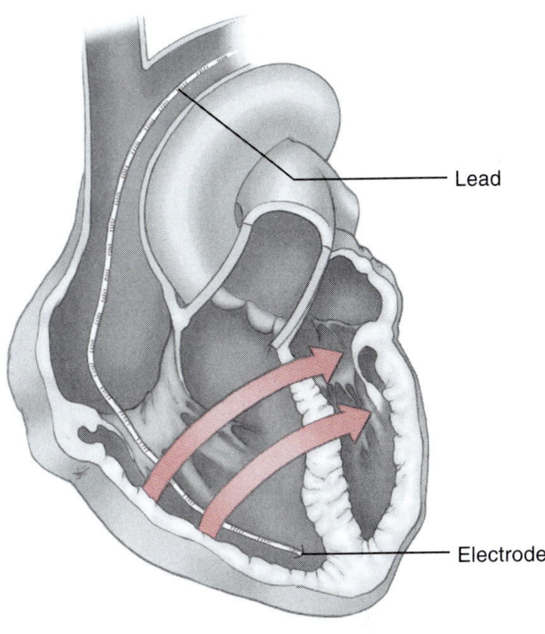

Recognizing the escape interval

To determine the escape interval for a ventricular pacemaker, measure from the end of the intrinsic QRS complex to the pacing spike. This interval represents the longest time period the pacemaker allows the heart to rest without contracting.

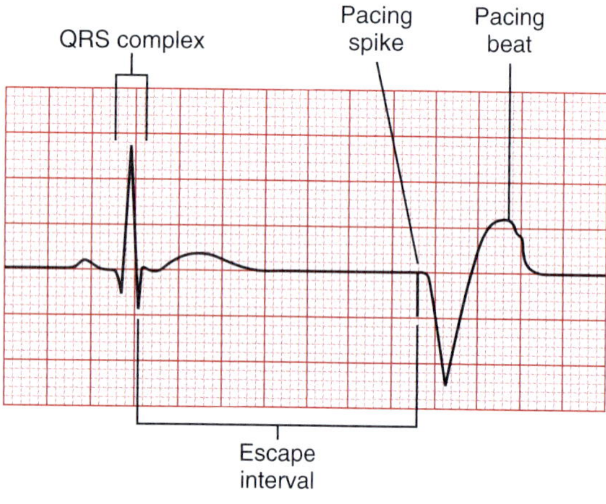

usually appears as a straight line called a pacemaker spike. If the pacemaker is functioning properly, this spike is followed by depolarization of the chamber that's being paced. If the electrode is pacing the atria, the spike occurs before the P wave; if the electrode is pacing the ventricles, the spike occurs before the QRS complex.

Normally, with a properly functioning pacemaker, the appearance of the pacing spike should remain constant. Unipolar pacing spikes are generally large; bipolar pacing spikes are not. Capture occurs with successful stimulation of the myocardium, indicated by QRS complexes following pacer spikes. And with a dual-chamber pacemaker, one spike appears before the P wave, and another appears before the QRS complex.

Typically, the pacemaker spike on the ECG is very short in duration and has no measurable width (unlike an intrinsic P or Q wave). If the pacemaker is set to fire asynchronously or if your patient has no intrinsic rhythm of his own, pacemaker spikes should appear at regular intervals. On the ECG, the rate is controlled by the pacemaker's rate setting. Most pacemakers are programmed to fire at 72 bpm, but this rate may vary with your patient's physiologic needs. Remember that rate-responsive pacemakers vary their firing rates according to the patient's activity level.

Typically, the QRS complex that follows a pacemaker spike is wider than normal (more than 0.12 second). This wide QRS complex occurs because the electronic pacemaker's impulse spreads through the ventricles slower than it would if the impulse were conducted through the heart's normal conduction system. If the impulse comes from an electrode placed in the right ventricle, it must travel across the septum to also depolarize the left ventricle. This conduction time is greater than that of an intrinsic impulse coming down the bundle branches and spreading to both the right and left ventricles at the same time.

Because pacemaker-initiated ventricular depolarization spreads abnormally, the resulting repolarization also differs from normal, intrinsic repolarization. The result is an abnormal ST segment and T wave following the QRS complex.

If the pacemaker is pacing the atria, expect to see the pacemaker spike before the P wave. P waves generated by an atrial pacemaker look somewhat odd, and the PR interval tends to be longer than normal. You may have difficulty evaluating whether an atrial pacing lead has depolarized the atria because the amplitude of the waveform is so much lower than that seen in ventricular depolarization. Sometimes, an atrial spike may be followed by a small bump, called a hump sign, that's best seen in leads V_1, V_2, and II.

Escape interval

All pacemakers have a setting for the escape interval, the time during which the pacemaker senses an intrinsic impulse and waits for the impulse to conduct. This escape interval also occurs after the pacemaker fires its own impulse.

For a patient with a simple single-chamber pacemaker, the escape interval usually equals the pacemaker's automatic rate. And if the heart isn't producing any of its own impulses, the heart rate equals the pacemaker's escape interval.

For an atrial pacemaker, the escape interval is measured from the intrinsic P wave to the next atrial pacemaker spike. For a ventricular pacemaker, the escape interval is measured from the intrinsic QRS complex to the next ventricular pacemaker spike (see *Recognizing the escape interval*).

Indications for pacing

Pacemakers may benefit patients who have insufficient CO, abnormal electrical impulse conduction, SA node dysfunction, an AV block, a bundle branch block, or a nervous system or blood pressure disorder. Typically, a physician determines the type of pacemaker a patient needs by considering the nature of the arrhythmia and factors such as the patient's overall health and activity level.

Inadequate cardiac output

As you know, bradycardia can reduce a patient's CO by decreasing the rate of his heart's contractions. For such a patient, a pacemaker may help improve CO, so he can maintain organ function and a desired activity level (see *Reviewing indications for pacing*).

A VVI-type pacemaker maintains a specific heart rate and prevents severe decreases in CO due to periods of asystole. However, the ventricular contractions initiated by VVI pacing are less effective than a patient's intrinsic sinus rhythm because they lack atrial kick. Many patients can feel the effects of VVI pacing because they notice this reduction in CO, a condition called pacemaker syndrome. Signs and symptoms of pacemaker syndrome include light-headedness and slight activity intolerance.

Dual-chamber pacing usually improves a patient's CO and exercise tolerance. And the AV synchrony provided by DDD-type pacing produces a normal atrial kick. But if the patient's atrial rate doesn't increase in response to sympathetic nervous system stimulation or increased metabolic needs, DDD pacing may fail to provide a normal CO.

Reviewing indications for pacing

Familiarize yourself with the following indications for temporary transcutaneous, temporary transvenous, and permanent pacing.

Type of pacing	Indications
Temporary transcutaneous pacing	• significant bradycardia unresponsive to atropine, or atropine not readily available • interim relief before transvenous pacing • drug-induced cardiac arrest, especially with profound bradycardia or pulseless electrical activity • asystolic cardiac arrest lasting less than 10 minutes
Temporary transvenous pacing	• hemodynamically unstable bradycardia including complete atrioventricular (AV) block, symptomatic second-degree AV block, sick sinus syndrome, drug-induced bradycardias, permanent pacemaker failure, idioventricular rhythm, and symptomatic atrial fibrillation with slow ventricular response • bradycardia with escape rhythms • overdrive pacing of tachycardia refractory to drugs and electric shock • bradyasystolic cardiac arrest
Permanent pacing	• permanent or incomplete AV block, especially second-degree AV block type II • sinoatrial (SA) node dysfunction, including severe sinus bradycardia, bradycardia-tachycardia syndrome, sinus arrest, and SA exit block

Inadequate impulse conduction

A physician may use a pacemaker to treat a patient whose heart doesn't consistently generate its own electrical impulses. A pacemaker also may be used for a patient whose heart doesn't conduct impulses to the atria or the ventricles.

Sinoatrial node dysfunction

About half of all pacemakers implanted each year are used to treat SA node dysfunction, or sick sinus syndrome. Examples of SA node dysfunction include bradycardia-tachycardia syndrome, sinus arrest, and sinus exit block.

Ventricular pacing and atrial flutter

Despite an underlying rhythm of atrial flutter (represented by the characteristic sawtooth waves), ventricular pacing controls the ventricular rhythm. Note that a pacemaker spike appears before each QRS complex.

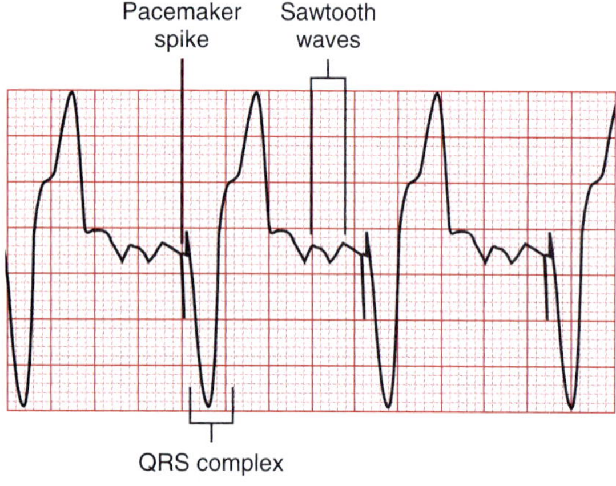

Atrioventricular block

With an AV block, a ventricular pacemaker may be used to bypass the conduction system disturbance. The pacemaker produces an impulse that stimulates the ventricles, causing them to contract and produce the needed stroke volume.

Most pacemakers can sense when an intrinsic impulse is generated, so they can inhibit pacemaker firing. However, when complete ventricular pacing is performed, the ventricular rhythm occurs independently of activity in the atria. And a single-chamber ventricular pacemaker can't sense what's going on in the atria. If your patient's pacemaker has only a ventricular lead, expect to see complete dissociation from any atrial rhythm (see *Ventricular pacing and atrial flutter*).

Bundle branch blocks

As you know, bundle branch blocks can produce observable patterns on the ECG. However, these signs and symptoms alone don't usually warrant treatment with a pacemaker.

Typically, a physician uses a pacemaker for a patient with a severe bundle branch block, such as a bifascicular or trifascicular block that causes syncope. He also may use a pacemaker if a bifascicular or trifascicular block occurs with an arrhythmia such as second-degree AV block type II.

Nervous system and blood pressure disorders

Because the heart interacts with the autonomic nervous system, syncope can result if this interaction is compromised. For example, pressure on the carotid sinus can inhibit cardiac function. With carotid sinus syndrome, this inhibition is so extreme that periods of asystole can result. If the pause is longer than 3 seconds and your patient is symptomatic, the physician will usually insert a pacemaker.

With vasovagal syndrome, a patient's sympathetic tone increases, and his parasympathetic tone decreases. This condition causes vasodilation of the peripheral blood vessels, resulting in bradycardia and hypotension. If the patient with bradycardia becomes symptomatic and his heart rate falls below 60 bpm, he may require artificial pacing.

A patient with dilated cardiomyopathy that doesn't respond to medical treatment may receive some hemodynamic benefit from a dual-chamber pacemaker.

Overdrive pacing

In some patients, a temporary pacemaker may be used to override rapid tachycardia. For such an arrhythmia, the physician programs the electronic pacemaker for a rate faster than that produced by the patient's irritable ectopic pacemaker. The electronic pacemaker takes control of the heart rate away from the ectopic site until the heart regains a more normal rate. A physician also may use this type of pacing to terminate reentrant tachycardia.

Pacemaker problems

Several problems can occur with pacemakers. Some result from limitations of a particular pacemaker. Others result from technical failure of one or more of the pacemaker's components.

Pacemaker syndrome

Pacemaker syndrome occurs when a pacemaker doesn't respond to a patient's need for increased CO. With this condition, if simple ventricular pacing is performed at a consistent, predetermined rate, a patient's CO won't change with variations in his activity level. For example, if such a pacemaker is set to pace at 72 bpm in a patient who has a slower intrinsic heart rate, the pacemaker will continue to pace the heart at 72 bpm, regardless of whether the patient is sitting quietly reading a book or running to catch a bus. The pacemaker doesn't increase the heart rate or CO in relation to increased activity, so the patient's physiologic need for more oxygenated blood can't be met.

Also, with ventricular pacing, atrial and ventricular contractions become asynchronous. And this asynchrony diminishes atrial kick.

Signs and symptoms of pacemaker syndrome include light-headedness, fatigue, and dyspnea. And they may occur even with mild exertion.

Implanting a pacemaker that responds to increased activity levels, such as a rate-responsive pacemaker, or one that provides atrial-ventricular synchrony, such as a dual-chamber pacemaker, can alleviate pacemaker syndrome.

Technical malfunction

Pacemaker malfunction can result from defects in the components of the pacing system. For the pacemaker to sense, pace, and capture effectively, the device must have the following components:

- adequate battery power
- appropriate settings
- intact wire and lead connections.

Of course, the heart also must be capable of responding to electrical stimulation.

Common pacemaker malfunctions include failure to pace, failure to capture, and failure to sense.

Failure to pace

Failure to pace or stimulate the heart occurs when the pacemaker doesn't deliver an electrical stimulus to the myocardium. Although the reason for this malfunction may be simple, the result can be life threatening.

The most common reason for failure to pace is failure of the power source. A permanent pacemaker must have sufficient battery power to produce the level of milliamperes needed to pace the heart. Also, a temporary pacemaker must be connected to a power source and turned on. In true failure to pace, no pacing spikes appear on the ECG.

Other reasons for failure to pace include an excessively high sensitivity setting and electromagnetic interference. If the pacemaker is too sensitive, its function can be inhibited by T waves or even by muscle artifact.

Electromagnetic interference can result from exposure to a magnetic resonance imaging (MRI) machine. A cellular telephone can cause problems with pacemaker function when the telephone is held over the pacemaker pocket, but not when it's held to the ear. Also, the ultrasonic and electrosurgical instruments used by dentists may inhibit the function of atrial and ventricular pacemakers.

Failure to capture

Capture, the depolarization of the atria or ventricles in response to a pacemaker's electrical stimulus, can be affected by physiologic problems in the myocardium or by mechanical problems with the pacemaker. Even the strongest pacemaker impulse won't produce depolarization if the myocardium is too weak to respond. Conversely, even the healthiest myocardium can't respond to a pacemaker whose signal is too weak or is delivered to the wrong area.

Mechanical reasons for failure to capture include problems with the power source, such as a failed battery or a low setting, and problems with the lead wires, such as fracture or dislodgment. In particular, atrial leads are easily dislodged.

Sometimes the lead wire pierces the myocardium, which prevents the pacemaker's impulse from pacing the heart. Insulation of the lead wire may break as well. The electrode tip may become dysfunctional if it's surrounded by edema or scarring. Also, a pacemaker setting that paced the heart effectively in the past may become ineffective over time as a result of electrolyte changes or a physiologic response to drug therapy.

With failure to capture, the ECG shows a pacing spike that isn't followed by a QRS complex or by a P wave, for ventricular pacing or atrial pacing, respectively (see *Recognizing a failure to capture,* page 164).

Recognizing a failure to capture

This electrocardiogram shows the difference between a captured pacemaker impulse and an uncaptured one. Note that the captured impulse produces a pacemaker spike followed by a QRS complex. The uncaptured impulse produces only the spike.

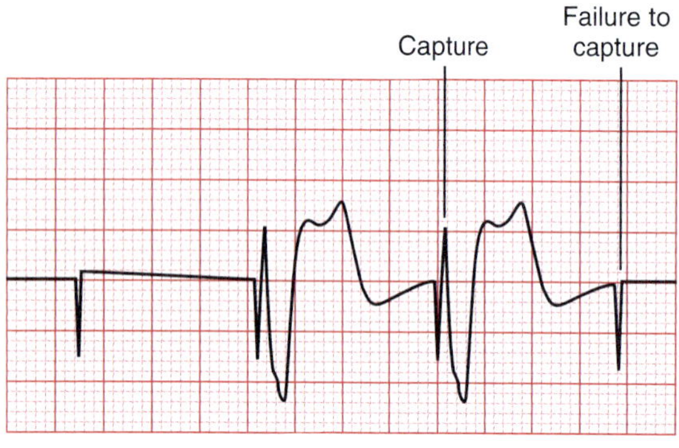

Failure to sense

Failure to sense may result from either undersensing or oversensing. With undersensing, the pacemaker fires impulses at inappropriate times. With oversensing, it's inhibited from firing.

Undersensing

The sensitivity setting on the pacemaker determines how strong an intrinsic impulse must be for the pacemaker to recognize it. If the pacemaker's sensitivity is set too low, it undersenses.

Many of the same problems that lead to failure to capture can also cause failure to sense. The most common problem is that the electrode tip moves out of the optimal position for sensing. Electrolyte disturbances, antiarrhythmic drugs, and physiologic changes within the myocardium, such as edema and fibrosis, may alter the pacemaker's sensitivity threshold. Also, the electronic components of the pacemaker's sensing system may fail.

Even a pacemaker that has been working consistently may suddenly develop problems if the battery fails or lead wires fracture. In such cases, the pacemaker would be able to pace and would probably capture, but it wouldn't be able to sense. If a pacemaker can't sense, it may fire at regular intervals (the pacemaker's automatic rate) regardless of the heart's intrinsic electrical activity.

Oversensing

Oversensing may occur because the pacemaker's sensitivity is set too high. Instead of appropriately detecting only the patient's intrinsic complexes (P waves for an atrial lead and QRS complexes for a ventricular lead), the pacemaker senses other electrical activity.

Oversensing may result from electromagnetic interference, such as when a patient has an MRI study or transcutaneous electrical nerve stimulation. Also, the pacemaker may sense an inappropriate component of the cardiac cycle. For example, a ventricular lead may become inhibited if it interprets a large T wave as a QRS complex, or an atrial lead may become inhibited if it senses ventricular activity.

Oversensing is a particular problem with unipolar electrodes. Such electrodes may even sense pectoral muscle contractions.

With oversensing, the ECG tracing shows a lack of pacemaker activity where you expect to see it. For example, the pacemaker spike doesn't appear, even though your patient's heart beats slower than the pacemaker's automatic interval. In such a case, you may have difficulty determining whether the malfunction is failure to pace or oversensing. A physician may have you try adjusting the pacemaker's sensitivity setting to try to correct the problem.

Pacemaker anomalies

Sometimes, normal pacemaker beats or interactions between pacemaker and intrinsic beats may look like pacemaker malfunctions on an ECG. However, anomalous pacemaker complexes such as fusion beats, pseudofusion, and hysteresis really represent correct pacemaker functioning. So you must be able to distinguish between an ECG that shows a real problem and one that only appears to be abnormal.

Fusion beats

Correct pacemaker function can be confusing on an ECG, particularly when the heart's intrinsic complexes are interspersed with those generated

Recognizing fusion beats

Fusion beats occur during the transition between pacemaker control of the heart and sinoatrial node control. This electrocardiogram shows four paced beats, followed by a fusion beat, followed by three normal sinus rhythms.

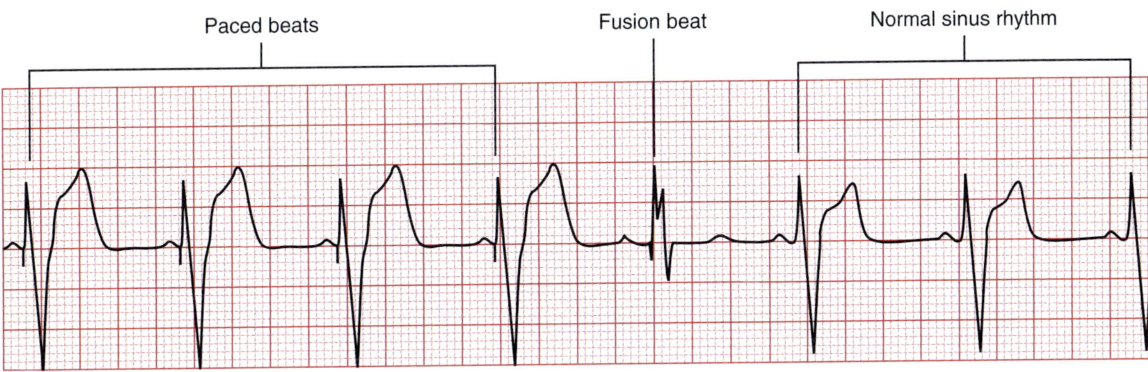

by a pacemaker. For instance, the ECG may show fusion beats, bizarre complexes that appear when a correctly functioning pacemaker generates an impulse at about the same time that an intrinsic impulse fires (see *Recognizing fusion beats*).

Usually, fusion beats occur because the SA node fires an impulse that's too weak for the pacemaker to sense. Though fusion beats may look odd, they can help you evaluate pacemaker function or determine a pacemaker's automatic interval.

Pseudofusion

Pseudofusion, another complex sometimes confused with pacemaker malfunction, occurs when the pacemaker's rate and the heart's intrinsic rate are similar. The difference between a fusion beat and pseudofusion is the presence of a clearly identifiable pacemaker spike on the ECG. In a pseudofusion beat, the pacemaker generates an impulse, but the heart's intrinsic impulse is the one that captures and depolarizes the myocardium.

You might see a pacemaker spike followed by a normal-looking intrinsic complex. This may look like a fusion beat, but in fact, it's pseudofusion because depolarization results from just the intrinsic impulse, not both the intrinsic and pacemaker impulses.

Hysteresis

Hysteresis, an impulse delay programmed into some pacemakers, allows more time for the heart to generate its own intrinsic impulse. Usually, such natural pacing is preferable to mechanical pacing.

The hysteresis setting of a pacemaker is somewhat slower than its programmed automatic rate. For example, if your patient has an intrinsic heart rate of 76 bpm and the pacemaker's automatic rate is 72 bpm, the pacemaker would usually fire after it senses a pause that would make the overall rate less than 72 bpm. But with hysteresis, the pacemaker may not fire until it senses a pause that corresponds to an overall rate of 60 bpm. Then, when the pacemaker does fire, it continues to do so at its preset rate of 72 bpm until the heart once again resumes control of the pacing.

On the ECG of a patient with such a pacemaker, hysteresis may resemble failure to pace.

Preventing and correcting pacemaker malfunctions

Usually, with proper setup, implementation, safety measures, and patient teaching, you can avoid many of the problems that can occur with pacemaker use. However, if a pacemaker malfunction should occur, be prepared to treat your patient for the malfunction and for the possible complications it may cause.

Setting a temporary pacemaker

Before initiating temporary pacing, insert a fully charged battery into the pulse generator. Mark the date and time that the battery was changed on a piece of tape and place it on the back of the pulse generator. Then, connect the proximal end of the leads to the generator.

Always wear gloves when touching the bare metal tips of the leads because electrostatic current can be transmitted across the wires. This current can depolarize your patient's heart just as a pacing stimulus can. It may also cause R-on-T phenomenon, predisposing your patient to ventricular fibrillation.

Ventricular settings

For ventricular settings, start with the output and sensitivity settings at the lowest possible levels. Then, determine the stimulation and sensitivity thresholds.

To determine the sensitivity threshold, watch the ECG monitor while gradually increasing the pacemaker's output setting, as ordered. When you see that each pacing stimulus results in capture, you have found the stimulation threshold.

For transvenous leads, you'll typically use a relatively low stimulation threshold (0.1 to 1 milliampere [mA]). However, for some patients, a physician may order a higher output setting to allow for the changes that may result from altered fluid, electrolyte, acid-base, and oxygenation levels.

For epicardial leads, you'll typically use a higher stimulation threshold (more than 1 mA). But be aware that with epicardial leads, you may not be able to increase the output more than 1 to 5 mA over the stimulation threshold without causing myocardial damage.

To determine the sensitivity threshold, set the pacemaker rate to a level less than your patient's intrinsic rate. Begin with the sensitivity control set to sense at 20 mA. At this setting, you should see a sensing light flash with each QRS complex on the ECG monitor. Gradually lower the sensitivity control until the pacemaker loses sensing. This is evident when the indicator light no longer flashes with each QRS complex. The lowest number at which you note consistent sensing is the sensitivity threshold.

After you determine the sensitivity threshold, return the sensitivity control to the setting ordered by the physician. Then, document with a rhythm strip your patient's intrinsic rhythm, the paced rhythm, the stimulation and sensitivity thresholds, and the actual settings used for output and sensing.

Atrial settings

For atrial output and sensitivity settings, take the same initial steps as described for ventricular settings. First, determine the stimulation and sensitivity thresholds. Then, adjust the output and sensing controls accordingly.

With atrial settings, you'll also need to set an upper pacing limit. Typically, this pacing limit should equal the longest normal PR interval, or 0.2 second. The upper pacing limit helps to control ventricular response if your patient's intrinsic atrial rate accelerates. It also prevents an excessive increase in the cardiac workload that could lead to ischemia.

When using an older temporary pacemaker, you also may need to set the postventricular atrial refractory period. This period is programmed into the pulse generator to prevent the heart rate from becoming too fast, which may happen if your patient has retrograde impulse conduction or an atrial arrhythmia such as atrial flutter.

To determine the postventricular atrial refractory period, first establish the total duration of the cardiac cycle. Then, determine how long each component of the cycle lasts. For example, if the patient's heart rate is 100 bpm, each cardiac cycle lasts 0.6 second. If the atria are paced at 0.22 second and the ventricles are paced at 0.14 second, then the refractory period cannot exceed the 0.24 second remaining in the cardiac cycle. Usually, the refractory period shouldn't be greater than half of the cardiac cycle.

Maintaining patient safety

After a temporary pacemaker has been set and is functioning, focus on monitoring your patient's safety. In particular, a patient with a transvenous pacemaker is at risk for microshock, which may occur if an electrostatic discharge crosses the lead wires and depolarizes the myocardium. If microshock occurs during the relative refractory period of the heart, ventricular tachycardia or fibrillation may result.

To protect your patient, always wear gloves when touching the pacemaker leads or connections. If the pacing wires aren't connected to your patient, cover the exposed metal leads with an insulating material such as a latex glove, a finger cot, or the rubber cap of a syringe. Tape the insulating material to the lead loosely so that it will come off easily if you need to reinitiate pacing.

Take measures to avoid static electricity. Always discharge electric current by touching metal before you touch your patient. If your patient with a temporary pacemaker is ambulatory, protect him from accidentally discharging electric current across the leads. The air should have adequate humidity to reduce the risk of electrostatic shock. Also, have any carpeting in the area treated with an antielectrostatic chemical or an undercarpet antielectrostatic device.

During transcutaneous pacing, you can safely touch your patient to provide care. For example, if your patient experiences cardiopulmonary arrest, you should perform cardiopulmonary resuscitation (CPR) as normal. However, remember that the pacing electrodes must remain firmly adhered to your patient's chest during the compressions. If the electrodes aren't secured, the impulse may be transmitted across his chest to your hands.

If your patient requires defibrillation, be sure to remove all conductive gel from his chest before reinitiating pacing. This gel can allow the transmission of electrical impulses to anyone who touches his chest during pacing.

Ensure that pacing is performed at the proper settings. Perform continuous cardiac monitoring of your patient. And use a systematic plan to evaluate his ECG (see *An approach to interpreting your patient's pacemaker electrocardiogram*).

Routinely check the pacing thresholds and any readjustments in settings at least every 8 hours. Be sure to document any changes made in the settings and include a rhythm strip in your patient's chart. If a problem with pacing arises, check the pacemaker immediately.

Protect the leads from dislodging. With transvenous pacing, the electrode must maintain contact with viable myocardial tissue. If a transvenous or epicardial lead becomes slightly repositioned, capture may be lost. When dressing the lead exit site, don't put any tension on the lead that might pull it out of position. And tell your patient to restrict movement of the arm on the side where a temporary transvenous pacemaker is placed to prevent dislodgment of the lead.

Preventing infection is crucial because the lead insertion site is a direct path to the heart. Use aseptic technique for dressing changes and follow the same guidelines as for the care of a central ve-

RESEARCH UPDATE

An approach to interpreting your patient's pacemaker electrocardiogram

Interpreting your patient's pacemaker electrocardiogram (ECG) can be a complex task. However, research into the common ECG characteristics of pacemakers has led to a checklist of questions that may help you evaluate your patient's pacemaker rhythm.

First, check the pacemaker codes. Then ask yourself the following questions:

- What is the intrinsic rate and rhythm? Are P waves present? If so, at what rate? Are QRS complexes present? If so, at what rate?
- Do you see atrial or ventricular pacemaker spikes? Can you determine the atrial rate? Is the pacing interval regular? What is its rate? Can you determine the ventricular rate? Is the pacing interval regular? What is its rate?
- What is the escape interval? What is the paced interval? Do you see evidence of hysteresis, atrial tracking, or rate responsiveness?
- Do you see evidence of atrial or ventricular capture?
- If your patient has a dual-chamber pacemaker, what is the atrial-ventricular interval, the postventricular atrial refractory period, and the ventricular-atrial interval?
- Is the atrial lead sensing properly? Is the ventricular lead sensing properly? Do you note oversensing or undersensing?

nous catheter. Temporary epicardial wire exit sites require more frequent dressing changes. Treat the exit sites as you do the incision. To avoid contamination, don't contain these wires under your patient's chest-tube dressing.

When the physician removes your patient's temporary pacemaker, be sure to monitor the patient's status. Observe the ECG monitor for arrhythmias that may result from myocardial irritation or valve damage. Continue monitoring your patient for several hours because he has a risk of cardiac tamponade occurring from injury during removal of the wire. Be alert for an increase in jugular venous pressure and a low pulse pressure (low systolic and high diastolic blood pressure).

Preventing problems with permanent pacemakers

Typically, a patient who undergoes permanent pacemaker insertion spends very little time in the hospital. During the day or two of hospitalization, monitor your patient carefully so that any pacemaker malfunction can be detected early and the device reprogrammed. Also, teach him how to prevent complications of the pacemaker insertion (see *Going home with a permanent pacemaker*).

Teach your patient the signs and symptoms that may indicate his pacemaker is oversensing environmental electrical signals. Have him avoid sources of electrical interference such as older microwaves, cellular telephones, car alternators, and large electrical towers. Tell him that if he feels light-headed and his radial pulse rate is less than the lower limit set on the pacemaker, he should leave the dangerous environment immediately.

Also, teach him how to care for the incision site. Warn him that infection of the incision could lead to sepsis and infective endocarditis. For the first few days after implantation of the device, he should limit use of the arm on the side of the pulse generator insertion to prevent the lead from dislodging. Some patients may require a sling to maintain arm position.

Later follow-up should focus on assessing your patient's activity tolerance. Rate-responsive VVI and DDD pacemakers can increase activity tolerance, so assess how much activity your patient performs. At times, the pacemaker rate may be decreased to preserve battery life. Include your patient in decision making when optimizing pacemaker function to improve his quality of life.

Correcting malfunctions

Most pacemaker malfunctions result from weak batteries and lead dislodgment, making repair the most common solution. Typically, medical or pharmacologic interventions aren't effective in treating pacemaker malfunctions. However, if a pacemaker fails and your patient's heart rate falls to a level that produces hemodynamic instability, you should initiate emergency therapy with drugs such as atropine, as prescribed. But remember that such drug therapy is just a short-term remedy. You must correct the problem with the pacemaker to provide a long-term solution.

For some patients, treatment may involve surgery to replace pulse generators or pacing leads. Such operations are generally performed under local anesthesia with small amounts of I.V. sedation, usually on an outpatient basis.

Remember that malfunctions can occur with both temporary and permanent pacemakers. And the proper way to correct a malfunction depends on the type of device.

Failure to pace

If your patient experiences failure to pace with a temporary pacemaker, check that the pacemaker is turned on and the battery has power. Sometimes, connections between the pulse generator and the lead wires become loose, so you may need to tighten them. For either temporary or permanent pacemakers, the pulse generator may need to be replaced. If your patient has a temporary pacemaker, simply disconnect the malfunctioning pulse generator and attach a new one. If your patient has a permanent pacemaker, he'll require surgery to replace the pulse generator.

Failure to capture

If your patient with a temporary transvenous pacemaker experiences failure to capture, you may need to replace the pulse generator and the pacing leads. Also, try positioning your patient on his left side, which may help move the pacemaker lead into a better position.

Check the setting for pacemaker output. If it's set too low, the pacemaker can be reprogrammed to gradually emit a stronger signal until capture is achieved.

Undersensing

If you detect pacemaker undersensing, you may need to replace the pulse generator. Occasionally,

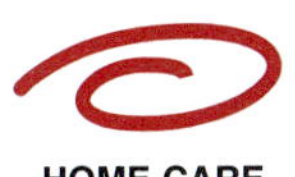

HOME CARE

Going home with a permanent pacemaker

Because your patient may have a limited hospital stay after undergoing permanent pacemaker insertion, teaching him to care for himself is vital for preventing complications after discharge. In particular, teach him to live with his pacemaker, care for the insertion site, and obtain follow-up care.

Living with a pacemaker

- Instruct your patient to take his pulse every morning when he wakes. Advise him to report a pulse rate that's slower than the pacemaker's set rate by at least 5 beats per minute.
- Tell your patient about the programmable features of his pacemaker. Warn him that his pulse may be somewhat irregular, with some spontaneous and paced beats.
- Teach him the signs and symptoms of pacemaker malfunction, including dizziness, fainting, chest pain, shortness of breath, fatigue, and sudden weight gain and puffy ankles caused by fluid retention.
- Tell him the expected life of the pacemaker battery.
- Encourage your patient to carry his pacemaker identification card at all times and to wear a medical identification bracelet or necklace stating that he has a pacemaker.
- Warn him that some electrical devices may cause electromagnetic interference with pacemaker function. Caution him to avoid areas with high voltage, magnetic fields, and radiation. Tell him to inform his dentist about the pacemaker because some ultrasonic and electrosurgical dental instruments may cause interference.
- Warn your patient that the pacemaker's metal casing and programming magnet may trigger metal detectors. Although this typically doesn't damage the pacemaker, he may find the situation embarrassing.

Caring for the insertion site

- Teach your patient to inspect the insertion site daily and to look for signs and symptoms of infection, including redness, tenderness, drainage, and increased soreness. Also, instruct him to take his temperature daily and to report a temperature above 100°F (37.7°C).
- If necessary, teach your patient to clean the insertion site and change his dressings.
- Two days after the insertion, encourage your patient to perform active and passive range-of-motion exercises with the affected arm and shoulder. Tell him to continue these exercises until he no longer feels discomfort.
- Advise him to avoid high-impact activities, including contact sports. Tell him to report any activity that may have injured the insertion site.

Following up

- Tell your patient about the need for regular follow-up so that his physician can evaluate pacemaker function and reprogram the pacemaker, as necessary.
- If appropriate, teach your patient to use telephone monitoring for evaluation of his pacemaker.

the leads may require adjustment. And the sensitivity settings may need to be increased.

Oversensing

If oversensing occurs, determine what is being sensed instead of the intrinsic complexes. If you can determine a source of electrical interference, take steps to eliminate it, such as removing unnecessary electrical equipment from the area.

Also, check the pacemaker's sensitivity setting. If it's too high, oversensing can occur. Or your patient may require a bipolar lead that's less likely to sense muscle activity.

Mechanical malfunctions

As with any mechanical device, the possibility of malfunction always exists. Remind your patient of this when he receives his limited-warranty information after the pacemaker is implanted.

Some pacemaker leads don't perform well initially, resulting in intermittent failure. Pay attention to safety alerts and advisories issued about pacemaker products. Remember that careful surveillance of your patient, such as with ambulatory ECG monitoring, helps reveal a lead that's beginning to malfunction. Such monitoring can be far more effective for preventing pacemaker mal-

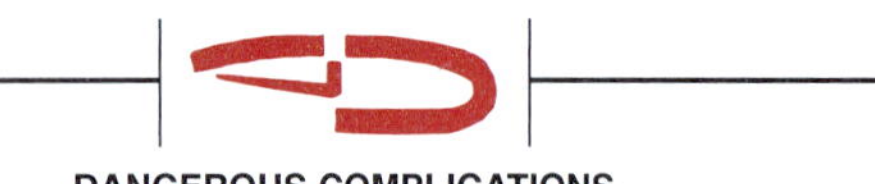

DANGEROUS COMPLICATIONS

Reviewing complications of pacemaker use

Type of pacemaker	Complications
Temporary transcutaneous	• pain from electrical stimulation of skin and muscles • tissue damage, including third-degree burns from prolonged or improper electrode placement
Temporary transvenous	• bleeding • infection • pneumothorax • arrhythmias • myocardial infarction • hematoma at insertion site • right ventricular perforation and cardiac tamponade • perforation of inferior vena cava, pulmonary artery, or coronary arteries from improper lead placement
Permanent	*Caused by implantation* • bleeding • pneumothorax • arrhythmias • air embolism • thrombosis • infection *Caused by pacing* • heart failure • pacemaker-induced arrhythmias • right ventricular perforation and cardiac tamponade

functions than routine pacemaker clinic follow-up.

Nursing considerations

To provide comprehensive nursing care, consider the problems your patient may experience in emotionally adjusting to a pacemaker. Also, be aware that your patient may experience acute and chronic complications caused by the pacemaker.

Psychological problems

A patient with a pacemaker may worry about the function of the device and fear that he's dependent on a battery-operated generator that could easily fail. He may be afraid to move or concerned about having others touch him. Explore any fears that your patient has regarding his pacemaker and answer any questions that he and his family have.

A patient may experience depression, anxiety, insomnia, loss of energy, and hypochondria after receiving the device. Adjusting to the implantation of a permanent pacemaker may significantly challenge your patient's psychological health.

Monitor your patient for these psychological problems and assess his adjustment throughout his period of care. If necessary, refer him to a mental health professional.

Acute complications

The various acute complications that can occur during and after pacemaker use depend on the type of pacemaker. For example, a transcutaneous pacemaker can cause uncomfortable muscle contractions because of the electrical stimulation from its externally applied electrodes.

Acute complications from transvenous pacemakers commonly arise during implantation. Such problems include infection, bleeding, and the possibility of pneumothorax, thrombosis, and air embolism. Also, a patient with a temporary transvenous pacemaker has a continuing risk of infection at the insertion site and electrical accidents. For example, stray electric current from static electricity or electrical devices in the immediate vicinity may travel to the heart through poorly insulated pacemaker electrodes, causing lethal arrhythmias (see *Reviewing complications of pacemaker use*).

Chronic complications

Permanent transvenous pacemakers, in particular, introduce the additional risk of chronic complications. The insertion site may become infected, or the pulse generator may become displaced. Sometimes, a patient consciously or unconsciously moves the pulse generator in a twisting fashion, so the leads become intertwined and the pacemaker malfunctions, a phenomenon called twiddler's syndrome.

Pacing leads may fracture and electrodes may become dislodged, potentially damaging the cardiac chamber in which they're placed. Also, perforation may lead to pericardial tamponade.

With a dual-chamber pacemaker, your patient may experience pacemaker-mediated tachycardia, or endless-loop tachycardia. Like reentry phenomenon, pacemaker-mediated tachycardia occurs when an intrinsic premature ventricular contraction conducts impulses to the atria in a retrograde fashion, outside of the postventricular atrial refractory period. The pacemaker senses this impulse and initiates ventricular pacing. The paced beat also conducts in a retrograde fashion, and the same process recurs. As long as this scenario is repeated, a continual tachycardia results.

Some pacemakers are designed to sense pacemaker-mediated tachycardia and to interrupt the cycle of this type of arrhythmia. However, if such a pacemaker isn't available for your patient, you may be able to increase his pacemaker's postventricular atrial refractory period so that retrograde P waves don't initiate ventricular pacing.

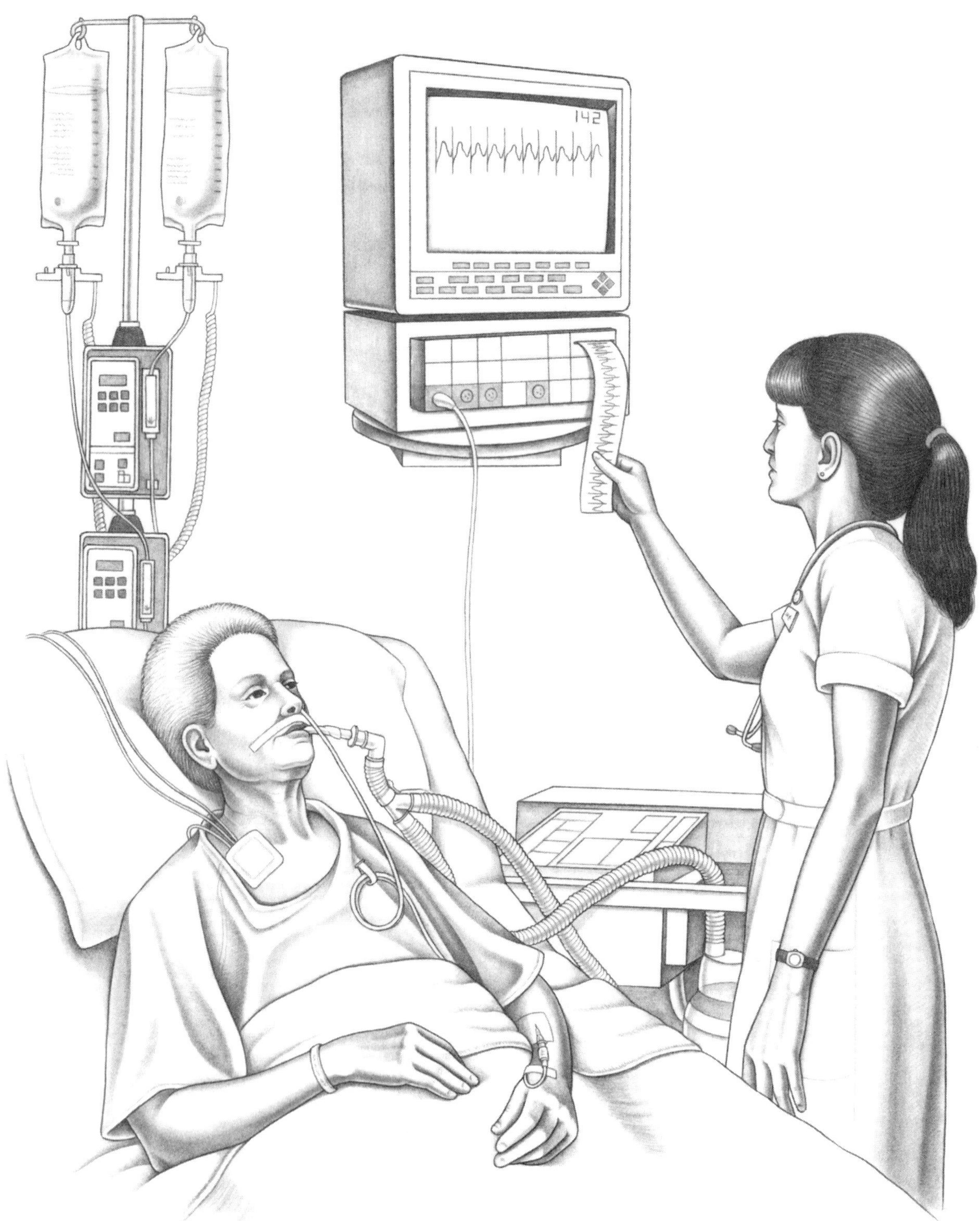
142

9

Conditions That Cause Arrhythmias

Patients can develop arrhythmias even though they don't have a cardiac problem. The arrhythmias may result from conditions such as adrenal insufficiency, anemia, anorexia, bulimia, asthma, thyroid dysfunction, and pulmonary embolism. Arrhythmias can also develop in elderly patients who take several drugs.

Typically, the best way to resolve such arrhythmias is to recognize and respond to their underlying cause. In this chapter, you'll find explanations of how certain fairly common conditions can lead to arrhythmias—and how you can detect and correct the conditions.

Adrenal insufficiency

Located at the top of the kidneys, the adrenal glands influence the activity of almost every body system, including the cardiovascular system, by secreting a number of powerful substances. In particular, the adrenal medulla secretes dopamine, norepinephrine, and epinephrine. And the adrenal cortex secretes glucocorticoids, mineralocorticoids, and androgens. Insufficient amounts of some of these chemicals can lead to cardiac arrhythmias.

In patients with primary adrenal insufficiency, high stress levels can trigger acute insufficiency and shock. In patients with secondary insufficiency, an acute episode commonly results from the abrupt withdrawal of glucocorticoid therapy.

Pathophysiology

Adrenal insufficiency may result from destruction of the adrenal glands—a condition called primary adrenal insufficiency or Addison's disease. This destruction can result from autoimmune forces, tuberculosis, metastatic cancer, fungal infection (such as histoplasmosis), cytomegalovirus, amyloidosis, hemochromatosis, and adrenal hemorrhage.

More commonly, adrenal insufficiency results from a disruption in the hypothalamic-pituitary axis that leads, in turn, to inadequate secretion of adrenocorticotropic hormone (ACTH) by the pituitary gland. This disorder, called secondary adrenal insufficiency, typically stems from hypopituitarism, withdrawal of long-term glucocorticoid therapy, or surgical removal of the pituitary gland.

Adrenal insufficiency that stems from hypofunction of the hypothalamic-pituitary axis can alter cortisol and aldosterone levels, which, in turn, can lead to severe cardiovascular compromise and lethal cardiac arrhythmias.

Role of cortisol

Cortisol, the most important glucocorticoid secreted by the adrenal cortex, regulates the metabolism of nutrients and controls the body's response to stress. It works by stimulating gluconeogenesis, mobilizing fatty acids, causing the release of vasoactive substances in vessels, and inhibiting the effects of insulin, which decreases cellular use of glucose.

If reduced levels of ACTH cause cortisol levels to fall, the body can't maintain its normal vascular response to vasoconstrictors or the integrity of its cell walls. Because cortisol has some mineralocorticoid effects, a deficiency can also influence the body's fluid and electrolyte levels. And the subsequent dehydration can decrease cardiac output (CO) sharply.

Role of aldosterone

Aldosterone is the principal mineralocorticoid secreted by the adrenal cortex. Produced in response to angiotensin II in the blood, it maintains extracellular fluid volume by causing the body to conserve sodium and excrete potassium. Thus, when aldosterone levels decline, the body excretes increased amounts of sodium, and its potassium levels rise.

As you know, potassium directly affects cardiac performance by influencing the resting potential and irritability of cells. Mild potassium elevations cause cells to repolarize more rapidly and to become more irritable, resulting in a lower resting potential, a rapidly initiated action potential, and an electrically unstable heart.

As aldosterone levels decrease and potassium levels increase, the resting potential can exceed the threshold potential. Cells can't repolarize or respond to excitation. And delayed repolarization and increased myocardial irritability can lead to ventricular arrhythmias and cardiac standstill.

If the resting phase of the action potential is prolonged, slower ectopic impulses from the atrioventricular (AV) node, bundle branches, or ventricles have more time to take over as the heart's pacemaker.

What's more, as extracellular potassium levels rise, more calcium crosses the cell membrane, and hydrogen ions flow into the cells. Hypercalcemia causes AV conduction delays, which may lead to heart block and cardiac arrest. It also delays repolarization and prolongs the QT interval, which may allow ectopic foci to take over as the heart's pacemaker, resulting in premature junctional contractions or premature ventricular contractions (PVCs).

Retention of hydrogen ions sets the stage for metabolic acidosis, a process that commonly leads to weakness, malaise, and headache and can progress to flaccid paralysis, seizures, cardiac arrhythmias, and death.

Also, because glucocorticoids potentiate the body's response to epinephrine and norepinephrine, a glucocorticoid deficiency depresses the effects of catecholamines, thus reducing the force and rate of myocardial contractions. As a result, your patient may develop peripheral vasodilation, hypotension, hypoglycemia, and decreased CO.

Signs and symptoms

A patient with adrenal insufficiency may have a wide range of signs and symptoms, which vary depending on whether the patient has primary or secondary adrenal insufficiency.

Primary adrenal insufficiency

If your patient has primary adrenal insufficiency, her signs and symptoms may include weakness, nausea, vomiting, weight loss, and orthostatic hypotension with syncope. Arterial hypotension develops in nearly all patients who have primary adrenal insufficiency. And your patient probably will complain of feeling dizzy and faint when changing positions.

As the disorder progresses, her signs and symptoms will intensify. She may report a salt craving, constipation, diarrhea, emotional disturbances, and a poor tolerance for stress. You may find that she has hypoglycemia, hyponatremia, hyperkalemia, and dehydration. You may notice skin changes characteristic of vitiligo. And you may detect cardiac rhythm conduction disturbances, which may involve the AV node or bundle branches.

Electrocardiogram (ECG) changes caused by primary adrenal insufficiency typically include sinus bradycardia, flattened or inverted T waves, and prolonged QT intervals.

Secondary adrenal insufficiency

A patient with secondary adrenal insufficiency typically has signs and symptoms related to decreased cortisol levels, such as anorexia, weight loss, nausea, vomiting, hypoglycemia, emotional disturbances, and decreased tolerance for stress.

If your patient becomes critically ill, her signs and symptoms may reflect severe metabolic, fluid, and electrolyte imbalances, such as hypoglycemia, hyponatremia, and hyperkalemia. Also, she may have tachycardia and tachypnea. She may be pale and dehydrated and may experience sudden, profound weakness; severe abdominal, bone, and leg pain; and hyperpyrexia followed by hypothermia.

Typically, secondary adrenal insufficiency causes hyperpigmentation in critically ill patients. As the insufficiency continues, your patient also may seem confused and lethargic. She may develop extreme hypotension and shock. And eventually, she may become unresponsive and decline into a coma.

The ECG changes that result from secondary adrenal insufficiency are typical of hyperkalemia, and their severity depends on the degree of your patient's potassium imbalance. Early ECG changes include tall, peaked T waves and shortened QT intervals. As potassium levels increase, the ST segments become depressed, PR intervals become prolonged, and QRS complexes widen. Bradyarrhythmias commonly occur, which can lead to ventricular fibrillation and cardiac arrest.

Diagnostic tests

To help determine the severity of your patient's condition, a physician may order radioimmunoassays of her blood and urine. Typically, blood and urine levels of cortisol, aldosterone, and 17-ketosteroid are low in a patient with cortisol deficiency.

Because patients with primary adrenal insufficiency have elevated levels of ACTH and those with secondary adrenal insufficiency have low levels of ACTH, measuring ACTH levels can help differentiate between primary and secondary forms of the disease. Your patient will probably undergo ACTH stimulation testing. During the test, your patient will receive a parenteral dose of synthetic ACTH; then her plasma cortisol levels will be measured. Normally, plasma cortisol levels rise dramatically after ACTH is administered. If your patient has secondary adrenal insufficiency, however, her plasma cortisol levels will remain low or undetectable. The lack of response to ACTH stimulation confirms acute adrenal insufficiency.

The physician also may test your patient's blood electrolyte levels. If your patient has adrenal insufficiency, her sodium levels probably will be low and potassium levels high. Her blood glucose levels may reveal hypoglycemia, and fluid volume depletion may raise her blood urea nitrogen (BUN) level and hematocrit.

Treatment

If your patient with primary or secondary adrenal insufficiency isn't critically ill, the physician may start her on hormone replacement therapy, which may continue permanently. Most patients take 12 to 15 mg/m^2 of hydrocortisone in divided oral doses. Adjust the dosage, as prescribed, until your patient becomes asymptomatic. Any ECG changes usually resolve with replacement therapy.

Some patients also take a mineralocorticoid replacement, typically 0.1 to 0.2 mg of fludrocortisone per day orally. However, because most glucocorticoids exert some mineralocorticoid effects, such therapy may not be necessary.

Teach your patient about her prescribed drug therapy and emphasize that it may continue for the rest of her life. Also, review any special precautions your patient should take to minimize stress and the risk of adrenal insufficiency recurring (see *Teaching your patient to manage adrenal insufficiency,* page 176).

Tell your patient that if she experiences physiologic stress—such as an infection, traumatic injury, or dental work—she may need to increase her glucocorticoid dose. Once the stressor has been treated, she can resume her standard dose.

Nursing considerations

If your patient develops acute adrenal insufficiency, she'll need prompt intervention to prevent circulatory collapse. Focus your care on supporting vital functions, providing hormone replacement, restoring fluid and electrolyte balances, and controlling arrhythmias.

Keep in mind that any patient with acute adrenal insufficiency is under great physiologic stress. Also, she has a decreased ability to tolerate external stressors. To minimize additional physiologic insult, keep her quiet, keep the lights dimmed, and stabilize the room temperature. Place your patient on bed rest and limit her activities. And explain

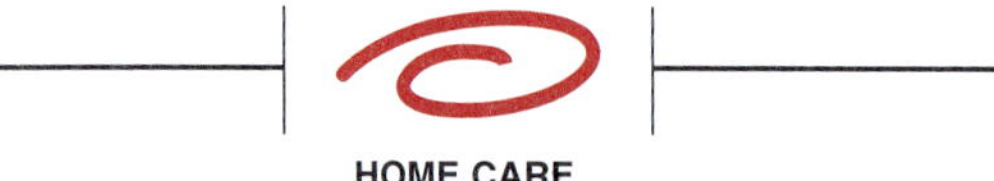

HOME CARE

Teaching your patient to manage adrenal insufficiency

To help your patient with adrenal insufficiency adapt to her hormone replacement therapy, make sure your teaching addresses these topics:

- actions and dosages of the prescribed hormones
- importance of taking hormones exactly as prescribed
- signs and symptoms of overdose and underdose
- signs and symptoms of adverse effects
- influence of stress on her condition (include examples of stressful situations)
- need to change hormone dosages during times of stress
- need to call the physician about exposure to stress that may require dosage adjustments
- diet plan that emphasizes increased fluids and salt intake during diaphoresis
- use of medical alert identification to warn health care providers about the patient's condition
- use of emergency self-injection kit.

any treatment she'll have to undergo before it starts.

Supporting vital functions

With acute adrenal insufficiency, metabolic, fluid, and electrolyte problems may increase your patient's risk of hypovolemia, shock, hypoperfusion, and lactic acidosis. As with any patient in crisis, first check her airway, breathing, and circulation. Immediately assess her vital signs, level of consciousness, and airway patency. She may be extremely hypotensive, tachycardic, and tachypneic. Her level of consciousness may be altered, affecting her ability to maintain a patent airway. If so, she's at risk for aspiration and respiratory distress. Anticipate the need for airway insertion or endotracheal intubation to ensure a patent airway.

Hypotension caused by decreased fluid volume can reduce tissue perfusion, including perfusion to the heart. Because of her unmet myocardial oxygen demands, your patient's ECG may reveal ventricular ectopia. Administer supplemental oxygen, as ordered, to prevent hypoxemia and subsequent arrhythmias. Use pulse oximetry to monitor your patient's oxygen saturation levels. And begin continuous cardiac monitoring to check for changes caused by hypoxemia and electrolyte imbalances, specifically hyperkalemia. Assess your patient's vital signs and level of consciousness every 15 minutes.

Obtain your patient's baseline body weight. And anticipate insertion of a large-bore I.V. catheter to administer fluids, hormone replacements, and emergency drugs to prevent circulatory collapse, if needed.

Acute adrenal insufficiency commonly causes hyperpyrexia, which may be followed by hypothermia. Keep in mind that temperature extremes alter metabolism and can further compromise your patient's already fragile status. Check your patient's temperature at least hourly, and be prepared to use cooling blankets followed by warming blankets, as needed. Also, monitor her ECG for the J waves commonly seen with hypothermia (see *How hypothermia affects a patient's electrocardiogram*).

As ordered, insert an indwelling urinary catheter so that you can keep precise hourly records of your patient's intake and output. Remember that severe fluid volume deficits can adversely affect renal function, worsening your patient's recurrent electrolyte imbalances. If your patient's urine output drops below 30 ml/hour (or 0.5 to 1 ml/kg/hour), report it right away.

Hemodynamic monitoring may be necessary to evaluate your patient's fluid volume status, its effect on cardiac function, and her response to therapy. As needed, assist with insertion of a central venous or pulmonary artery catheter. Track your patient's hemodynamic status carefully by monitoring central venous pressure (CVP) or pulmonary artery pressure. Check mean arterial pressure (MAP) hourly. To maintain cerebral and renal perfusion, MAP should be 60 mm Hg or higher. Keep in mind that glucocorticoid deficiency can worsen your patient's fluid volume deficit and her CO by decreasing her body's ability to respond to stress.

Obtain laboratory tests as ordered, including

How hypothermia affects a patient's electrocardiogram

On a normal electrocardiogram (ECG) waveform, the J point appears at the junction of the QRS complex and the ST segment. If your patient develops hypothermia, her ECG may show a characteristic J wave.

Normal electrocardiogram

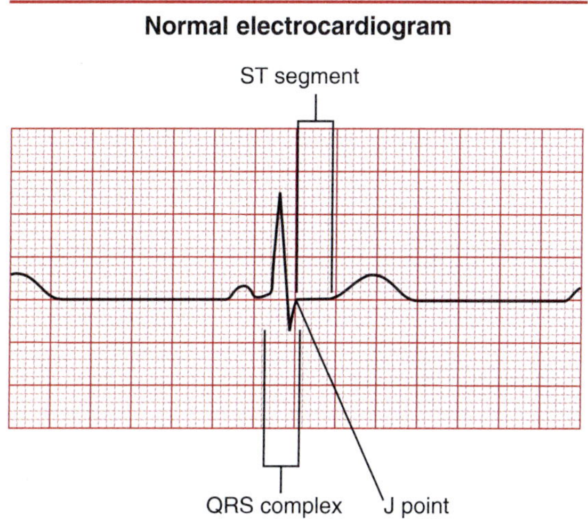

Electrocardiogram with J wave

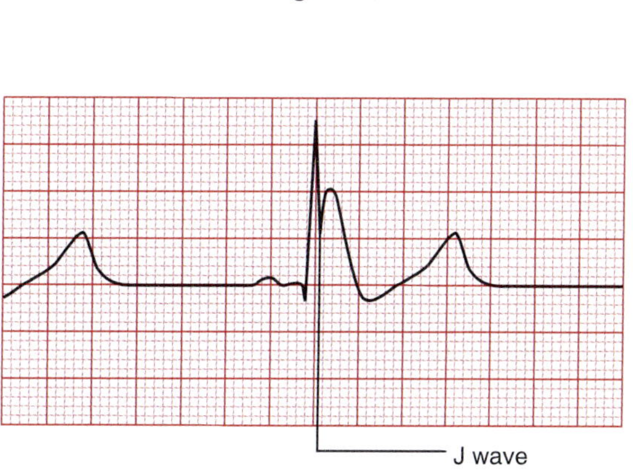

hematocrit, blood electrolyte levels, and blood glucose levels. Your patient's severe fluid volume deficit raises her risk of lactic acidosis from poor tissue perfusion—another possible cause of cardiac arrhythmias. Use serial arterial blood gas (ABG) levels to monitor her respiratory and acid-base status.

Providing hormone replacement

Initially, your patient with acute adrenal insufficiency may receive a 100-mg bolus of hydrocortisone I.V. or an equivalent drug. Then she'll either receive a continuous infusion at a rate of 25 mg/minute, or she'll continue to receive bolus doses every 6 to 8 hours. As your patient's condition improves, her dose will be tapered, eventually reaching an oral maintenance dose of about 20 mg in the morning and 10 mg at night. Keep in mind that hydrocortisone can cause edema, hypertension, and heart failure, possibly leading to cardiac arrhythmias.

If your patient's diagnosis hasn't been confirmed, you may administer 1 to 4 mg of dexamethasone I.V. instead of hydrocortisone because dexamethasone doesn't interfere with the results of an ACTH stimulation test. After administering it, watch your patient for tachycardia, an adverse effect of dexamethasone. Also, you may give fludrocortisone orally. But it, too, may induce cardiac arrhythmias.

Restoring fluid and electrolyte balance

For a patient with acute adrenal insufficiency, begin fluid volume replacement quickly and in large amounts. Start by giving 1 L of 0.9% sodium chloride solution I.V. over 60 minutes, as prescribed. Then infuse 1 to 2 L over 4 to 8 hours or 2 to 3 L over 2 to 3 hours, depending on the severity of the fluid deficit. If your patient is hypoglycemic, infuse dextrose 5% in 0.9% sodium chloride solution, as prescribed. If she's hyperkalemic, make sure that none of her I.V. solutions contain potassium.

Usually, vigorous fluid replacement together with large doses of glucocorticoids can correct a fluid deficit and hypotension. A physician may prescribe volume expanders and sympathomimetic

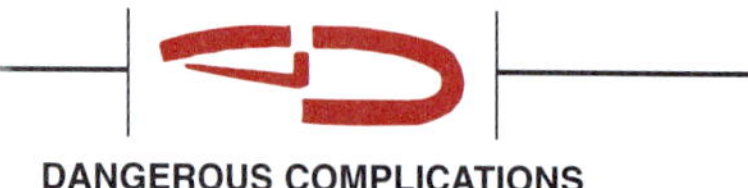

DANGEROUS COMPLICATIONS

Warning signs and symptoms of fluid overload

Anytime you administer fluids to correct a patient's fluid deficit, monitor her carefully to make sure she doesn't develop fluid overload. Look for these early warning signs and symptoms:

- a full, bounding pulse
- crackles on auscultation
- jugular vein distention
- shortness of breath
- tachycardia.

Other signs and symptoms may include nausea, vomiting, weakness, and neurologic changes, but remember that they also may result from your patient's adrenal insufficiency.

drugs as well, although the latter won't be effective unless glucocorticoids have been replaced. When administering fluids, remember to monitor your patient's hemodynamic status carefully to catch early warning signs and symptoms of fluid overload (see *Warning signs and symptoms of fluid overload*).

Throughout fluid replacement therapy, document your patient's intake and output hourly and weigh her daily. Monitor her blood electrolyte levels closely, watching for blood sodium levels to increase and potassium levels to decrease. Monitor her ECG for changes that suggest improving electrolyte balance. As balance is restored, your patient's myocardial irritability should decrease, and her arrhythmias should become less frequent. Her blood glucose level should begin to rise, and her BUN level and hematocrit will decrease as fluid volume returns to normal. Check your patient's complete blood count (CBC) for underlying anemia, and confirm her renal status with repeat BUN testing.

Controlling arrhythmias

Typically, ECG changes caused by cortisol deficiency resolve with glucocorticoid treatment; those caused by hyperkalemia resolve with mineralocorticoid therapy. If your patient's hyperkalemia continues, anticipate administering calcium gluconate to stabilize the myocardium, sodium bicarbonate to correct acidosis, or an infusion of glucose and insulin to drive extracellular potassium back into the cells, as ordered.

Anemia

When the number of circulating red blood cells (RBCs) decreases or the quantity or quality of hemoglobin declines, blood loses some of its oxygen-carrying capacity. The resulting condition, called anemia, typically stems either from a loss of RBCs or decreased production of RBCs.

Loss of RBCs may result from bleeding or from hemolysis. Decreased or defective RBC production may result from a deficiency of the nutrients needed for hemoglobin or deoxyribonucleic acid synthesis. This situation can arise after exposure to toxic substances that cause RBC production in bone marrow to fail.

Typically, anemias are classified by the structure, or morphology, of the RBCs (see *Classifying anemias*). All anemias, however, have a common characteristic: they reduce the oxygen-carrying capacity of blood. This reduction leads to ischemic changes in the body, especially the heart. And as you know, myocardial ischemia increases the risk of arrhythmias.

Pathophysiology

Normally, stem cells differentiate into RBCs in the bone marrow, producing oxygen-carrying hemoglobin as part of the process. Mature RBCs circulate for about 120 days, after which they're cleared by macrophages from the liver and spleen. Hemoglobin breaks down into globin and heme. Globin further breaks down into amino acid; heme breaks down into carbon monoxide and iron. The lungs excrete the carbon monoxide in the form of carboxyhemoglobin. And most of the iron returns to the bone marrow for use in new RBCs.

Usually, RBC production and destruction is a relatively constant process that's controlled by erythropoietin, a hormone manufactured by the kidneys and released in response to tissue hypoxia. Possible triggers include changes in atmospheric oxygen, decreased oxygen in arterial blood, and decreased hemoglobin concentration. Erythropoietin causes erythropoiesis, a compensatory increase in RBC production and hemoglobin concentration. When adequate oxygen saturation of the tissues has been restored, erythropoietin secretion decreases.

Erythropoiesis requires an adequate supply of protein, vitamins, and minerals. If any are lacking, RBC production slows, leading to anemia and, possibly, to myocardial ischemia and its resulting arrhythmias. The type and severity of arrhythmia that develops depends on the severity of the patient's anemia, the speed at which it develops, and the body's ability to compensate. If the anemia is mild and begins slowly, the patient may be able to compensate fairly well. If anemia begins suddenly and becomes severe, however, compensatory mechanisms may be inadequate. As a result, life-threatening arrhythmias can develop, profoundly affecting CO.

A decrease in circulating RBCs also can lead to arrhythmias by changing blood viscosity and volume. When RBCs decline, fluid moves into the vascular space to expand the blood volume. As a result, viscosity decreases. Blood flows more rapidly and more turbulently through the vessels and heart. Turbulent blood flow increases vascular resistance, possibly leading to ventricular dysfunction, cardiac dilation, and valvular insufficiency. All of these conditions can affect cardiac conduction and contractility, resulting in arrhythmias.

What's more, hypoxia caused by anemia can lead to vasoconstriction, which increases the rate of blood flow. The higher flow rate increases venous return to the heart, which, in turn, increases tissue demands and the risk of cardiopulmonary congestion. Ischemia and arrhythmias can stem from the resulting increase in myocardial demand.

Severe or sudden anemia leads to hypovolemia and hypoxemia. As a result, peripheral vasoconstriction diverts blood away from the kidneys to the heart and brain. In response, the kidneys release renin, which converts to angiotensin II and becomes a potent vasoconstrictor. Angiotensin II causes the body to retain water and sodium. It also stimulates the release of aldosterone from the adrenal cortex, causing an increase in the absorption of sodium, chloride, and water. These compensatory attempts to restore vascular volume can compromise your patient's fragile cardiac status.

Classifying anemias

Types of anemia	Characteristics of red blood cells
Macrocytic normochromic anemia • vitamin B_{12} deficiency (pernicious) anemia • folic acid deficiency anemia	• Large stem cells develop into unusually large red blood cells (RBCs) with normal hemoglobin content.
Microcytic hypochromic anemia • iron deficiency anemia • sideroblastic anemia • thalassemia	• Abnormally small RBCs contain decreased amounts of hemoglobin.
Normocytic normochromic anemia • aplastic anemia • posthemorrhagic anemia • hemolytic anemia • anemia of chronic disease	• Normal RBCs with normal hemoglobin content are reduced in number.

Signs and symptoms

Anemia can cause a wide range of signs and symptoms, depending on its severity and the speed at which it develops. If your patient has mild anemia that begins slowly, she may have no signs or symptoms. Or she may have them only when she exerts herself, raising her body's demand for oxygen.

If your patient has pronounced anemia or if it begins quickly, she'll probably have such signs and symptoms as pallor, weakness, vertigo, malaise, shortness of breath, and palpitations. Check her carefully for evidence of arrhythmias. Start with her heart rate and rhythm. Then ask her

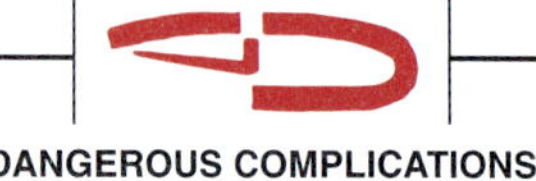

DANGEROUS COMPLICATIONS

When anemia leads to myocardial ischemia

If your patient's anemia leads to myocardial ischemia, you'll see telltale signs on her electrocardiogram, including inverted T waves, particularly in leads I, aV_L, and V_1 through V_6.

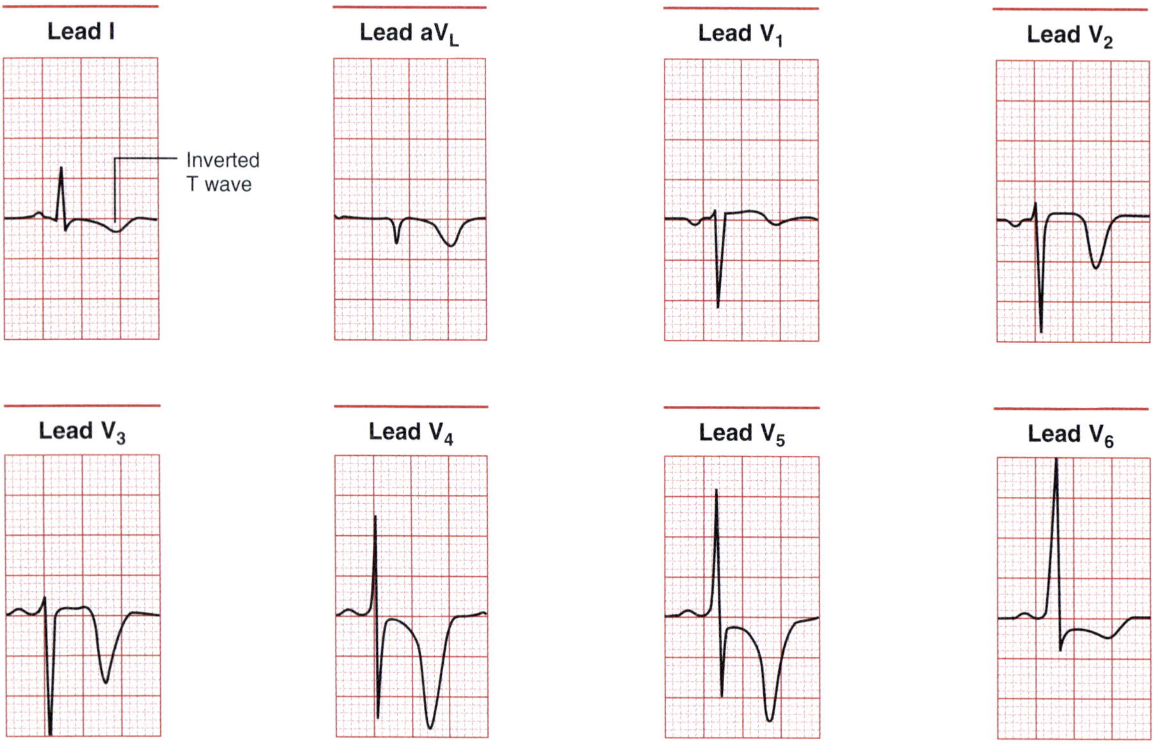

Lead I

Inverted T wave

Lead aV_L

Lead V_1

Lead V_2

Lead V_3

Lead V_4

Lead V_5

Lead V_6

about complaints that may stem from an arrhythmia, such as palpitations, chest pain on exertion, a rapid heart rate, and swollen ankles and feet.

To help confirm an arrhythmia, check your patient's chest X-rays for cardiomegaly. Listen for bruits. Also, look for ischemic changes on her ECG (see *When anemia leads to myocardial ischemia*).

With severe anemia caused by a sudden loss of a large amount of blood, your patient may have signs and symptoms of hypovolemia and circulatory collapse.

Diagnostic tests

To confirm your patient's anemia, its severity, and its type, her physician will order blood studies, especially a CBC. Typically, your patient's hemoglobin level, hematocrit, and RBC count will be low.

A physician also may order a reticulocyte count to provide more information about the cause and type of anemia. For example, in hemolytic anemia, the count is high; in aplastic anemia, it's abnormally low. Other laboratory tests, such as serum folate, vitamin B_{12}, and iron levels, may be performed to confirm a deficiency. Bone marrow aspiration may be necessary to evaluate bone marrow function.

Treatment

Treatment for anemia typically focuses on resolving or controlling the underlying cause and relieving hypoxia. Such treatment usually involves replacing a missing nutrient. For example, if your patient has pernicious anemia, she'll probably receive 30 µg of vitamin B_{12} by intramuscular (I.M.) injection daily for 5 to 10 days, followed by 100 to 200 mg monthly. Most patients respond dramatically within 48 hours.

If your patient has a folic acid deficiency, she'll receive folic acid, up to 1 mg daily by the oral route. For a severe deficiency, she may receive the drug I.V., I.M., or subcutaneously until her blood counts improve.

If your patient has iron deficiency anemia, she'll take oral iron supplements or receive iron parenterally by deep, I.M. Z-track injection. Usually, the parenteral route is used only if a patient can't or won't take the oral form in sufficient amounts or if she has a physiologic problem that interferes with iron absorption from her gastrointestinal (GI) tract.

If your patient's anemia results from exposure to toxic chemicals or radiation, her treatment will first aim to stop the exposure. Then she'll probably receive blood transfusions to replace her RBCs and prevent new arrhythmias. Her physician may prescribe corticosteroids and androgens to stimulate the function of her bone marrow. If function doesn't return, she may need a bone marrow transplant.

Nursing considerations

No matter what kind of treatment your patient with anemia receives, you'll need to monitor her blood studies carefully. Expect to monitor her hemoglobin level, hematocrit, and RBC and reticulocyte counts at least daily. Also, evaluate laboratory tests that demonstrate the effectiveness of treatment, such as total iron-binding capacity and serum folate, vitamin B_{12}, ferritin, and transferrin levels.

One of the most important measures to help alleviate hypoxia and its adverse effect on your patient's myocardium is the use of supplemental oxygen. It increases the oxygen available to blood and tissues without increasing the heart's workload. When giving oxygen, monitor your patient's oxygen saturation levels via pulse oximetry. Also, obtain ABG measurements, as ordered, to evaluate your patient's partial pressure of arterial oxygen ($Pa{O_2}$) and acid-base status.

Begin continuous cardiac monitoring to watch for signs of ischemia and cardiopulmonary congestion.

Because of existing hypoxia, work to minimize any activities that could increase oxygen demand. For example, if your patient is short of breath or tachypneic, help her into the semi-Fowler or high-Fowler position to maximize chest expansion and decrease the work of breathing. Teach your patient to take slow, controlled, deep breaths. If necessary, breathe with her to show her how to do it.

Plan frequent rest periods and try to minimize distractions and disruptions. Pace any procedures and treatments as much as possible to prevent overtaxing your patient. Because eating increases energy use, schedule rest periods before mealtimes. Provide small, frequent meals throughout the day. Assess your patient's skin color and monitor her oxygen saturation levels and ECG in response to her activity. Use your observations to guide your care.

Keep in mind that marked temperature changes increase the body's demand for oxygen. Make sure to monitor your patient's temperature closely and take necessary action to keep it within normal limits.

Monitor all of your patient's body systems to help detect the effects of hypoxia and arrhythmias. For example, assess your patient's neurologic status frequently for evidence of cerebral ischemia, which may indicate persistent anemia or reduced CO caused by an arrhythmia. Also, auscultate your patient's bowel sounds, noting any increase or decrease. And monitor her intake and output. Remember that decreased urine output may reflect decreased renal perfusion.

If ischemia and arrhythmias develop, your patient may need transfusion therapy to increase her circulating RBCs. You'll probably administer packed RBCs, which replace RBCs without increasing blood volume, thus reducing the risk of circula-

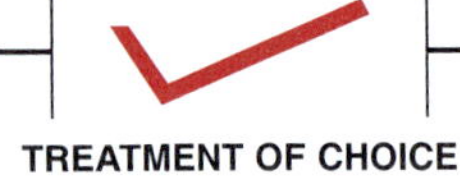

TREATMENT OF CHOICE

Administering a blood transfusion

If your patient develops severe anemia, she may need a blood transfusion. If you assist with or perform the procedure, keep these tips in mind.

Before the transfusion

To ensure compatibility, obtain a blood sample for typing and crossmatching, as ordered. Confirm that your patient has given her informed consent in writing. If she doesn't already have an I.V. catheter in place, prepare to insert one—preferably an 18-gauge catheter—in a large vein. Make sure you have filtered tubing and 0.9% sodium chloride solution on hand for the infusion. When the blood is available, follow your facility's policy for checking the patient's identity and confirming that the blood has been correctly crossmatched.

During the transfusion

Obtain your patient's vital signs. Then start infusing the blood slowly, at about 2 ml/minute. Stay with your patient for about 30 minutes to make sure she doesn't have an allergic reaction to the blood product. Check her vital signs every 15 minutes.

If your patient doesn't have signs or symptoms of a transfusion reaction, such as flushing, itching, hives, chills, fever, or low back pain, increase the infusion to the prescribed rate. Usually, you'll infuse a unit of blood over 2 to 4 hours. During that time, continue to assess your patient for signs and symptoms of a transfusion reaction. Also, monitor her vital signs, according to your facility's policy, until the transfusion is complete.

If your patient does have an acute transfusion reaction, she may be in imminent danger. The reaction could lyse her red blood cells in minutes, robbing her blood of its oxygen-carrying capacity. Without immediate intervention, she may experience overwhelming cardiac ischemia followed by lethal arrhythmias. Usually, treatment involves administering oxygen, a diuretic, and, possibly, epinephrine.

After the transfusion

Follow-up laboratory studies can help you evaluate the effectiveness of the transfusion. However, to avoid falsely elevated results, don't perform a hemoglobin test for at least 2 hours after the transfusion.

Continuous monitoring of your patient's electrocardiogram can also help by showing the effects of increased oxygenation on her myocardium.

tory overload and increased myocardial workload. If your patient also needs volume replacement, you may administer whole blood instead (see *Administering a blood transfusion*).

Anorexia and bulimia

Two eating disorders, anorexia and bulimia, affect mainly girls between ages 13 and 20. No one knows exactly why such eating disorders arise. However, some of the patients affected by them have neuroendocrine problems. Also, some have abusive, overprotective, or otherwise dysfunctional family backgrounds. But all typically have reduced self-esteem and an overwhelming preoccupation with weight.

Some patients develop anorexia nervosa. Others develop bulimia nervosa. And some develop both disorders at once. Although both disorders are distinct, they share similar psychological and physiologic components, treatments, and dangers (see *Comparing anorexia and bulimia*).

Cardiac arrhythmias form one of the most ominous dangers of eating disorders. They can result from changes in basal metabolism, hypothermia, and electrolyte disturbances.

Pathophysiology

Eating disorders interfere with the body's ability to use nutrients. With anorexia, the interference usually results from inadequate food intake. With bulimia, it typically results from eating junk food and then removing that food from the body prematurely. Both disorders can cause serious metabolic disturbances.

Comparing anorexia and bulimia

Distinguishing between anorexia and bulimia can be difficult because they have some similar characteristics, but the differences listed here can help you tell them apart.

Characteristic	Anorexia	Bulimia
Weight	• < 85% of expected body weight for age and height	• usually within normal limits; may be slightly overweight or underweight
Behavior	• refusal to maintain body weight • intense fear of gaining weight • preoccupation with food and food-related activities • severe restriction of food intake and excessive exercise or purging to prevent weight gain	• binge eating • lack of control over eating episodes • guilt, remorse, and self-contempt after binge episode • purging by self-induced vomiting; misuse of laxatives, diuretics, enemas, or other drugs • fasting or excessive exercise
Body image	• feeling of being fat even when emaciated	• undue influence of body weight in self-evaluation • disturbed view of body, weight, or shape

Inadequate nutritional intake causes the body to use stored nutrients. Glycogen stored in the liver breaks down into glucose. Noncarbohydrate sources—such as lactate, amino acids, and glycerol—also produce glucose. As the process of glucose production continues, it begins to deplete the body's store of nutrients. Eventually, if nutritional intake continues to be inadequate, glucose production will exhaust the body's supply of stored nutrients.

If necessary, the body may use fatty acids, ketones, and protein to create energy. Poor nutritional intake results in protein wasting and metabolic acidosis caused by the breakdown of stored fats, fatty acids, and ketones. Eventually, metabolic acidosis depresses myocardial contractility, lowers the fibrillation threshold, and interferes with the normal pressor response to catecholamines, placing your patient at risk for atrial and ventricular fibrillation.

Fluid volume deficit

Eating disorders—especially bulimia—also raise the danger of fluid volume deficit. Your patient with an eating disorder can lose a large volume of fluid through self-induced vomiting or the overuse of diuretics or laxatives.

When extracellular fluid volume declines, the body tries to compensate. Baroreceptors and osmoreceptors stimulate the release of antidiuretic hormone to increase water resorption in the distal tubules. Sympathetic stimulation triggers vasoconstriction to increase blood pressure and venous return to the heart, thereby increasing CO.

These events increase the workload of the heart, leading to an increase in the myocardial demand for oxygen. With available nutrient stores depleted, your patient has a reduced ability to adapt to these changes, predisposing her to abnormalities of cardiac contractility and conduction.

Electrolyte imbalances

Anorexia and bulimia commonly cause electrolyte imbalances. Excessive fluid losses caused by vomiting, diuretics, or laxatives can lead to hyponatremia. Because depolarization and repolarization rely in part on the action of sodium, decreased sodium levels combined with a fluid volume deficit can adversely affect cardiac conduction and contractility.

Most minerals, such as potassium, calcium, and magnesium, are supplied through diet. Thus, a person with an eating disorder may develop an electrolyte imbalance from poor dietary intake and excessive losses of electrolytes from vomiting and laxative abuse. The use of potassium-wasting diuretics compounds the risk of hypokalemia. As you know, hypokalemia increases the resting potential of cardiac cells, delays ventricular repolarization, and heightens myocardial excitability, raising the risk of ventricular tachycardia and fibrillation.

Your patient may also develop hypomagnesemia, hypophosphatemia, and hypocalcemia or hypercalcemia.

Like potassium, magnesium plays a role in neuromuscular excitability and ventricular repolarization. And a magnesium imbalance can lead to arrhythmias.

Generally, RBCs require phosphate to release oxygen from hemoglobin. With hypophosphatemia, RBCs have a diminished ability to provide oxygen to tissues, possibly leading to hypoxia. Phosphate deficits also may lead to decreased cardiac contractility and decreased sensitivity to inotropic and vasoconstrictive drugs. Together these events can predispose your patient to arrhythmias.

Hypocalcemia results from inadequate dietary intake of calcium that causes electrolyte and metabolic disturbances, including hypomagnesemia, alkalosis, and inadequate intestinal absorption. It also prolongs the myocardial action potential and slows AV and intraventricular conduction. Hypercalcemia can stem from hypophosphatemia or the overuse of thiazide diuretics. It decreases myocardial automaticity and shortens mechanical systole.

Vomiting and misuse of diuretics and laxatives also can lead to metabolic acidosis. As the body attempts to compensate by decreasing the respiratory rate, hypoventilation can lead, in turn, to hypoxemia, compounding the risk of arrhythmias.

Also, hyperexcitability of the parasympathetic nervous system—caused by increased vagal stimulation from vomiting—can slow the heart rate. Coupled with an electrolyte imbalance, this further increases your patient's risk of cardiac arrhythmias.

Signs and symptoms

A patient's weight is the most common sign of an eating disorder. In fact, the diagnosis of anorexia nervosa specifies that the patient weigh less than 85% of the expected weight for her age and height. Typically, a patient with anorexia is extremely thin and cachectic. However, be aware that such patients may attempt to hide their thinness under layered clothing.

A patient with anorexia may show a severe loss of subcutaneous fat. Her core body temperature, blood pressure, and heart rate probably will be decreased. If she developed anorexia before puberty, you may notice a lack of secondary sexual features. She also may experience menstrual irregularities, including amenorrhea.

Other physical findings may include intolerance to cold, lethargy, muscle weakness, hypotension, hypothermia, extremely dry skin, bradycardia, and complaints of abdominal pain and constipation.

A patient with bulimia may be slightly underweight as well, but she'll more likely have a normal or slightly increased weight. She may have such physical problems as esophageal tears and tooth erosion from frequent, self-induced vomiting.

Whether your patient has anorexia or bulimia, she'll probably have a history of being overweight. She may be depressed or anxious, socially withdrawn, overly restrained, or irritable. She may complain of insomnia. She may abuse or be dependent on alcohol, stimulants, or other substances. Also, she may have the following characteristic behavioral signs and symptoms:

- preoccupation with food
- concerns about eating in public
- feelings of ineffectiveness
- a need for control.

Diagnostic tests

For your patient with an eating disorder, blood studies commonly reveal metabolic and electrolyte disturbances. Expect to see the following conditions:

- elevated BUN level
- elevated liver function studies
- electrolyte imbalances
- metabolic acidosis or alkalosis
- decreased levels of thyroid hormones
- low blood estrogen level
- anemia
- elevated blood amylase level (with bulimia)
- elevated cholesterol levels (with anorexia).

Cardiac findings include bradycardia, which results from a reduced metabolic rate, and ECG abnormalities, which reflect underlying metabolic or electrolyte disorders. For example, if your patient has a potassium imbalance, you may see prominent U waves on her ECG (see *Identifying common electrolyte imbalances*).

Identifying common electrolyte imbalances

Use this table to review the three most common electrolyte imbalances caused by eating disorders, the electrocardiogram changes they cause, and their characteristic signs and symptoms.

Imbalance	Electrocardiogram changes	Signs and symptoms
Hypokalemia	• depressed ST segment • flat or inverted T wave • U wave • ventricular tachycardia or ventricular fibrillation	• weak, slow pulse • hypoventilation • muscle weakness and tenderness • drowsiness • confusion • abdominal cramps • adynamic ileus
Hypomagnesemia	• prolonged QT interval • broadened T wave with decreased amplitude • shortened ST segment	• muscle weakness • tremors • vertigo • ataxia • positive Chvostek's and Trousseau's signs • generalized muscle spasticity • depression and psychosis
Hypocalcemia	• prolonged ST segment • prolonged QT interval	• numbness and tingling in limbs • circumoral paresthesia • muscle cramps • tetany • laryngeal stridor • hyperreflexia • abdominal cramps • seizures

Treatment

Treatment focuses on restoring nutritional balance and correcting any metabolic and electrolyte disturbances. Your patient will also need psychological treatment. Nutritional therapy and psychotherapy may take place simultaneously because of the close connection between food intake and body image. Treatment for underlying fluid, metabolic, and electrolyte imbalances usually resolves arrhythmias and ECG changes.

Nursing considerations

To care for your patient with an eating disorder, you'll need to help increase and stabilize her oral intake, restore normal electrolyte balances, prevent or control arrhythmias, and assist with her psychological treatment.

At the start of treatment, weigh your patient to obtain a baseline. Then continue to weigh her on a prescribed schedule. Keep in mind, however, that your patient's intense focus on weight control may make it unwise to obtain daily weights or to announce the weight when you obtain it. Anxiety can induce the release of excessive catecholamines, leading to tachycardia.

Also, keep in mind that because of your patient's impaired nutritional status, she may be weak, fatigued, and intolerant of activity. If so, minimize her activity level until her condition improves. Then gradually increase her activity, as tolerated. As ordered, use pulse oximetry to monitor changes in oxygen saturation caused by activity.

Restoring nutritional status

A patient with an eating disorder, particularly one with anorexia, typically is in a state of starvation.

Thus, your first step in treating her will probably involve improving her oral nutrient intake.

A physician probably will prescribe a diet that contains 1,200 to 1,500 calories daily, divided into several meals and snacks. If your patient can't or won't eat that much, you may need to provide her with liquid protein supplements. If possible, ask a dietitian to help with meal planning and food selection.

Also, monitor your patient's intake carefully to make sure that she actually eats and retains the food. Remember that she may try to throw food away or purge when you're not around. If your patient's condition fails to improve with oral feedings, she may need enteral or total parenteral nutrition (TPN).

As you know, enteral nutrition involves delivering solutions of variable concentration into the stomach or small intestine through a tube. Whenever you administer such a feeding, assess your patient's GI function closely. Monitor your patient's vital signs, bowel sounds, and hydration. Giving a hypertonic solution too quickly can slow gastric emptying and lead to gastric distention, nausea, and vomiting. It also could cause diarrhea, especially when delivered to the small intestine, which may increase the loss of electrolytes. Also, giving the feeding too quickly may cause large amounts of fluid to shift into the small intestine, diluting its hypertonic contents and possibly worsening an already compromised fluid volume status.

Your patient may require TPN, which provides carbohydrates, fats, proteins, vitamins, minerals, trace elements, and water. When administering it, use an in-line filter. Also, use sterile technique when caring for the insertion site. The patient's impaired nutritional status places her at high risk for infection—a risk compounded by the fact that glucose in the TPN solution creates an excellent medium for bacterial growth.

Replacing fluids

In many cases, I.V. fluid therapy is administered to restore fluid balance. If your patient is dehydrated or hypotensive, anticipate additional fluid replacement and administration of drugs to support her vital functions. If your patient doesn't have an I.V. catheter in place, prepare to insert one. If she has a double-lumen or multilumen catheter for TPN, you may be able to use it to replace fluids rather than perform another venipuncture. But make sure to keep track of which lumen carries the TPN solution and which one carries the fluids.

The type of fluid used depends on your patient's fluid volume status. Commonly used solutions include dextrose 5% in water, 0.9% sodium chloride solution, and lactated Ringer's solution. Lactated Ringer's solution may be used to treat a patient with mild metabolic acidosis. For severe acidosis, administer sodium lactate or sodium bicarbonate, as prescribed. Don't administer sodium lactate to a hypoxic patient, however, because her body can't convert the lactate to bicarbonate. If a physician prescribes sodium bicarbonate, infuse it slowly and use a volume-control device. Monitor your patient's serial ABG levels for changes.

When replacing fluids, monitor your patient's intake and output frequently. Obtain laboratory studies, as ordered, including serum osmolality to evaluate her fluid status and BUN and creatinine levels to check her renal function.

Keep in mind that a fluid volume deficit can easily become a fluid volume overload, especially in a patient debilitated by her eating disorder. To detect a possible overload, auscultate your patient's heart and breath sounds often. Also, listen for complaints of shortness of breath. Check your patient's mucous membranes, skin turgor, and urine specific gravity for changes. If your patient has a severe volume depletion, anticipate insertion of a central venous catheter or pulmonary artery catheter to monitor her hemodynamic status.

Replacing electrolytes

At the start of your patient's treatment, monitor her serum electrolyte levels. A patient with chronic anorexia may have a stable potassium level as low as 2.8 mEq/L, yet have no signs or symptoms. Continue monitoring your patient's electrolyte levels periodically throughout treatment. Even minor shifts in electrolyte status can result in ventricular tachycardia or ventricular fibrillation.

Depending on your patient's initial and ongoing electrolyte levels, you may administer fluids that contain varying concentrations of electrolyte replacement. If necessary, her physician may prescribe oral or parenteral electrolytes as well (see *Responding to electrolyte imbalances*).

Obtain a 12-lead ECG and inititate continuous cardiac monitoring, as ordered, to confirm your patient's electrolyte imbalance and track her response to therapy.

Any patient who needs electrolyte replacement therapy faces a high risk of neurologic and cardiac

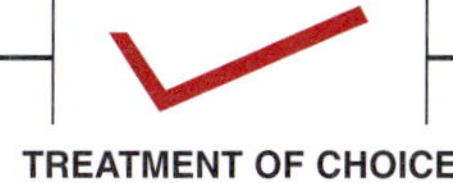

TREATMENT OF CHOICE

Responding to electrolyte imbalances

Electrolyte imbalances commonly result from eating disorders. Review these guidelines for treating hypokalemia, hypomagnesemia, hypocalcemia, and hypophosphatemia.

Hypokalemia

Expect to administer potassium either orally or I.V. If the oral route is prescribed, mix the potassium replacement with at least 4 ounces of water or with food to prevent gastric irritation.

If your patient has a blood potassium level of 3 mEq/L or below, you'll probably administer potassium I.V. Dilute and mix it thoroughly with an I.V. solution.

To minimize the risk of toxic effects, administer it at a concentration of 40 to 60 mEq/L. Infuse the solution at 200 to 250 mEq/day, as prescribed. Use an infusion pump to ensure an accurate flow rate.

Assess your patient's I.V. site frequently for evidence of infiltration. Also, remember that potassium is highly irritating to the vein. Stay alert for complaints of localized pain or burning.

Assess your patient's urine output hourly to track potassium excretion. If her urine potassium level drops while potassium replacement continues, she could develop hyperkalemia.

Hypomagnesemia

Administer magnesium boluses at no more than 1.5 ml of a 10% solution per minute. Run a continuous infusion at no more than 3 ml/minute. Too rapid a rate can cause cardiac arrest.

Check your patient's blood magnesium level after each bolus or at least every 6 hours during a continuous infusion. As ordered, discontinue therapy when levels return to normal.

Closely assess your patient's urine output before, during, and after therapy. It should be at least 100 ml every 4 hours. Also, assess her deep tendon reflexes before each bolus injection and at least every 4 hours during a continuous infusion. If they're decreased, notify a physician and hold the bolus injection or stop the infusion. Decreased deep tendon reflexes suggest hypermagnesemia, a warning of respiratory failure.

Because hypomagnesemia commonly causes muscle weakness, tremors, vertigo, and ataxia, keep the side rails raised on your patient's bed. Place the call bell within reach and help her with walking, as necessary.

Hypocalcemia

A patient with an eating disorder is at risk for hypocalcemia from other disturbances, such as hypomagnesemia and metabolic alkalosis. If she has hypomagnesemia, she'll also require magnesium replacement because hypocalcemia usually doesn't respond to calcium therapy alone.

As prescribed, administer a bolus of calcium gluconate or calcium chloride diluted in dextrose 5% in water. Follow that with a slow infusion given with the hypomagnesemia treatment. Don't mix calcium with 0.9% sodium chloride solution because sodium and chloride in the solution increase calcium excretion by the kidneys.

Hypophosphatemia

If your patient's blood phosphate level drops below 1 mg/dl, you'll give potassium phosphate or sodium phosphate I.V. to help raise it. The dosage may range from 0.6 to 0.9 mg/kg/hour based on whether the imbalance is recent and simple or long-standing and complicated.

Typically, when your patient's blood phosphate level reaches 2 mg/dl, you'll switch to an oral replacement.

Because of the inverse relationship between phosphate and calcium, watch your patient for signs and symptoms of hypercalcemia.

If she develops hypercalcemia in response to hypophosphatemia, common treatments include hydration and forced diuresis. For a severe imbalance, hemodialysis or peritoneal dialysis may be necessary. A physician also may prescribe a corticosteroid and calcitonin to inhibit bone resorption.

Throughout treatment for hypophosphatemia, take precautions to keep the patient safe and reduce her risk of injury. Take seizure precautions in response to central nervous system dysfunction.

problems. Monitor her level of consciousness, vital signs, and output frequently for changes. Take steps to keep her safe, and institute seizure precautions, as needed. If your patient has a severe imbalance, keep emergency equipment readily available in case she has respiratory failure or a cardiac arrest. Stay alert for inadvertent rebound electrolyte excess.

Keep in mind that your patient's intense fear and anxiety about food may make her overly anxious about fluid and electrolyte therapy. Take time to explain the reason for the therapy and the dangerous problems it can help resolve.

Assisting with psychotherapy

Your patient will probably need psychotherapy to address the root of her misperceptions about her body and her appearance. Therapeutic techniques may involve identifying the triggers to disordered eating, using self-monitoring and awareness training, and interrupting the binge-purge cycle. Such techniques will help improve your patient's self-esteem, decrease her anxiety, facilitate coping, decrease denial and social isolation, and improve compliance. Overall, therapy is focused on fostering the development of a positive self-image and a regular eating pattern.

As prescribed, administer an antidepressant to help minimize obsessive thinking about food and weight and to help decrease the effects of depression on her continued recovery. Selective serotonin reuptake inhibitors, especially fluoxetine, may be most helpful during the maintenance phase. However, keep in mind that such drugs may cause nausea and anorexia, which may worsen signs and symptoms of your patient's disorder. Likewise, the anticholinergic effects of tricyclic antidepressants can worsen constipation and cardiotoxicity.

Throughout therapy, be sensitive to your patient's needs and allow her to talk about her anxiety. Don't be surprised if her anxiety increases as she nears her target weight. Stay aware of her fears and anxiety while correcting any misconceptions to help her handle this next step.

Asthma

A frightening disorder, asthma occurs when a patient's airways overreact to certain stimuli. And the consequences of severe asthma, such as diminished airflow and reduced gas exchange, can lead easily to cardiac compromise and arrhythmias.

Pathophysiology

When certain allergenic or trigger substances enter the airways of a patient with asthma, the reaction can be swift and dramatic. First, the allergen binds with mast cells in the lungs. Then the mast cells degranulate, releasing inflammatory mediators such as histamines, prostaglandins, leukotrienes, and bradykinin.

Because of the inflammatory effects of these mediators, smooth muscles in the airways constrict and spasm. They also increase vascular permeability, which leads to mucosal edema, and increase mucus secretion, which leads to mucus plugs, overinflation, and, possibly, atelectasis.

As airflow declines through the narrowed, plugged airways, gas exchange is compromised, and the signs and symptoms of an acute asthma attack become apparent: coughing, shortness of breath, and, possibly, wheezing and hyperventilation. The patient's heart rate increases as her cardiovascular system tries to compensate for the decrease in airflow. As it does, however, her $Pa{O_2}$ may continue falling while her partial pressure of arterial carbon dioxide ($Pa{CO_2}$) continues to rise—a situation that can lead to hypoxemia, acidosis, and cardiac arrhythmias

What's more, drugs used to treat asthma, especially theophylline, can increase the risk of arrhythmias. In particular, patients over age 50 who have asthma and underlying heart disease or a pulmonary disease, such as emphysema or bronchitis, face a much greater risk. Typically, the most serious arrhythmias result from acute asthma combined with aggressive therapy and underlying cardiovascular disease.

Signs and symptoms

If your patient is having an asthma attack, you'll note that she's pale and having trouble breathing. Her respiratory rate may exceed 30 breaths per minute. Watch for retraction of the sternocleidomastoid muscle; you'll probably notice that she's using accessory muscles to breathe. Your patient may experience palpitations or the sensation of a racing heart. If the asthma attack is severe, she may develop cyanosis, status asthmaticus, and respiratory failure.

Your patient with asthma is at risk for arrhythmias, including sinus tachycardia in which the heart rate exceeds 120 beats per minute (bpm) and life-threatening ventricular arrhythmias. Elderly patients, especially those with coexisting heart disease or underlying emphysema or bronchitis, may complain of chest pain or pressure.

Treatment

Treatment for an asthma attack typically starts with an inhaled beta agonist to relieve bronchospasm and dilate the airways. Beta agonists are easy to administer and are rapidly absorbed. Also, they inhibit inflammatory mediators.

However, a difficulty with beta agonists is their nonselectivity: they stimulate both $beta_1$ and $beta_2$ receptors. While stimulation of these receptors relieves bronchospasm by relaxing smooth muscles in the bronchioles, it also causes compartmental shifts in calcium. Subtle changes in intracellular ion gradients may affect myocardial action potentials, stimulate the heart, and increase CO, cardiac workload, and myocardial oxygen consumption. The stimulating effects of beta agonists, together with hypoxia-induced irritability, predispose the myocardium to atrial and supraventricular tachycardias.

Keep in mind that different drugs have different selectivity. For example, the commonly prescribed bronchodilators albuterol and metaproterenol are relatively $beta_2$ selective, depending on the dose. Albuterol, which is generally the least cardiotonic, may produce atrial fibrillation if higher-than-normal doses are delivered.

Subcutaneous epinephrine can relieve bronchospasm in 5 to 15 minutes, but it stimulates both $beta_1$ and $beta_2$ receptors. Thus, it can cause palpitations and tachyarrhythmias.

Certain disorders and the simultaneous use of other drugs can limit the usefulness of bronchodilators. For example, cardiac and hepatic dysfunction increase the likelihood of a toxic reaction, as does the simultaneous administration of such drugs as ciprofloxacin, erythromycin, clarithromycin, and cimetidine.

Indeed, combinations of asthma drugs can produce serious arrhythmias. For example, aminophylline and epinephrine given together may cause supraventricular and ventricular tachyarrhythmias. Isoproterenol and albuterol infusions cause ischemia and ventricular tachycardia. And I.V. aminophylline given with terbutaline can cause ventricular arrhythmias, multifocal PVCs, and ventricular tachycardia. Because astemizole increases the risk of arrhythmias, it shouldn't be used with ketoconazole or erythromycin. It also shouldn't be given to a patient with hepatic disease.

Nursing considerations

If your patient is having an asthma attack, take steps to soothe and calm her. Doing so will help her breathe better; it also will help you assess her condition more accurately. As much as possible, stay with your patient to provide emotional support, comfort, and reassurance. Help her into the high-Fowler position to provide optimal ventilation and keep her airway as open as possible.

When your patient is relatively calm and positioned properly, perform a physical assessment, a respiratory assessment, and hemodynamic and ECG monitoring. Also, perform blood tests to measure your patient's ABG, electrolyte, and drug levels. Provide her with appropriate treatments for easing her asthma attack as well as for resolving any arrhythmias that arise (see *Treating arrhythmias in an asthma patient,* page 190).

Assessing your patient

During your physical examination, evaluate your patient's pulmonary status by assessing her for coughing, chest tightness, wheezing, dyspnea, prolonged expiration, accessory muscle use, cyanosis, and altered level of consciousness. Also, check her ABG levels. A Pao_2 level below 60 mm Hg indicates hypoxemia. A $Paco_2$ level above 45 mm Hg indicates that airway resistance may be increasing. As the $Paco_2$ level rises, the pH falls, indicating acidosis.

Use pulse oximetry to measure your patient's oxygen saturation. A measurement of less than 91% indicates hypoxemia. Monitor her serum potassium level for hypokalemia.

Also, watch for these signs of worsening hypoxia:
- hypotension from reduced CO
- regular or irregular tachycardia
- a respiratory rate above 30 breaths per minute
- a paradoxical pulse that exceeds 12 mm Hg.

Treating arrhythmias in an asthma patient

If your patient with asthma develops an arrhythmia, you may need to administer the following treatments:

- supplemental oxygen at 2 to 3 L/minute by nasal cannula to correct hypoxia
- a bronchodilator, a corticosteroid, or both to relieve bronchospasm and inflammation
- an antiarrhythmic drug, such as digoxin or a calcium channel blocker, to help restore a stable rhythm
- sodium bicarbonate to correct acidosis
- antibiotics, if necessary.

Because beta-blockers have bronchoconstrictive effects, you won't use them for a patient with asthma. Also, avoid antihistamines during acute episodes. These drugs increase heart rate, elevate blood pressure, and cause vasoconstriction, which can lead to further bronchospasm. And keep in mind that inhaled mucolytics may worsen airway obstruction.

Monitor your patient's fluid and electrolyte replacement to maintain her hydration and correct hypokalemia, as necessary. Also, monitor your patient for adventitious breath sounds. Anticipate the need for mechanical ventilation to correct worsening hypoxia and respiratory distress.

Depending on the type of arrhythmia your patient has, she may need cardioversion or defibrillation. For example, if your patient develops supraventricular tachycardia and becomes hemodynamically unstable, she'll need cardioversion.

Assist with pulmonary function tests, as needed, to gain information about the severity of your patient's bronchospasm and airway obstruction. Keep in mind, however, that during an acute asthma attack, she may not be able to exert the respiratory effort that these tests require.

Other tests may include a chest X-ray to rule out pneumonia or other disease, a sputum culture to detect infection, and a CBC. Use your patient's baseline ECG to detect the development of arrhythmias during the course of her treatment. Stay alert for signs and symptoms of toxic or adverse reactions.

Detecting cardiac compromise

Observe your patient for jugular vein distention, which can result from lung overinflation that increases negative pleural pressure and pulmonary vascular resistance. Increased intrathoracic pressures may promote increased venous return to the right atrium and ventricle. The thin-walled chambers of the right side of the heart may overfill and enlarge from too much blood.

Assess your patient's ECG for evidence of strain and enlargement on the right side such as right axis deviation and an abnormally tall and symmetrically peaked P wave (P pulmonale) in leads II, III, and aV_F. Right ventricular hypertrophy creates R waves of 7 mm or more in lead V_1, along with deeper-than-normal S waves in leads I and V_4 through V_6. The R waves will not be as high as S waves are deep in lead V_6.

Throughout your patient's asthma treatment, continue pulse oximetry.

Pinpointing adverse drug effects

Carefully monitor your patient's drug levels to help identify arrhythmias resulting from a toxic reaction.

Beta agonists

A beta agonist helps reduce bronchospasm; however, without supplemental oxygen therapy, it also may worsen hypoxemia by further reducing $Pa{O_2}$. This occurs because, in reducing bronchospasm, the drug stimulates pulmonary blood flow to poorly ventilated lung tissue, which increases the delivery of unoxygenated blood. This effect typically occurs about 5 minutes after inhalation and lasts for 30 minutes.

Hypokalemia, another adverse effect of beta-agonist therapy, tends to cause PVCs. Multifocal atrial tachycardia may arise as well during beta-agonist therapy.

Theophylline

The therapeutic range for theophylline is 10 to 20 µg/ml. Toxic effects begin when drug levels exceed 20 µg/ml. As needed, check your patient's baseline and serial theophylline levels to detect evidence of a toxic reaction. Also, monitor your patient's ECG for arrhythmias.

A toxic reaction to theophylline can cause multifocal atrial tachycardia, paroxysmal atrial tachycardia, atrial fibrillation, ventricular tachycardia, and PVCs. Acute overdose tends to cause arrhythmias more than long-term overdose does.

Multifocal atrial tachycardia arises most commonly in patients who have severe obstructive lung disease, especially if they also have bronchospasm or infection. As ordered, treat your patient's signs and symptoms by administering digoxin or verapamil, which has a weak bronchodilating effect. You may also administer digoxin or verapamil to slow the increased heart rate in paroxysmal atrial tachycardia or atrial fibrillation.

Ventricular tachycardia is most common in patients with asthma who have heart disease, emphysema, or bronchitis or who have suffered a drug overdose. If the blood theophylline level exceeds 100 µg/ml, this arrhythmia can progress rapidly to ventricular fibrillation. It also may occur after rapid central venous infusion of aminophylline. To treat it, administer lidocaine or procainamide I.V., as prescribed. If the arrhythmia doesn't resolve, assist with cardioversion, as needed.

In elderly patients, PVCs usually occur as a result of a severe toxic reaction to theophylline. Typically, the occurrence of PVCs declines as toxic levels decline.

Hyperthyroidism

The thyroid gland, one of the largest of the endocrine glands, is shaped like a butterfly and wraps loosely around the front of the trachea, just below the cricoid cartilage. It controls cellular metabolism by producing the hormones thyroxine (T_3) and triiodothyronine (T_4) in response to thyroid-stimulating hormone (TSH) released by the pituitary gland. The thyroid gland also produces calcitonin, a hormone that decreases plasma calcium levels by increasing calcium deposition in bone.

If your patient's thyroid gland produces too much thyroid hormone, she will enter a hypermetabolic state that can alter cardiovascular, GI, and neuromuscular function. Commonly, this condition causes a cardiac arrhythmia to develop. Likewise, hyperactivity of the parathyroid glands, which are tucked just behind the thyroid, can cause arrhythmias (see *How hyperparathyroidism causes arrhythmias,* page 192).

Although hyperthyroidism doesn't always have an identifiable cause, it can result from various factors, including an autoimmune reaction, excessive TSH secretion, thyroiditis, a tumor, and an overdose of synthetic thyroid hormones.

Pathophysiology

Hyperthyroidism is a complex syndrome characterized by increased levels of T_3, T_4, or both. It mostly appears in the form of Graves' disease, a disorder that may be caused when autoimmune activity is triggered by emotional stress. Graves' disease is 10 times more common in women, especially those under age 40, than in men.

Increased circulation of thyroid hormones increases your patient's response to catecholamines. It also increases metabolism of carbohydrates, proteins, and lipids. Heightened protein catabolism results in a negative nitrogen balance, depleted lipids, and lowered glucose tolerance. Over time, the hypermetabolic effects of hyperthyroidism result in caloric and nutritional deficiencies, increased oxygen consumption, increased heat production, alterations in fluid and electrolyte balance, and an overall catabolic state. Cardiac demand increases, resulting in a hyperdynamic state. As a result, CO and peripheral blood flow increase.

Indeed, a person with hyperthyroidism is at high risk for altered CO. Excess thyroid hormone directly affects the heart, increasing stroke volume and heart rate. Increased metabolism raises the oxygen demand of peripheral tissues, increasing the heart's workload as a result. This increase in metabolic demand can lead to systolic hypertension, angina, arrhythmias, and cardiac failure.

Signs and symptoms

Characteristic signs and symptoms of hyperthyroidism reflect both an increased level of circulating thyroid hormone and an increased level of sympathetic stimulation. For example, you may see or feel a diffuse enlargement of your patient's thyroid gland (goiter). Her eyes may seem to protrude from their sockets (exophthalmos). The patient may report weight loss, heat intolerance, and an increase in nervousness, irritability, and

How hyperparathyroidism causes arrhythmias

Tiny parathyroid glands embedded in the back of the thyroid help to maintain homeostasis by regulating calcium levels. When calcium levels drop, these glands secrete parathyroid hormone (PTH), which increases calcium resorption in the kidneys and gastrointestinal tract while stimulating the release of calcium from bone.

If the parathyroid glands secrete too much PTH, a patient may develop hyperparathyroidism. This condition elevates calcium to abnormally high levels. And as you know, hypercalcemia commonly causes arrhythmias.

With hypercalcemia, the amount of calcium available for exchange during the action potential increases, delaying repolarization. As a result, the patient may develop bradycardia, atrial flutter, atrial fibrillation, varying degrees of atrioventricular (AV) block, ventricular tachycardia, and ventricular fibrillation.

Evidence of hypercalcemia on the patient's electrocardiogram begins with a shortened QT interval. As the condition worsens, T waves may widen—a warning sign of ventricular arrhythmias and AV block.

restlessness. She may experience palpitations and easily become short of breath and fatigued. Keep in mind, however, that your patient may not show all of these signs and symptoms.

Your patient's pulse rate may be between 90 and 160 bpm. She may look flushed and have trouble sitting still. Your patient may also have a fine hand tremor.

If she has pronounced hyperthyroidism or underlying cardiac disease, she may develop an arrhythmia, such as sinus tachycardia, atrial fibrillation, ventricular fibrillation, or a second-degree or third-degree AV block.

Tachycardia develops even at rest in about 40% of patients with hyperthyroid disease. It may result from an accelerated rate of diastolic depolarization and a shortened action potential in the sinus node.

Atrial fibrillation arises in about 15% of patients with hyperthyroidism. Extremely rapid atrial impulses bombard the AV node, resulting in an irregular ventricular response pattern. Atrial fibrillation may occur suddenly and recur, or it may persist as a chronic disturbance. Signs and symptoms stem from the ventricular response rate and may include a decreased CO and impaired tissue perfusion from the loss of atrial kick.

An excessive level of thyroid hormone has a direct effect on the cardiac conduction system, specifically on the AV node and bundle of His. Second-degree and third-degree AV block develop in about 15% of patients with hyperthyroidism, especially those with Graves' disease. With such a patient, you'll see a prolonged or notched P wave or evidence of right bundle branch block on her ECG. Such an AV block may resolve when the primary endocrine problem resolves.

If a patient with hyperthyroidism doesn't receive treatment, she could develop an acute hyperthyroid crisis, commonly called thyroid storm. If that happens, she may experience an abrupt fever, sweating, tachycardia, pulmonary edema, heart failure, trembling, and restlessness. Thyroid storm is an emergent condition that can be fatal without proper treatment.

Treatment

Treatment commonly includes an antithyroid drug such as propylthiouracil or methimazole, an iodine or iodide compound to reduce hormone release and the size of the gland, and, possibly, a beta-blocker to reduce sympathetic nervous effects. Your patient may undergo radiation therapy with iodine 131 to destroy overactive thyroid cells. If she can't tolerate radiation therapy, she may undergo surgery to have most of the gland removed.

Treatment for thyroid storm typically involves administration of a beta-blocker, such as propranolol. Treatment for any cardiac arrhythmias that may develop varies according to the specific arrhythmia.

Nursing considerations

Because your patient with hyperthyroidism has an increased risk of decreased CO, focus your care on detecting and limiting alterations in CO. For example, assess your patient's cardiovascular status often. Monitor her blood pressure, heart rate and rhythm, respiratory rate, and breath sounds. Assess her for peripheral edema and jugular vein distention. Document her intake and output and regulate her fluid replacement. And check her level of consciousness often.

Anticipate the administration of a beta-blocker to reduce the effects of catecholamines and reverse supraventricular tachycardias, such as atrial fibrillation. Maintain a cool room temperature and keep your patient calm to minimize circulating catecholamines and their effects. Also, provide frequent rest periods to conserve her energy and minimize the demand for oxygen.

If your patient is elderly or has coronary artery disease, be aware that she has an increased risk of cardiovascular collapse. Stay alert for such signs and symptoms as hypotension, tachycardia that deteriorates into bradycardia, a decreased CO, low pulmonary artery and occlusive pressures, oliguria, and a decreasing level of consciousness.

If your patient develops sinus tachycardia, administer a beta-blocker, as prescribed. If she develops atrial fibrillation, focus your treatment on converting the arrhythmia to a normal sinus rhythm. Be prepared to respond promptly to any arrhythmias that may arise. Remember that although atrial fibrillation is common in patients with hyperthyroidism, such patients also may experience ventricular fibrillation and AV block.

Atrial fibrillation

If your patient with hyperthyroidism experiences atrial fibrillation, determine whether it's a controlled fibrillation. If it is, your patient will have a normal level of consciousness, adequate blood pressure, sufficient urine output, and warm, dry skin. As prescribed, administer a beta-blocker (such as esmolol, metoprolol, or labetalol), a calcium channel blocker (usually diltiazem or verapamil), digoxin, magnesium, or amiodarone.

If your patient is hypotensive, has an altered level of consciousness, complains of chest pain, or has mottled skin (a sign of poor tissue perfusion), suspect an uncontrolled fibrillation. In that case, focus your treatment on controlling the ventricular response rate rather than restoring a sinus rhythm immediately. As prescribed, administer drugs to block the AV node, such as a beta-blocker, calcium channel blocker, digoxin, amiodarone, or magnesium.

If drug therapy is unsuccessful, your patient may require electrical cardioversion. If so, administer a sedative, as prescribed, before the procedure. Remember that cardioversion doesn't establish atrial contractions immediately. Rather, they usually don't resume for a few hours, even though the heart has been restored to a sinus rhythm electrically. Remember, the failure rate for electrical cardioversion is 20% to 50%, depending on the duration of the atrial fibrillation.

Ventricular fibrillation and atrioventricular block

If your patient develops ventricular fibrillation, follow advanced cardiac life support guidelines. If she has a first-degree or second-degree AV block, assess her closely for progression to third-degree AV block. Be prepared to administer atropine or isoproterenol I.V., and anticipate insertion of a transvenous pacemaker.

Hypothyroidism

In hypothyroidism, known as myxedema in its most severe form, the thyroid gland fails to secrete adequate amounts of thyroid hormone. Primary hypothyroidism, the most common type, usually stems from damage or dysfunction of the gland itself. It may result from autoimmune activity (such as Hashimoto's disease), iodine deficiency, surgical removal of the thyroid gland, cancer of the thyroid gland, radiation therapy with iodine 131, thyroiditis (usually viral or immune mediated), withdrawal of thyroid hormone replacement, and the use of antithyroid drugs. Primary hypothyroidism is two to four times more common in women, especially those between ages 40 and 60, than in men.

In secondary hypothyroidism, the thyroid gland is healthy, but it receives inadequate stimulation to secrete thyroid hormone. This condition may result from a pituitary tumor or a deficiency in pituitary hormones. In tertiary hypothyroidism, the hypothalamus fails to secrete thyrotropin-releasing hormone.

Severe hypothyroidism occurs most commonly in elderly people during the winter months. It usually follows exposure to cold, an abrupt withdrawal of thyroid hormone, an illness, or a traumatic injury. Severe hypothyroidism may trigger the development of cardiac arrhythmias and may cause myxedema coma, a rare but serious end-stage complication of progressive hypothyroidism.

Pathophysiology

When thyroid hormone levels decline, all metabolic processes also decline. The force of myocardial contractions decreases, and the heart rate becomes irregular. As a result, CO drops.

Hypothyroidism also decreases fat metabolism. As a result, mucopolysaccharides—a major protein polysaccharide complex—accumulate in the interstitial space rather than being metabolized. With myxedema, an excessive amount of mucopolysaccharides accumulate, causing them to infiltrate surrounding connective tissue. This condition alters capillary membrane permeability: body fluids leak into the interstitial space and edema results.

The change in cell membrane permeability also leads to a loss of intravascular sodium (hyponatremia). Thus, fluid, proteins, and electrolytes leak into the interstitium, causing a major fluid shift that affects every body system. Cardiac arrhythmias and pericardial effusion may develop. And severe hyponatremia can lead to seizures.

As you know, sodium plays an essential role in the sodium-potassium pump, which is necessary for normal cardiac conduction. The natural exchange gradient between sodium and potassium produces an ionic flow across cardiac cell membranes that results in electrical activity. When this ionic flow declines, the number of action potentials available for cardiac conduction declines, resulting in severe bradycardia.

Signs and symptoms

If your patient has untreated hypothyroidism, she may experience unexplained weight gain, dry skin, hair loss, a deepening voice, and intolerance to cold. She'll probably complain of fatigue and may report sleeping 14 to 16 hours a day. She may also experience menstrual irregularities, although many patients wrongly assume this is related to menopause.

As hypothyroidism progresses, your patient will develop a puffy appearance, including periorbital edema, although her edema will be nonpitting. Her skin will be cool and dry with a yellow tinge, her hair will look dry and coarse, and her nails will be thick and brittle. Her body temperature may be 94°F (34.4°C) or lower. Capillary refill may be prolonged greater than 2.5 seconds because of peripheral vasoconstriction. You also may note that your patient has orthopnea and dyspnea on exertion. Her voice may sound husky, and her speech may seem slowed by a thick tongue.

Physical examination may reveal a significant delay in deep tendon reflexes. Visible inspection of your patient's neck may reveal an enlarged thyroid gland—a result of increased levels of TSH released from the pituitary gland in response to reduced levels of thyroid hormone. If your patient's thyroid is visibly enlarged, don't palpate it; doing so could cause the release of thyroid hormone.

Keep in mind that the decreased metabolism caused by hypothyroidism leads to increased cholesterol levels and increased atherosclerosis. If your patient's coronary arteries are narrowed, decreased perfusion may lead to myocardial ischemia, cardiac arrhythmias, and infarction—especially when treatment for hypothyroidism increases her metabolism. Your patient's ECG may reveal depressed T waves, hyperacute changes in the ST segment, and a prolonged QT interval.

Auscultate your patient's heart sounds. If they're muffled, suspect a pericardial effusion, which can be confirmed with an echocardiogram or a chest X-ray.

If your patient is obtunded because of severe hypothyroidism, obtain her medical history from her medical records or, if necessary, from family members.

Diagnostic tests

A physician may order tests for blood levels of TSH, T_3, and T_4. Increased blood levels of TSH along with decreased levels of T_3 and T_4 confirm hypothyroidism. Also, TSH levels can help differentiate between primary and secondary hypothyroidism.

Other laboratory findings for a patient with hypothyroidism may include decreased T_3 resin uptake, hyponatremia, and decreased plasma osmolality. An ABG analysis will reveal increased $Paco_2$, decreased Pao_2, and decreased pH (respiratory acidosis).

Because your patient's slowed metabolism affects organ function, she'll probably have hypoglycemia, anemia, and increased creatine kinase, carotene, and total blood cholesterol levels. A decreased hemoglobin level, an increased total cholesterol level, and hyponatremia increase your patient's risk of cardiac arrhythmias.

Treatment

Treatment for hypothyroidism typically includes reversing the underlying hypothyroid condition with synthetic thyroid hormones and correcting any complications.

As prescribed, give one of several synthetic thyroid hormones to reverse your patient's hypothyroidism. Typically taken once daily, these oral drugs include levothyroxine sodium, the most common; liothyronine sodium; and liotrix, a combination of T_3 and T_4. If your patient is under age 50, full replacement therapy calls for 1.7 µg/kg/day. Elderly patients may require less than 1 µg/kg/day. A child may need up to 4 µg/kg/day.

During treatment, weigh your patient daily. Remember that 1 kg of weight equals 1 L of fluid. Auscultate her heart sounds; they may seem distant. Check her peripheral pulses and assess her level of peripheral edema. Also, check your patient's blood pressure; it may be normal or slightly low (see *Cardiac evidence of hypothyroidism*).

As necessary, your patient may require treatment for respiratory and cardiac complications of hypothyroidism. She may also require close monitoring of her fluid and electrolyte levels.

Respiratory and cardiac interventions

Assess the quality and rate of your patient's respirations. Inhibited central ventilatory drive and respiratory muscle weakness may cause an abnormal breathing pattern. Hypercapnia and hypoxia can lead to myocardial ischemia and changes in level of consciousness. An ischemic myocardium, with its delayed action potentials, increases the risk of escape rhythms.

If your patient has a compromised respiratory status or acidosis, anticipate endotracheal intubation and mechanical ventilation, as needed. Remember that a decreased hemoglobin level affects the ability of blood to transport oxygen. Further, oxygen deprivation can lead to worsened myocardial ischemia and ventricular arrhythmias from myocardial irritability.

Assist your patient in maintaining proper body alignment to ensure adequate chest-wall expansion. Prepare to administer supplemental oxygen, if indicated. Keep emergency resuscitation equipment nearby, and maintain seizure precautions.

Keep in mind that increased total cholesterol levels increase your patient's risk of atherosclerotic cardiovascular disease and subsequent cardiac arrhythmias. If your patient's total cholesterol level rises above acceptable levels, help her modify her diet to reduce cholesterol intake. Respond quickly to any complaints that could have a cardiac origin, such as chest pain.

Review your patient's ECG, looking for QT intervals longer than 0.44 second. If you find a prolonged QT interval, report it immediately. If untreated, the rhythm could progress to ventricular fibrillation and asystole.

If your patient has severe bradycardia, she may temporarily need an external transcutaneous pacemaker or a percutaneous transvenous pacemaker to ensure adequate CO. Administer atropine I.V. and epinephrine I.V., as prescribed. Dopamine, a potent vasoconstrictor, may also be needed to maintain adequate blood pressure.

Fluid and electrolyte monitoring

Monitor your patient's blood electrolyte tests for changes in her sodium level. If she has marked hyponatremia, administer hypertonic sodium chloride solution I.V., as prescribed.

Although pericardial effusion may develop, pericardiocentesis is rarely necessary. That's because serous fluid accumulates slowly in the pericardium, and the body usually can accommodate the gradual change. Eventually, however, pericardial effusion restricts myocardial contractions, leading to an overall decrease in CO. Compensatory mech-

---

Cardiac evidence of hypothyroidism

Typically, cardiac signs and symptoms of hypothyroidism include the following:

- bradycardia
- cardiomegaly
- decreased stroke volume
- decreased cardiac output
- flattened or inverted T waves
- prolonged QT and PR intervals.

anisms may cause tachycardia if your patient develops a significant pericardial effusion.

Patient teaching

When you teach your patient about hypothyroidism and the cardiac arrhythmias it can cause, focus on the treatment prescribed for her underlying thyroid disorder. Remind your patient to take her thyroid replacement hormone regularly and not to skip doses.

When you discuss risk factors for severe hypothyroidism, emphasize methods to reduce stress. Review your patient's normal activity level and coping mechanisms. Remind her that physical and emotional stress can trigger severe hypothyroidism even if she follows her drug regimen faithfully. Caution your patient to increase physical activity slowly as treatment improves activity tolerance.

Patients with hypothyroidism typically are sensitive to changes in environmental temperatures. Instruct your patient to wear warm clothing, as needed. Also, because hypothyroidism slows metabolism, warn your patient that she may need to restrict her daily caloric intake to avoid gaining weight.

Tell your patient that once replacement thyroid hormone is administered, cardiac signs and symptoms tend to resolve quickly. Also, explain the importance of routine follow-ups. All patients who receive treatment for a thyroid condition should have a yearly examination, including evaluation of blood thyroid hormone levels.

Pulmonary embolism

When part of a thrombus dislodges, usually from a site in the leg, it floats through the systemic circulation until it reaches a vessel too small to pass—typically the pulmonary artery or one of its branches. The thrombus then lodges in the vessel, partially or fully obstructing blood flow to distal lung tissue. This disorder, called a pulmonary embolism, can quickly become life threatening. Of the more than 500,000 Americans who develop a pulmonary embolism each year, about 50,000 die within 1 hour of its onset.

The cardiovascular effects of pulmonary embolism depend on the degree to which it obstructs pulmonary blood flow. These effects also vary with the patient's underlying cardiopulmonary status. In all cases, however, pulmonary embolism increases the risk of cardiac arrhythmias.

Pathophysiology

Almost all pulmonary emboli begin as thrombi in veins of the thigh, calf, or pelvis. However, thrombi also may originate in the right side of the heart, the venae cavae, or the arms. Other possible sources of pulmonary embolism include amniotic fluid, tumor cells, air introduced through an intravascular catheter, and a fat embolism released from a fractured long bone.

Although a piece of a thrombus may detach spontaneously, it usually detaches in response to a mechanical force, such as standing suddenly after prolonged bed rest or performing Valsalva's maneuver, which alters the rate of blood flow. Other conditions may increase the risk of pulmonary embolism as well (see *Risk factors for pulmonary embolism*).

Once the thrombus detaches (becoming an embolus), it begins to move through the systemic circulation to the right side of the heart and into the pulmonary artery. Along the way, it may break into smaller emboli that can occlude more than one small vessel. Of course, occlusion reduces or stops blood flow through the blocked vessels, which inhibits oxygen from reaching the lung tissues supplied by those vessels. The greater the degree of occlusion, the greater the reduction in circulation.

Coating the surface of an embolus is a mesh of fibrin, RBCs, and platelets that degrades when it becomes lodged in a vessel. Degradation of platelets releases substances that constrict the pulmonary arteries and arterioles. Those substances include catecholamines, prostaglandins, serotonin, histamine, and thromboxane. They also affect receptors in the bronchioles, alveoli, and smooth muscles of the airway normally supplied with blood by the occluded vessel.

The release of these substances, combined with mechanical obstruction and vasoconstriction caused by hypoxemia, leads to an increase in pulmonary vascular resistance and pulmonary hypertension. This process may occur even in patients who have no underlying cardiac disease, especially when the obstruction affects 30% or more of the lung tissue. The right ventricle must work harder to exert enough pressure to continue moving blood. If pulmonary hypertension becomes severe, the right ventricle may fail, resulting in tachycardia and reduced CO.

The release of catecholamines also stimulates alpha and beta receptors. Stimulation of $beta_2$ receptors increases heart rate, atrial and ventricular contractility, and the speed of electrical conduction through the AV node. Consequently, it commonly causes sinus tachycardia.

Also, the obstruction created by a pulmonary embolism causes increased dead space in the lung and ventilation-perfusion mismatches. Typically, ventilation is adequate, but perfusion isn't. In response, platelets in the obstructed area release serotonin or histamine, causing bronchoconstriction, which acts as a compensatory mechanism to balance ventilation and perfusion. However, it also can cause hypoxemia and impaired pulmonary blood flow, which decreases surfactant levels and may allow alveoli to collapse. Alveolocapillary shunting results, causing tissue hypoxia that leads to myocardial irritability and PVCs.

Risk factors for pulmonary embolism

The following factors raise your patient's risk of pulmonary embolism:
- acute injury to a vessel wall
- advanced age
- atrial fibrillation
- hypercoagulable state
- immobility
- mitral valve stenosis
- obesity
- pregnancy
- recent surgery
- traumatic injury
- use of oral contraceptives
- venous stasis.

Of these factors, venous stasis is the most significant. Also, remember that women have a greater risk of pulmonary embolism than men.

Signs and symptoms

A patient with a pulmonary embolism may complain of sudden shortness of breath and sharp chest pain that varies with breathing or position changes. Unless your patient has a large embolus, they may be her only symptoms. However, you may notice a subtle deterioration in her condition without any apparent cause.

Besides sudden dyspnea and pleuritic chest pain, some patients may experience the following signs and symptoms of a pulmonary embolism:
- restlessness, apprehension, and a sense of impending doom
- tachycardia
- third heart sound (S_3) and fourth heart sound (S_4) gallop rhythm
- increased intensity of pulmonic component of the second heart sound (S_2)
- crackles
- pleural friction rub
- tachypnea
- hemoptysis
- coughing or wheezing
- slightly elevated temperature
- swelling and tenderness in a leg.

Keep in mind that obstruction of more than half of the total pulmonary blood flow may cause cardiac decompensation. Your patient will be hypotensive and cyanotic. You'll probably see transient, nonspecific changes on her ECG. She may have abnormal QRS complexes, elevated ST segments, and inverted T waves. Pulmonary embolism also may cause the following ECG changes:
- ST-segment depression
- tall, peaked T waves
- right axis deviation
- right bundle branch block of new onset
- atrial flutter or fibrillation.

Diagnostic tests

Typically, a physician uses pulmonary angiography to identify pulmonary perfusion defects. Ventilation and perfusion scans, although inconclusive alone, may be used to assist the diagnosis if they are evaluated for ventilation-perfusion mismatches. The patient also may undergo Doppler ultrasonography, impedance plethysmography, or venography to detect venous thrombosis.

Although ABG levels help confirm pulmonary embolism, they aren't diagnostic on their own. However, don't assume that normal ABG levels rule out a pulmonary embolism; the embolus may not be large enough to significantly alter gas exchange. If it is large, abnormal results may include a Pao_2 under 80 mm Hg and a $Paco_2$ under 36 mm Hg.

Typically, the patient's chest X-ray will be normal. However, results that may suggest a pulmonary embolism include an enlargement of one or both chambers on the right side of the heart, an enlarged pulmonary artery, linear basal atelectasis, infiltrates, pleural effusion, and an elevated diaphragm on the side of the embolism. If your patient's diaphragm is elevated on the left side, the left ventricle may be under considerable external pressure. Such pressure could reduce her myocardial contractility and CO, leading to thrombus formation and atrial flutter.

Treatment

If your patient develops a pulmonary embolism, she'll need rapid treatment to support her vital functions, prevent further thrombosis, and prevent or halt cardiac arrhythmias. She may receive anticoagulant and thrombolytic therapy. If necessary, she may undergo surgery.

If your patient develops signs and symptoms of a pulmonary embolism, be especially alert to the rate, depth, and character of her respirations. If she develops dyspnea or tachypnea, elevate the head of her bed to promote chest expansion and ease the work of breathing. Auscultate her breath sounds for crackles and her heart sounds for S_3 or a pleural friction rub. As prescribed, give your patient supplemental humidified oxygen to decrease hypoxemia. Also, assess her skin color and oxygen saturation levels continuously.

Use ABG measurements to monitor trends in your patient's acid-base status. A decreasing $Pa{O_2}$ indicates that her respiratory status is worsening. If her level of consciousness changes at the same time and she seems overly anxious or describes a sense of impending doom, watch her carefully for changes in her respiratory condition. If she develops respiratory distress or failure, anticipate the use of endotracheal intubation and mechanical ventilation.

If your patient isn't hypotensive, admininster morphine, as prescribed, to reduce her anxiety and pleuritic chest pain. Morphine eases bronchoconstriction and dilates coronary arteries, improving myocardial circulation and oxygenation. However, because morphine depresses respiratory function, you'll need to reassess your patient's level of consciousness and her respiratory rate and pattern before and after administering the drug.

If your patient has a large or severe pulmonary embolism, inotropic drugs, such as dopamine and vasopressors, can help maintain her CO. Otherwise, systemic hypotension and shock may result from the reduction in CO caused by right ventricular failure. Fluid volume loading may be prescribed to increase pulmonary blood flow.

Anticipate insertion of a central venous catheter or pulmonary artery catheter to evaluate your patient's hemodynamic status. She also may receive an indwelling urinary catheter to allow precise evaluation of urine output. Document your patient's intake and output carefully.

Be prepared to obtain a 12-lead ECG to rule out an MI. Also, initiate continuous cardiac monitoring, as prescribed, to evaluate your patient's cardiac function. Be especially alert for a rapid increase in heart rate, indicating atrial tachycardia.

Preventing further thrombus formation

To help reduce your patient's risk of further thrombus formation, you may assist with one of more of these treatments: anticoagulant therapy, thrombolytic therapy, and, in severe cases, surgery.

Anticoagulant therapy

Heparin administered by continuous I.V. infusion is the treatment of choice for acute pulmonary embolism. As you know, heparin inhibits formation of thrombi and clots by preventing conversion of prothrombin to thrombin and by preventing the release of thromboplastin from platelets.

Excessive bleeding is the most common adverse effect of heparin therapy. Hemorrhage increases the demand on your patient's already stressed cardiopulmonary system, predisposing her to tachycardia, paroxysmal atrial tachycardia, atrial flutter, and shock. If she develops an atrial arrhythmia, anticipate administering digoxin, as prescribed. Because digoxin can potentiate the effects of heparin, however, you'll want to keep protamine sulfate, the antidote to heparin, readily available.

Before stopping your patient's heparin therapy, begin giving her an oral anticoagulant such as warfarin, as ordered. Warfarin interferes with the synthesis of vitamin K–dependent clotting factors II, VII, IX, and X. As these factors become depleted, clotting time becomes prolonged.

Initially, administer 10 to 15 mg of warfarin daily. Then adjust the dosage to keep her prothrombin time or international normalized ratio at 2 to 2.5 times above the control.

Once warfarin reaches therapeutic levels, a process that typically takes 2 to 3 days, you'll dis-

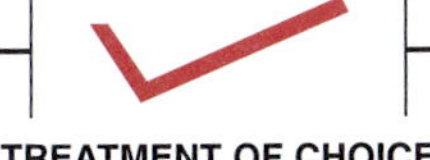

TREATMENT OF CHOICE

How a Greenfield filter works

A Greenfield filter reduces the risk of recurring pulmonary embolism by straining emboli from the blood as it flows through the inferior vena cava. The filter is an inverted cone-shaped device that traps emboli while allowing blood to flow relatively freely through it.

Usually, a physician inserts a Greenfield filter percutaneously, using fluoroscopic guidance. At the end of the procedure, the filter rests above the common iliac vein and below the renal veins. Hooks at the open end of the filter hold the device in place. Complications of the procedure include perforation of the vena cava, migration of the filter, and recurrent emboli, which develop in about 5% of patients.

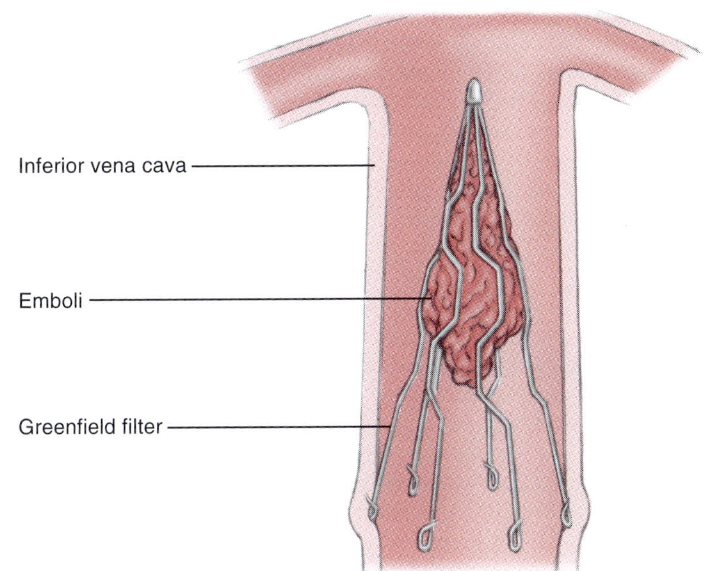

continue the heparin, as ordered. Your patient will continue taking warfarin for 3 months or more. Be sure to teach her about the drug, including measures to reduce the risk of bleeding and the need for follow-up blood tests. Provide your patient with a list of foods rich in vitamin K and encourage her to eat consistent amounts of those foods to avoid interfering with the warfarin therapy.

Thrombolytic therapy

If your patient has a massive pulmonary embolism and is hemodynamically unstable, she'll probably receive thrombolytic therapy with streptokinase, urokinase, or alteplase. These drugs convert plasminogen to plasmin, a fibrinolytic enzyme that actively lyses thrombi and emboli.

If she receives thrombolytic therapy, you won't administer heparin until after the therapy begins and your patient's coagulation studies have returned to a level less than twice the upper normal limit. Thrombolytic therapy is contraindicated in patients with bleeding disorders or recent cerebrovascular hemorrhage.

During and after thrombolytic therapy, watch for reperfusion arrhythmias. You might see sinus bradycardia, PVCs, an accelerated idioventricular rhythm, or ventricular tachycardia. Be prepared to provide antiarrhythmic drugs or emergency life support if your patient develops ventricular bradycardia or ventricular irritability.

Surgery

On rare occasions, a patient with a pulmonary embolism requires surgery. Indications for surgery include the following:

- a massive embolism that obstructs total pulmonary blood flow by 50% or more
- a contraindication to thrombolytic therapy
- ineffective thrombolytic therapy
- life-threatening complications.

Two surgical methods used to relieve the effects of pulmonary embolism are embolectomy and the placement of a filter in the vena cava. Because as many as 70% of patients who undergo embolectomy die, the surgical treatment of choice is to place a Greenfield filter in the vena cava to prevent more emboli from reaching the pulmonary circulation (see *How a Greenfield filter works*).

After surgery, anticoagulant therapy typically continues for several months. Teach your patient how to recognize the signs and symptoms of complications, such as recurrent embolism, venous insufficiency, air embolus, and migration of the filter.

Controlling arrhythmias

Typically, ECG changes—such as sinus tachycardia—that arise during a pulmonary embolism will resolve as the effects of the embolism resolve with treatment. If necessary, administer propranolol, as prescribed, to help slow your patient's tachycardia. A physician also may prescribe verapamil to slow SA node discharge.

Drug therapy in the elderly

In the United States, people over age 65 make up about 12% of the population, but they use about 33% of all prescription drugs. Most patients over age 65 take two or more prescription drugs daily. And typically, those who live in long-term-care facilities take three or more drugs daily. Taking several drugs each day is termed *polypharmacy,* a condition that raises the risk of serious adverse effects, including cardiac arrhythmias.

Elderly patients are more likely to share drugs, hoard drugs, store drugs improperly, mix several drugs in the same container, fail to take a drug, or save a leftover drug and take it at an improper time or for an unintended purpose. Such patients are also more likely to misunderstand a drug's purpose, forget its name, and not comply with a drug regimen because of scheduling difficulties, adverse effects, and physical limitations.

Elderly patients also take a disproportionate percentage of over-the-counter (OTC) drugs, including analgesics, anti-inflammatories, laxatives, decongestants, antihistamines, and vitamins.

They're also more likely to see several physicians, each for a different health problem. If each of these physicians prescribes one or more drugs without fully checking the patient's prescription and OTC drug list, the chance of harmful interactions—including cardiac reactions and arrhythmias—rises dramatically.

Pathophysiology

For patients of all ages, taking more than one drug at a time raises the risk of adverse effects and interactions. For elderly patients, however, the risk is even greater, partly because of the natural effects of aging on the body. An older patient's ability to respond to illness, injury, and disease is naturally reduced, further compounding the problem (see *How age-related changes alter drug effects*).

Elderly patients face an increased risk of adverse cardiac effects, in part because of age-related changes that alter cardiac function, such as the generation and conduction of impulses. Common changes include the following:

- sclerosis and fibrosis of heart valves
- reduced myocardial efficiency and contractility
- decreased stroke volume and CO
- prolonged isometric contraction and relaxation of the left ventricle
- increased vessel-wall rigidity
- narrowed vessel lumens
- diminished baroreceptor sensitivity
- decreased sinoatrial (SA) node rate
- reduced parasympathetic and sympathetic tone.

Although the heart rate doesn't change significantly with age, it takes longer to speed up and return to normal during periods of stress. What's more, atrial and ventricular arrhythmias occur more commonly among elderly patients. And the risk of arrhythmias is further increased by drug interactions. (see *Common effects of drug interactions in the elderly,* page 202).

Altered drug effects

As discussed, age-related changes can alter the intended effects of certain drugs. For example, physicians commonly prescribe digoxin for elderly patients. Digoxin inhibits the transport of sodium and potassium across cell membranes, thereby increasing the force of contractions, slowing the heart rate, and decreasing conduction through the AV node and intraventricular bundle. As a result, bradycardia and heart block may occur. And age-related cardiac changes may further enhance this effect.

An age-related decrease in renal excretion, especially if your patient takes a diuretic, raises her risk of a toxic reaction to digoxin. This condition may first appear as an arrhythmia. Some elderly patients are more sensitive to the effects of digoxin than others. With impaired renal function, however, even therapeutic doses can be toxic. Also, keep in mind that laxatives can contribute to electrolyte imbalances, which further increases the risk of arrhythmias when combined with digoxin and diuretics.

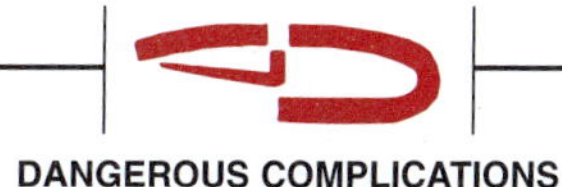

DANGEROUS COMPLICATIONS

How age-related changes alter drug effects

Characteristic	Age-related changes	Effects
Absorption	• decreased gastric acid secretion • decreased absorptive surface and blood flow to small intestine • slower gastric emptying • diminished blood flow through the viscera • decreased gastric motility	• delay in rate of absorption
Distribution	• increased body fat • decreased body water • decreased level of albumin • loss of lean body mass	• accumulation of drug • delayed drug effect • changes in protein binding, which can increase levels of unbound drug
Metabolism	• decreased liver mass • reduced hepatic blood flow • decreased enzyme activity	• decreased metabolism and delayed breakdown, leading to prolonged action, accumulation, and toxic effects
Elimination	• decreased renal blood flow • decreased glomerular filtration rate	• decreased rate of elimination • increased risk of prolonged action, accumulation, and toxic effects
Drug activity	• decreased efficiency of receptor function	• diminished response to drug • increased risk of toxic effects
	• decrease in neurotransmitters (dopamine and acetylcholine)	• increased susceptibility to adverse effects
	• increased sensitivity to depression	• increased risk of sedation and decreased cognitive function
	• deterioration of blood-brain barrier	• increased risk of drug-induced behavioral changes
	• decreased cardiac output and increased total peripheral resistance	• increased risk of adverse drug effects • increased levels of circulating norepinephrine • decreased sensitivity and function of baroreceptors
	• decline in glucose tolerance	• increased risk of hypoglycemia or hyperglycemia
	• diminished thyroid function	• slowed drug metabolism

Physicians also commonly prescribe diuretics for elderly patients who have heart failure or hypertension. Potassium sparing diuretics increase the risk of hyperkalemia—a common cause of arrhythmias. Thiazide diuretics increase the risk of hypokalemia, which also can lead to arrhythmias.

Diuretics also affect the metabolism and half-lives of other drugs, such as calcium channel blockers, quinidine, and amiodarone. In many cases, cardiac arrhythmias, especially AV blocks, are the first sign of a toxic reaction to a drug.

Beta-blockers may be prescribed as antihypertensive therapy. But in elderly patients, their beta-receptor response may be reduced. Such an age-

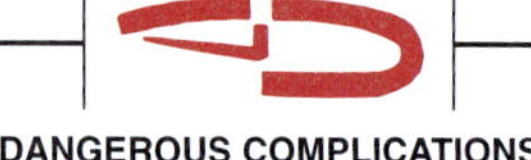

DANGEROUS COMPLICATIONS

Common effects of drug interactions in the elderly

This table highlights the physiologic effects of interactions between drugs commonly prescribed to elderly patients.

Drug	Interacting drugs	Effects
Digoxin	• thiazide and loop diuretics • certain broad-spectrum antibiotics	• increased risk of toxic effects from hypokalemia
	• calcium channel blockers • quinidine • indomethacin • hydralazine • anticholinergics	• increased blood levels of digoxin • increased risk of toxic effects
	• beta-blockers	• increased conduction through the atrioventricular (AV) node, leading to bradyarrhythmias, including third-degree AV block
	• macrolide antibiotics	• digoxin metabolism slowed, increasing risk of toxic effects
	• inhaled beta$_2$ agonists	• increased risk of hypokalemia, leading to tachyarrhythmias
Beta-blockers	• cimetidine	• increased beta-blocking effect, leading to bradycardia
	• theophylline salts	• slowed rate of theophylline metabolism, increasing risk of theophylline's toxic effects and subsequent arrhythmias
	• inhaled beta$_2$ agonists	• increased vagal tone, leading to bradycardia
Systemic corticosteroids	• loop and thiazide diuretics	• increased potassium excretion, leading to severe hypokalemia

related change alters the patient's response to the drug, increasing the risk of a toxic reaction, hypotension, bradycardia, and SA or AV node block.

Electrolyte imbalances

Chronic health problems and adverse drug effects can interfere with an older patient's nutritional status, placing her at risk for dehydration and an electrolyte imbalance. As in any patient, an electrolyte imbalance can lead to arrhythmias.

Imbalances common among elderly patients include hypokalemia, hyperkalemia, hypocalcemia, and hypercalcemia. Hypokalemia may result from dehydration, vomiting, gastric suction, overuse of thiazide or loop diuretics, overuse of laxatives, or decreased sodium levels. Hyperkalemia may result from potassium sparing diuretics, angiotensin-converting enzyme inhibitors, or reduced renal function. Hypocalcemia may result from loop diuretics, osteomalacia, hypoparathyroidism, or respiratory alkalosis. And hypercalcemia may result from adrenal insufficiency, hyperparathyroidism, renal failure, or cancer.

Signs and symptoms

Commonly, the adverse effects of drug therapy go undetected until a health care professional obtains a patient's complete health history. For your admission assessment, encourage your elderly patient to bring all her drugs with her, or have a family member bring them in later. The patient may report receiving one or two drugs from her primary physician, another one or two from a cardiologist, one from a gastroenterologist, and so on. When asked what each drug is for, she may have trouble answering or say that she doesn't remember (see *Obtaining a drug history from an elderly patient*).

Further investigation may reveal the use of duplicate drugs. The patient may not know that one is a generic form and the other is a brand name of the same drug. Generic equivalents may not be similar in color or shape.

Be sure to question your patient about any allergies she has to drugs or foods. Also, investigate her use of OTC drugs, such as antacids, enemas, analgesics, laxatives, diuretics, and vitamin and mineral supplements. Your patient may not consider them to be drugs and may not mention them unless asked specifically. Then, she may report that she uses OTC drugs for aches and pains, constipation, or heartburn.

Perform a physical examination to evaluate your patient's overall health status. Identify any age-related changes that could influence drug therapy. Confirm the existence and extent of any disorders or chronic health problems. And determine your patient's risk for problems caused by drug therapy.

Also, consider the results of recent laboratory tests, such as a CBC, blood electrolyte and glucose levels, renal function tests (including BUN and creatinine levels), and liver enzyme levels.

Signs and symptoms of a problem resulting from drug therapy include the following:
• bradycardia
• syncope
• hypotension
• hypokalemia or hyperkalemia
• hypocalcemia or hypercalcemia
• neurologic changes.

If your patient takes digoxin, she may have signs and symptoms of a toxic reaction, including:
• cardiac arrhythmias
• mental status changes
• abnormal visual sensations
• headache or irritability
• peripheral neuritis
• muscle weakness
• anorexia
• nausea, vomiting, or diarrhea.

Obtaining a drug history from an elderly patient

When obtaining a drug history from your elderly patient, take the time to gather as much information as possible. But be cautious not to tire or overwhelm her. Proceed at a relaxed pace, allowing your patient enough time to respond comfortably. Remember that she may have such age-related changes as a slowed response time, a hearing or visual deficit, a decreased attention span, and an impaired memory.

Gather the following information for all prescription and over-the-counter drugs your patient is taking as well as for all vitamin, mineral, and herbal supplements:
• drug name
• reason for taking it
• current dosage
• regimen specifics (for example, whether she takes the drug with food)
• length of time she has been taking it
• relief obtained
• name of person who prescribed or recommended the drug
• complaints, if any
• dosage changes, if any, and the reason she made them.

On her ECG, you may see signs of electrolyte imbalance. If she has hypokalemia, for example, you'll see flattened T waves and prominent U waves. The magnitude of the changes depends on the degree of potassium deficiency. Hypercalcemia may cause supraventricular or ventricular tachycardias.

Treatment

Care of an elderly patient at risk for arrhythmias from her drug therapy involves minimizing the number of drugs, supporting vital functions, maintaining fluid balance, controlling arrhythmias, and teaching her about her drug regimen.

Supporting vital functions

The degree of support your patient needs depends on the adverse reactions or interactions she's ex-

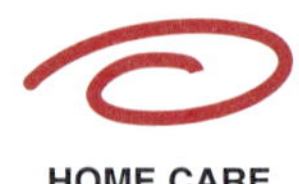

HOME CARE

Teaching an elderly patient to manage her drug therapy

When teaching an elderly patient who takes several drugs, make a special effort to help her avoid problems that may result from her drug regimen. Start by finding out what your patient already knows about her drugs. Clarify her misconceptions and misunderstandings while you provide new information. And use terms that she can understand, such as *teaspoons* instead of *milliliters.*

Remember that your elderly patient may have a decreased attention span. Use short, discrete teaching steps, allowing time for her to respond and ask questions. And repeat information, as necessary.

Also, give your patient written instructions. Use handouts with large print, if necessary. And make sure that she's using any assistive devices she may need, such as eyeglasses or a magnifying glass. As needed, include one or more members of the patient's family in your teaching sessions so that they can help her remember and comply with your instructions.

Assess your patient's ability to open drug containers, read labels, and handle and pick up pills. If necessary, arrange for her to obtain her drugs in easy-to-open containers. And help her devise a reminder system to ensure that she takes the correct drugs at the correct times.

Urge your patient to inform all of her health care providers about all of the drugs she takes, including prescription drugs, over-the-counter (OTC) drugs, and supplements. Assist her with making a list of her drugs and their dosages. Tell her to change the list anytime one of her drugs or dosages changes. And encourage her to bring the list to all medical appointments.

Review any adverse effects or drug interactions that may occur with her regimen. And tell her to call her physician before taking any OTC drugs.

Advise your patient to obtain all of her drugs from one pharmacy. And tell her that she should choose one that keeps her drug profile on record, so when she starts a new drug or changes the dosage of an old one, the pharmacist can alert her and her physician about any possible interactions.

periencing and on the underlying conditions. Be alert for bradycardia, hypotension, and adventitious breath sounds.

Obtain blood pressure readings with your patient lying down, sitting, and standing up. Note a decrease of 10 mm Hg or more between readings, which may indicate orthostatic hypotension. Complaints of dizziness or light-headedness with position changes may further confirm this condition. Caution your patient to change positions slowly and to use her call bell to request assistance in getting out of bed. Also, instruct her to dangle her legs over the edge of the bed for a few minutes before standing up.

If your patient has tachypnea or complains of shortness of breath, anticipate the need for supplemental oxygen to prevent hypoxemia. Auscultate her heart sounds for extra systoles, which could indicate PVCs, while simultaneously checking her radial pulse to determine whether the extra systoles are perfusing peripheral vessels adequately.

Provide continuous cardiac monitoring, if indicated. Elevate the head of your patient's bed 30 to 45 degrees to maximize lung expansion and decrease the work of breathing, thus minimizing metabolic oxygen demand. Monitor your patient's oxygen saturation levels using pulse oximetry. Also, evaluate her ECG for ischemic changes and other abnormalities that may result from her drug therapy. Obtain ABG measurements, as ordered, to evaluate your patient's respiratory status and acid-base balance.

If your patient has an altered level of consciousness, take safety precautions to reduce her risk of injury. Keep in mind that age-related neurologic changes increase the risk of neurologic adverse effects. Reorient your patient, as necessary, and perform frequent neurologic checks to detect changes.

Plan activities based on your patient's condition, oxygen saturation levels, and tolerance. Keep in mind that activity increases metabolic and myocardial oxygen demands. An elderly patient with arrhythmias caused by drug therapy may not be able to meet those demands. Therefore, plan frequent rest periods and pace your patient's activities to prevent her from becoming exhausted. Provide clear, simple explanations about treatment measures and care activities. Remember that anxiety increases metabolic oxygen demands as well.

Maintaining fluid balance

Assess your patient's skin turgor and mucous membranes for evidence of hydration. If she's dehydrated, begin I.V. fluid replacement using a volume-control device, as prescribed. Anticipate therapy that replaces deficient electrolytes or removes excess ones.

Monitor your patient's fluid therapy closely to prevent fluid overload. Elderly patients have an increased risk of overload because of a diminished reserve capacity. Such a reduction, together with decreased myocardial efficiency, reduced contractile strength, and increased vessel-wall rigidity, increases the workload of the heart, worsening existing cardiovascular problems.

Signs and symptoms of fluid overload include increasing shortness of breath, dyspnea, and jugular vein distention. Document your patient's weight daily, along with her intake and output. Report any sudden increases or decreases.

Increased urine output may cause further volume deficits and electrolyte losses. Decreased urine output may reflect renal dysfunction. Both conditions can worsen existing electrolyte imbalances or enhance preexcitation or conduction delays. Continue to monitor your patient's blood electrolyte levels, as ordered, to evaluate the effectiveness of treatment.

Controlling arrhythmias

The key to controlling arrhythmias lies in correcting the underlying cause. The physician may decrease the dosage of one or more of your patient's drugs. Or your patient may need to stop taking one or more of her drugs to avoid or minimize adverse cardiac effects. Also, take steps to reduce or prevent arrhythmias by making sure your patient remains fully hydrated and has no electrolyte imbalances.

If cardiac decompensation occurs, be prepared to intervene quickly. Monitor your patient's ECG continuously for changes that indicate adverse drug effects, increased cardiac workload, or ischemia. Intervene based on those ECG findings. Keep emergency equipment and drugs readily available in case your patient has a cardiac arrest.

If you think your patient may have a toxic reaction to digoxin, stop the drug and notify her physician immediately. You'll probably continue to withhold digoxin until blood drug levels return to the therapeutic range. Administer potassium supplements to reverse hypokalemia. Also, investigate your patient's other prescribed drugs, and anticipate dosage reduction or discontinuation, as needed. Monitor her ECG continuously for a return to the baseline tracing. If arrhythmias continue, especially AV blocks, your patient may need a temporary pacemaker (see *Teaching an elderly patient to manage her drug therapy*).

Suggested Readings

Andersen HR, Nielsen JC, Thomsen PE, et al. Atrioventricular conduction during long-term follow-up of patients with sick sinus syndrome. *Circulation.* 1998;98(13):1315-1321.

Anderson JL. Contemporary clinical trials in ventricular tachycardia and fibrillation: implications of ESVEM, CASCADE, and CASH for clinical management. *J Cardiovasc Electrophysiol.* 1995;6(10 Pt 2):880-886.

Armstrong ML. *Electrocardiograms: A Systematic Method of Reading Them.* New York: McGraw-Hill Book Co; 1997.

Atlee JL. *Arrhythmias and Pacemakers: Practical Management for Anesthesia and Critical Care Medicine.* Philadelphia: WB Saunders Co; 1996.

Atwood S, Stanton C, Storey J. *Introduction to Basic Cardiac Dysrhythmias.* 2nd ed. St Louis: Mosby, Inc; 1996.

Bennett DH. *Cardiac Arrhythmias: Practical Notes on Interpretation and Treatment.* 5th ed. Oxford; Boston: Butterworth-Heinemann Publishing; 1997.

Breithardt G, Shenasa M, Camm J, Borggrefe M, Rosen MR. *Antiarrhythmic Drugs: Mechanisms of Antiarrhythmic and Proarrhythmic Actions.* New York: Springer-Verlag New York; 1995.

Brembilla-Perrot B, Beurrier D, de la Chaise AT, et al. Significance and prevalence of inducible atrial tachyarrhythmias in patients undergoing electrophysiologic study for presyncope or syncope. *Int J Cardiol.* 1996;53(1):61-69.

Canobbio MM. *Mosby's Handbook of Patient Teaching.* St Louis: Mosby, Inc; 1996.

Carelton PF, Bodlt MA. Anatomy of the cardiovascular system. In: Price SA, Wilson LM. *Pathophysiology: Clinical Concepts of Disease Processes.* 5th ed. St Louis: Mosby, Inc; 1996.

Chung EK. *Pocket Guide to ECG Diagnosis.* Boston: Blackwell Scientific Pubns; 1996.

Clochesy JM, Breu C, Cardin S, Whittaker AA, Rudy EB. *Critical Care Nursing.* 2nd ed. Philadelphia: WB Saunders Co; 1996.

Conover MB. *Pocket Guide to Electrocardiography.* 4th ed. St Louis: Mosby, Inc; 1997. Mosby's Pocket Guide Series.

Conover MB. *Understanding Electrocardiography.* 7th ed. St Louis: Mosby, Inc; 1996.

Davis D. *Differential Diagnosis of Arrhythmias.* Philadelphia: WB Saunders Co; 1997.

Dracup K, Meltzer LE. *Meltzer's Intensive Coronary Care: A Manual for Nurses.* 5th ed. Stamford: Appleton & Lange; 1995.

Drzewiecki GM, Li JK, eds. *Analysis and Assessment of Cardiovascular Function.* New York: Springer-Verlag New York; 1998.

Fenstermacher K. *Dysrhythmia Recognition and Management.* 3rd ed. Philadelphia: WB Saunders Co; 1998.

Fontaine G, Fontaliran F, Andrade FR, et al. The arrhythmogenic right ventricle: dysplasia versus cardiomyopathy. *Heart Vessels.* 1995;10(5):227-235.

Frantz ID Jr, Dawson EA, Kuba K, Brewer ER, Gatewood LC, Bartsch GE. The Minnesota coronary survey: effect of diet on cardiovascular events and deaths. *Circulation.* 1995;52(Suppl 2);II-4.

Grauer K, Cavallaro D. *Arrhythmia Interpretation: ACLS Preparation and Clinical Approach.* St Louis: Mosby, Inc; 1997.

Gross Cohn E, Gilroy-Doohan M. *Flip and See ECG.* Philadelphia: WB Saunders Co; 1995.

Hampton JR. *The ECG Made Easy.* New York: Churchill Livingstone, Inc; 1997.

Hampton JR. *100 ECG Problems.* New York: Churchill Livingstone, Inc; 1997.

Hashiba K, Centurion OA, Shimizu A. Electrophysiologic characteristics of human atrial muscle in paroxysmal atrial fibrillation. *Am Heart J.* 1996;131(4):778-789.

Huff J. *ECG Workout: Exercises in Arrhythmia Interpretation.* Philadelphia: Lippincott-Raven Pubs; 1997.

Khan MG. *Rapid ECG Interpretation.* Philadelphia: WB Saunders Co; 1997.

Klein GJ, Prystowsky EN. *Clinical Electrophysiology Review.* New York: McGraw-Hill Book Co; 1996.

Kowey PR, Podrid PJ, eds. *Cardiac Arrhythmia: Mechanisms, Diagnosis, and Management.* Baltimore: Williams & Wilkins Co; 1995.

Kowey PR, Podrid PJ, eds. *Handbook of Cardiac Arrhythmia.* Baltimore: Williams & Wilkins Co; 1996.

Kroll MW. *Implantable Cardioverter Defibrillator Therapy: The Engineering-Clinical Interface.* Hingham, Mass: Kluwer Academic Publishers; 1996.

Lewis SM, Collier IC, Heitkemper MM. *Medical-Surgical Nursing: Assessment and Management of Clinical Problems.* St Louis: Mosby, Inc; 1995.

Mackay L. *Cardiac Rehabilitation.* Gaithersburg, Md: Aspen Pubs, Inc; 1997.

Mandel W. *Cardiac Arrhythmias: Their Mechanisms, Diagnosis, and Management.* 3rd ed. Philadelphia: Lippincott-Raven Pubs; 1995.

Mark JB. *Atlas of Cardiovascular Monitoring.* New York: Churchill Livingstone, Inc; 1997.

Marriott HJL, Conover MB. *Advanced Concepts in Arrhythmias.* 3rd ed. St Louis: Mosby, Inc; 1998.

McDermott MM, Feinglass J, Sy J, Gheorghiade M. Hospitalized congestive heart failure patients with preserved versus abnormal left ventricular systolic function: clinical characteristics and drug therapy. *Am J Med.* 1995;99:629-35.

Meluzín J, Cerny J, Frelich M. Prognostic value of the amount of dysfunctional but viable myocardium in revascularized patients with coronary artery disease and left ventricular dysfunction. *J Am Coll Cardiol.* 1998;32(4):912-920.

Ochs GM. *Recognition and Interpretation of ECG Rhythms.* 3rd ed. Stamford: Appleton & Lange; 1997.

Phalen T. *The 12-Lead ECG in Acute Myocardial Infarction.* St Louis: Mosby, Inc; 1995.

Pinsky MR. *Applied Bedside Cardiovascular Physiology.* Berlin; New York: Springer-Verlag New York; 1997.

Price SA, Wilson LM. *Pathophysiology: Clinical Concepts of Disease Processes.* St Louis: Mosby, Inc; 1996.

Purdie RB, Earnest SL. *Pure Practice for 12-Lead ECGs.* St Louis: Mosby, Inc; 1997.

Ramajah LS, Knilans TK. *Electrocardiography in Clinical Practice: Adult and Pediatric.* Philadelphia: WB Saunders Co; 1996.

Raviele A. Cardiac Arrhythmias 1997: Proceedings of the 5th International Workshop on Cardiac Arrhythmias (Venice, 7-10 October 1997). New York: Springer-Verlag New York; 1997.

Reiffel JA. Prolonging survival by reducing arrhythmic death: pharmacologic therapy of ventricular tachycardia and fibrillation. *Am J Cardiol.* 1997;80(8A):45G-55G.

Rosamond WD, Chambless LE, Folsom AR, et al. Trends in the incidence of myocardial infarction and in mortality due to coronary heart disease, 1987 to 1994. *N Engl J Med.* 1998;339(13):861-867.

Singer I. *Interventional Electrophysiology.* Baltimore: Williams & Wilkins Co; 1996.

Skidmore-Roth, L. *Mosby's 1999 Nursing Drug Reference.* St Louis: Mosby, Inc; 1998.

Stillwell SB. *Mosby's Critical Care Nursing Reference.* 2nd ed. St Louis: Mosby, Inc; 1996.

Taylor GJ. *Practice ECGs: Interpretation and Board Review.* Boston: Blackwell Scientific Pubns; 1997.

Taylor RL. *Advanced Cardiac Care in the Streets.* Philadelphia: Lippincott-Raven Pubs; 1997.

Thaler MS. *The Only EKG Book You'll Ever Need.* 2nd ed. Philadelphia: Lippincott-Raven Pubs; 1995.

Vardas PE, ed. *Cardiac Arrhythmias, Pacing and Electrophysiology: The Expert View.* Hingham, Mass: Kluwer Academic Publishers; 1998.

Vasan RS, Benjamin EJ, Levy D. Prevalence, clinical features and prognosis of diastolic heart failure: an epidemiologic perspective. *J Am Coll Cardiol.* 1995;26(7):1565-1574.

Walraven G. *Basic Arrhythmias.* 5th ed. Englewood Cliffs, NJ: Prentice-Hall; 1998.

Weinberg AD, Paturas JL. *Easy ACLS: Pocket Guide.* Boston: Jones & Bartlett Pubs, Inc; 1995.

Williamson EM, Somberg JC. *Control of Cardiac Rhythm.* Philadelphia: Lippincott-Raven Pubs; 1998.

Zaloga G. *The Critical Care Drug Handbook.* St Louis: Mosby, Inc; 1996.

Index

i indicates an illustration; t indicates a table.

B

C

D

i indicates an illustration; t indicates a table.

E F

G H

I J

L M N O

i indicates an illustration; t indicates a table.

P Q

R S

T

U V W

i indicates an illustration; t indicates a table.